VECTORCARDIOGRAPHY 3

VECTORCARDIOGRAPHY 3

Proceedings of the Symposium on Clinical Vectorcardiography 1975, *New York 1975.*
held in New York City, May 10-11, 1975

IRWIN HOFFMAN, *Editor*
ROBERT I. HAMBY, *Co-editor*

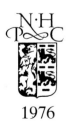

1976

NORTH-HOLLAND PUBLISHING COMPANY - AMSTERDAM · OXFORD

North-Holland ISBN: 0 7204 4523 X
American Elsevier ISBN: 0 444 10919 6

Published by:

North-Holland Publishing Company - Amsterdam
North-Holland Publishing Company, Ltd. - Oxford

Sole distributors for the U.S.A. and Canada:

American Elsevier Publishing Company, Inc.
52 Vanderbilt Avenue
New York, N.Y. 10017

PRINTED IN THE NETHERLANDS

PREFACE

This volume presents the papers presented at "Clinical Vectorcardiography 1975", a meeting held in New York City, May 10-11, 1975, and sponsored jointly by the Long Island Jewish Hillside Medical Center, and the American College of Cardiology.

The editors wish to acknowledge the patience and devotion to this project of the Communities Relations Department of the Long Island Jewish Hillside Medical Center, particularly Mrs. June Lewis, Mrs. Lola Sher and Mrs. Ruth Cook. The authors especially wish to thank Dr. Robert K. Match, President of the Long Island Jewish Hillside Medical Center, Dr. James E. Mulvihill, Dean of the Clinical Campus of the State University of New York at Stony Brook, and Dr. Edward Meilman, Chairman of the Department of Medicine, LIJH, and Professor of Medicine at Health Sciences Center, State University of New York at Stony Brook, for their encouragement and invaluable help in preparing and organizing the symposium and its publication.

Irwin Hoffman, M.D., Editor

Robert I. Hamby, M.D., Co-Editor

v

LIST OF CONTRIBUTORS

The papers comprising this volume were presented at "Clinical Vectorcardiography 1975" on May 10-11, 1975 in New York City. The scheduled speakers for that program, and their academic titles and affiliations, are listed below. Their cooperation in organizing the meeting, and in submission of manuscripts, is gratefully acknowledged by the editors.

J.A. ABILDSKOV, M.D., F.A.C.C., Professor of Medicine and Director of Cardiovascular Research and Training Institute, University of Utah College of Medicine, Salt Lake City, Utah

ALBERTO BENCHIMOL, M.D., F.A.C.C., Director, Institute for Cardiovascular Diseases, Good Samaritan Hospital, Phoenix, Ariz.

MARY JO BURGESS, M.D., Associate Professor of Medicine, Cardiovascular Division, University of Utah College of Medicine, Salt Lake City, Utah

AGUSTIN CASTELLANOS, JR., M.D., F.A.C.C., Professor of Medicine and Director, Clinical Electrophysiology, University of Maimi School of Medicine, Maimi, Fla.

TE-CHUAN CHOU, M.D., F.A.C.C., Professor of Medicine, University of Cincinnati College of Medicine, Cincinnati, Ohio

ROLF M. GUNNAR, M.D., F.A.C.C., Professor of Medicine and Chief, Section of Cardiology, Loyola University of Chicago, Stritch School of Medicine, Maywood, Ill.

ROBERT I. Hamby, M.D., F.A.C.C., Attending in Charge, Cardiology Division, Long Island Jewish-Hillside Medical Center, New Hyde Park; Associate Professor of Medicine, School of Medicine, Health Sciences Center, State University of New York at Stony Brook, Stony Brook, N.Y.

JOSEPH HILSENRATH, M.D., Internist and Cardiologist, Department of Medicine, Long Island Jewish-Hillside Medical Center, New Hyde Park; Assistant Professor of Clinical Medicine, School of Medicine, Health Sciences Center, State University of New York at Stony Brook, Stony Brook, N.Y.

IRWIN HOFFMAN, M.D., F.A.C.C., Attending in Charge, Electrocardiography-Vectorcardiography, Long Island Jewish-Hillside Medical Center, New Hyde Park; Associate Professor of Clinical Medicine, School of Medicine, Health Sciences Center, State University of New York at Stony Brook, Stony Brook, N.Y.

RICHARD J. KENNEDY, M.D., F.A.C.C., Director, Electrocardiographic Department, St. Vincent's Hospital and Medical Center of New York; Clinical Professor of Medicine, New York University-Bellevue Medical Center, New York, N.Y.

FRED KORNREICH, M.D., Director, Unit for Cardiovascular Research, University of Brussels, Brussels, Belgium

HENRI E. KULBERTUS, M.D., F.A.C.C., Associate Professor of Cardiology, Institute of Medicine, University of Liege School of Medicine, Liege, Belgium

JEROME LIEBMAN, M.D., F.A.C.C., Professor of Pediatrics, Case Western Reserve University School of Medicine; Director of Pediatric Cardiology, University Hospitals of Cleveland, Cleveland, Ohio

B. LYNN MILLER, M.D., F.A.C.C., Assistant Professor of Pediatrics, University of Florida College of Medicine J. Hills Miller Health Center, Gainesville, Fla.

HUBERT V. PIPBERGER, M.D., F.A.C.C., Professor of Clincial Engineering and Medicine, The George Washington University Medical Center ; Chief, Veterans Administration Research Center for Cardiovascular Data Processing, Veterans Administration Hospital, Washington, D.C.

PENTTI RAUTAHARJU, M.D., Ph.D., Professor-Director, Department of Physiology and Biophysics, Dalhousie University Faculty of Medicine, Halifax, Nova Scotia

HAROLD G. RICHMAN, M.D., F.A.C.C., Associate Professor of Medicine, University of Minnesota, Minneapolis, Medical School; Staff Physician, Cardiovascular Division and Director, Electrocardiography Laboratory, Veterans Administration Hospital, Minneapolis, Minn.

BORYS SURAWICZ, M.D., F.A.C.C., Professor of Medicine and Director, Cardiology Division, University of Kentucky College of Medicine, Lexington, Ky.

OLGA ZONERAICH, M.D., Associate Attending in Medicine and Cardiology, Long Island Jewish-Hillside Medical Center, Queens Hospital Affiliation, Jamaica; Associate Professor of Medicine, State University of New York at Stony Brook, Health Sciences Center, School of Medicine, Stony Brook, N.Y.

SAMUEL ZONERAICH, M.D., F.A.C.C., Head, Division of Cardiology, Long Island Jewish-Hillside Medical Center, Queens Hospital Center Affiliation, Jamaica; Associate Professor of Medicine, State University of New York at Stony Brook, Health Sciences Center School of Medicine, Stony Brook, N.Y.

CONTENTS

CONTENTS

SECTION 4.   COMPUTER APPLICATIONS

INTRODUCTION

Vectorcardiography 3 I. Hoffman and R.I. Hamby eds.

DEFENSIVE VECTORCARDIOGRAPHY

Irwin Hoffman

From the ECG-VCG Department, Long Island Jewish Hillside Medical Center,
New Hyde Park, N.Y. and The Health Sciences Center,
State University of New York at Stony Brook

Vectorcardiography is a powerful diagnostic tool, facilitating the recognition of myocardial infarction, ventricular conduction disturbances, and ventricular hypertrophies. However, the QRS and T-loop alterations in various disease states overlap considerably, leading to inevitable diagnostic error. Such mistakes are most easily detected when the vectorcardiogram is followed up by a complete hemodynamic investigation in the invasive cardiac laboratory.

In general, infarction shifts portions of the QRS loop away from the damaged area, while conduction disorders or hypertrophies shift the QRS forces towards the affected zones. These shifts may occur in any of the six directions of the XYZ orthogonal lead system employed. Unfortunately, the timing, shape and magnitude of loop displacements may be very similar in widely different disease states, making precise anatomic diagnosis of the VCG extremely difficult.

Nevertheless, the information content in the vectorcardiogram can and should be used by the cardiologist. Based on current and always changing knowledge in this field, certain precautions are herein proposed which may serve to protect the vectorcardiographer and his patient from the hazards implicit in diagnostic error.

(1) The patient has a normal vectorcardiogram, but has been submitted for study because of clinical suspicion of heart disease. The normal VCG does not rule out cardiac pathology. Indeed, coronary disease of single, double or triple extent may be present, as well as ventricular asynergy, mitral stenosis or hypertrophic subaortic stenosis. The principle to remember is that a normal vectorcardiogram does not rule out heart disease.

(2) The patient under study for cardiac disorder has small or absent anterior QRS forces on the Z-axis, resembling the picture of anterior wall infarction. Non-cardiac causes must also be considered. Left ventricular hypertrophy of any etiology, but especially aortic stenosis, should come first to mind. Chronic obstructive lung disease may result in a very similar VCG picture. Cardiomyopathies of any etiology, including amyloidosis, may result in decreased or absent anterior forces. Less commonly, mitral valve stenosis or prolapse of the mitral valve may cause a similar picture. Indeed, in the presence of left ventricular hypertrophy, any initial anterior forces should call the diagnosis of anterior wall infarction into question.

(3) Large anterior forces on the Z-axis are observed in a patient undergoing cardiovascular examination. These large forces may suggest the diagnosis of dorsal wall infarction or right ventricular hypertrophy. In this 1975 VCG symposium, the concept of anterior conduction delay as a cause for prominent anterior QRS forces was proposed [1]. If this concept is confirmed in the future, it is likely that many degrees of anterior conduction delay will be observed, similar to various degrees of right ventricular conduction delay which are so commonly encountered. When the diagnosis of true dorsal infarction is suspected, the diagnosis is more difficult in the absence of QRS or T-wave evidence of lateral or inferior wall infarction.

(4) Left bundle branch block is diagnosed from the vectorcardiogram and initial anterior forces are not seen, suggesting anterior wall infarction. Occasionally, in left bundle branch block in patients completely free of heart disease, no anterior forces are visible even with amplification. Occasionally, such anterior forces are present but are so small that even amplified loops do not reveal the initial QRS forces which are superimposed upon the E-point or on the P or T-loop. A high amplitude Z-axis lead, swept in a scalar manner, will occasionally reveal such small initial anterior forces.

(5) The patient under investigation for heart trouble has right bundle branch block. Under these circumstances, especially if the anterior conduction delay theory holds up, many right bundle branch blocks with anterior displacement on the Z-axis will represent combinations of right bundle branch block with mid-septal (anterior) branch block of the left division. Therefore, it seems likely that the diagnosis of true dorsal wall infarction will simply not be possible in patients with right bundle branch block. It is presently known that the combination of right bundle branch block and left anterior hemiblock, readily diagnosable from the frontal plane vectorcardiogram, presents as two families of loops in the horizontal plane--one anterior and one posterior. It seems likely that the anterior family of loops represents additional involvement of the left mid-septal branch.

Also, in right bundle branch block, Q-waves of small magnitude are commonly seen in leads V-1 and V-2 which, in the vectorcardiogram, are written as initial direct posterior forces. Goldman et al. [2] have clearly shown that such posterior initial QRS forces are frequently not correlated with the presence of anterior wall infarction at postmortem examination.

(6) The patient under investigation for heart trouble has a right anterior T-loop in the horizontal plane which rotates clockwise. This abnormality is not specific for coronary artery disease, although it may occur in that condition. Such clockwise right anterior horizontal T-loops have been seen in left ventricular hypertrophy, left bundle branch block, and right ventricular pacing. They frequently reflect severe underlying disease and may at times represent a combination of ventricular hypertrophy and ischemia, secondary to coronary obstruction. However, the clockwise rotation itself is not specific for coronary artery disease.

(7) The patient under investigation for heart pathology has a VCG interpreted as inferior wall myocardial infarction. The cardiologist must consider non-coronary conditions which may mimic inferior wall infarction. The commonest of these are hypertrophic subaortic stenosis, and aortic insufficiency. Occasionally right ventricular hypertrophy will present with initial superior forces meeting criteria for inferior wall M.I. Rarely, a similar picture is seen in the syndrome of mitral valve prolapse.

(8) Technical problems occur in vectorcardiography as well as in standard ECG studies. Reversal of electrodes, especially the A and I electrodes, may occur. This interchanges the voltages from the left and right axillae and results in a deep negative deflection in lead X, and therefore a rightward horizontal and frontal loop resembling right ventricular hypertrophy. Since there is no internal check in the vectorcardiogram, the XYZ leads observed will be consistent with the vectorcardiographic loops. However, comparison with the 12-lead tracing in the particular case should give the clue that a technical error has occurred. Similarly, if the VCG leads are placed too high or too low around the chest wall, significant changes in magnitude and direction of the XYZ leads resulting are very likely.

(9) Do not deprive a patient of cardiac catheterization and possible surgical help on VCG evidence alone of complicating disease. Specifically, if a patient is studied for valve disorder with left ventricular hypertrophy, but the VCG indicates anterior or inferior M.I., this latter diagnosis should be confirmed by coronary angiography. Pseudoinfarction patterns in LVH are very common and should not deprive a patient of his needed valve replacement.

(10) If a patient is perfectly normal clinically and has no chest pain, heart murmur or other cardiac symptomatology, but an ECG and VCG are somewhat bizarre, do not perform cardiac catheterization. Rarely, if ever, is significant pathology uncovered under these circumstances, and the patient is submitted to a procedure which is not without hazard.

(11) Any cardiologist reading vectorcardiograms should have some continuing contact with an invasive cardiac lab. In this way his VCG diagnoses will be subject to hemodynamic and anatomical confirmation. In no other way will the vectorcardiographer realize all the surprises, combinations and errors that are possible using the technique of vectorcardiography.

(12) Vectorcardiograms should not be read "cold." Even very simple preliminary information as the patient's underlying symptoms such as chest pain or dyspnea, or perhaps heart murmur, is sufficient to start the interpretation in the correct direction.

References

[1]   I. Hoffman et al., Anterior conduction delay-- A possible cause for pseudodorsal infarction, in present volume.
[2]   M. Goldman and H. Pipberger, Analysis of the orthogonal electrocardiogram and vectorcardiogram in ventricular conduction defects with and without myocardial infarction, Circulation 39 (1969) 243.

SECTION 1.
MYOCARDIAL INFARCTION AND HYPERTROPHY

Vectorcardiography 3 I. Hoffman and R.I. Hamby eds.

VECTORCARDIOGRAPHIC DIAGNOSIS OF MYOCARDIAL INFARCTION
AND LEFT VENTRICULAR HYPERTROPHY

Rolf M. Gunnar, John F. Moran, M. Ziad Sinno, and Dilip Shah

From the Sections of Cardiology, Departments of Medicine, Loyola University
Stritch School of Medicine, Maywood, Illinois, and the Veterans
Administration Hospital, Hines, Illinois

In order for the vectorcardiogram to be a useful diagnostic tool in patients with myocardial infarction, we must understand the genesis of the QRS loop and how infarction, by removing electrically active tissue, will deform that loop. Although the lower left septal endocardium and the apical anterior endocardium are the earliest areas of the heart to be activated, much of the cavity of the left ventricle has been activated by 25 msec. By 30 msec, the entire cavity, even the posterobasal segment, is activated. Thus, infarction of any area of the left ventricle will tend to deform the early forces of the QRS loop. Since the loop defines the resultant instantaneous vectors, infarction of any particular area will tend to enlarge the resultant vector, and, therefore, the QRS loop, in a direction away from the infarcted area.

There is additional information relating to myocardial infarction in the later portions of the QRS loop. Attempts have been made to analyze these terminal forces, but the value of criteria derived from these analyses remains to be proven. Since the velocity of movement of the wave of depolarization through the myocardium is much more variable than the direction of the initial forces, it is more difficult to codify the effects of loss of myocardium on terminal forces than it is to derive criteria for infarction from the initial forces.

Hugenholtz, working in Dr. Harold Levine's laboratory, proposed and tested criteria for myocardial infarction based on the deformity of the initial portion of the QRS loop [2]. These criteria have been re-tested and expanded. This has led to a better understanding of the accuracy of the various criteria and conditions other than myocardial infarction which may lead to similar deformities of the QRS loop [3, 4].

Anteroseptal Infarction (figure 1)

The loss of the lower portion of the septum and of the adjacent anterior wall of the left ventricle destroys the early forces whose vector is right and anterior. Thus, in anteroseptal infarction, the

Supported, in part, by NIH Grant #HL-15040, and NIH Training Grant #HL-05971.

initial QRS forces move quickly posterior and to the left so that the .02 sec vector is behind the null point. This deformity of the QRS loop can occur with marked fibrosis of the septum and anterior wall as well as with infarction, or with replacement of this area with amyloid [4]. The presence of marked posterobasal hypertrophy in patients with severe aortic stenosis or hypertrophic cardiomyopathy can also overwhelm the normal anterior forces generated by the septum and cause the .02 sec vector to move posteriorly. Loss of early anterior forces has been described in patients with severe emphysema [5]. The effect of emphysema may be particularly evident in the Frank lead system, since the correcting resistances do not allow for the imposition of a great deal of lung tissue between the anterior chest wall and the left ventricle (table 1).

Anterolateral Infarction (figure 2)

An infarct involving the anterior and lateral free wall of the left ventricle, but leaving the septum mostly intact, will allow the early septal vectors directed anteriorly and to the right to persist until the forces from the posterior free wall turn the loop posteriorly and to the left. This will allow the initial portion of the QRS loop to rotate in a clockwise direction in the horizontal plane. If the area of involvement of the lateral wall is extensive, the entire loop may rotate in a clockwise direction. Thus, anterolateral wall infarction is diagnosed by clockwise rotation of the initial QRS loop around the E point in the horizontal plane. This rotation is a rather specific deformity having a small number of false-positives, when severe fibrosis of the lateral wall occurs in patients with marked left ventricular hypertrophy [4]. Right bundle branch block and severe right ventricular hypertrophy will rotate the loop clockwise around the null point in the horizontal plane. In this deformity, the entire loop lies anterior while in anterolateral infarct the loop is directed posteriorly and to the left. Two additional criteria have been proposed. Though not well tested, they may give strength to the diagnosis of anterolateral infarction. The initial rightward forces may exceed the upper limits of normal of 0.16 mv [6]. The loop in the frontal plane may rotate in a counterclockwise direction when the maximal QRS vector is greater than 40°. This abnormal rotation in the frontal plane would be a reflection of the clockwise rotation in the horizontal plane if the loop did, indeed, remain vertical.

Extensive Anterior Infarction (figure 3)

The loop begins posteriorly and to the right, and the loop has a counterclockwise rotation. This is reflected in the frontal plane loop by prolongation of the initial rightward forces. In the standard electrocardiogram, it is seen as QS deformity over much of the precordium with large Q waves in leads V_5 and V_6 and standard leads I and AVL.

Table 1

Comparison of vectorcardiographic measurements in patients
with emphysema and patients with anteroseptal infarction.
Adapted from the report of Watanabe et al. [5]

	N	$R_x + R_z$	0.025 sec Z	$S_x/R_x + S_x$	QRS Duration	Comb.
		Emphysema VS ASI (m $\pm$ S.D.)				
Emphysema	52	0.85 ± 0.36	$.087 \pm 0.25$	0.42 ± 0.29	93.6 ± 20.5	88%
Anteroseptal Infarction	35	1.64 ± 0.68	0.35 ± 0.35	0.25 ± 0.26	105.5 ± 14.0	91%
Discrimin.		1.12mv	0.10mv	0.33mv	100.7	

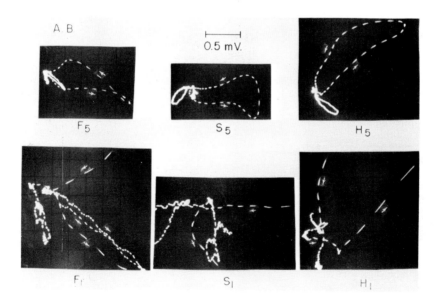

Fig. 1. Anteroseptal infarction with the 0.02 sec vector posterior. Interruptions are at 400 per sec (0.0025 sec per dot).

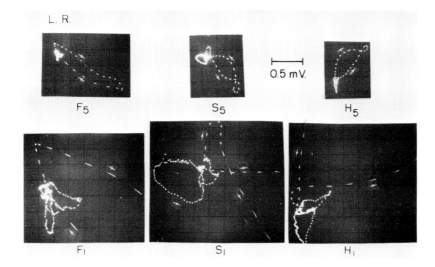

Fig. 2. Anterolateral infarction with clockwise initial forces in the horizontal plane. Also meets criteria for inferior infarction: 0.025 sec vector superior and left maximal superior vector > 0.4 mv with a clockwise QRS_F.

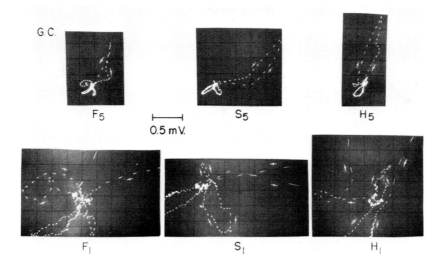

Fig. 3. Extensive anterior infarction with clockwise rightward and posterior rotation of the initial QRS_H and the entire QRS_H rotates in a clockwise manner.

Inferior Wall Infarction (figures 4 and 5)

Infarction of the inferior wall of the left ventricle shifts the initial forces superiorly and prolongs
the duration of the initial superior forces. It is reflected in changes in the frontal and sagittal leads.
The three most important criteria for diagnosis of
this deformity, as tested against autopsy data, are:
(1) the .02 and .03 second vectors superior to the X
axis; (2) the point at which the initial superior forces
traverse the X axis (left maximal superior voltage) >
0.4 mv to the left; and (3) persistence of clockwise rotation of the initial QRS forces when the maximal QRS
vector is shifted to the left of 0° [4].

If two of these three criteria are met, the incidence of inferior infarction, as proven at autopsy,
approaches 100%. These criteria, however, have a
false-negative incidence of 23%.

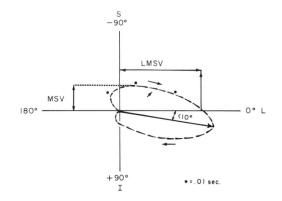

Fig. 4. Diagram of the QRS_F loop in inferior infarction. The left maximal vector is at less than 10°.
LMSV = left maximal superior voltage. MSV = maximum superior voltage.

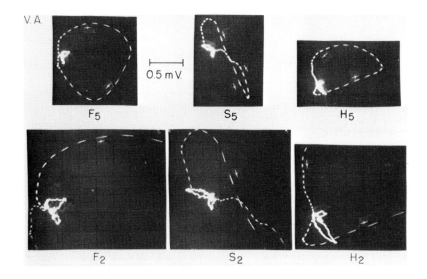

Fig. 5. Inferior infarction meeting the following criteria: 0.02 and 0.03 sec vectors superior. LMSV > 0.4 mv,
clockwise QRS_F with left maximal vector above 0°, and maximum superior voltage > 0.1 mv, and a $Q_y:R_y$ ratio >
1:5.

The criterion of LMSV = or > 0.4 mv is an extension of the findings of Hoffman et al. [7] who found the LMSV = or > 0.3 mv in 63 of 76 (83%) patients with documented previous inferior myocardial infarction, and proposed this as the criterion to be used for this measurement. However, they only decreased their yield slightly to identify 59 (78%) patients when the criterion was changed to LMSV = or > 0.4 mv. There have been instances of normal patients with frontal QRS loops meeting the less stringent criterion. These authors also tested the 0.025 second vector superior, and this identified 66 of the 76 patients (87%). The combination of these two criteria identified 72 (95%) of the patients. However, there was no control group to test how many patients without infarction would be identified by using these combined criteria.

Young and Williams proposed the following criteria for inferior infarction [8]:

(1) Clockwise initial superior forces in an upward convexity and > 0.02 sec in duration, and = or > 0.25 mv leftward in magnitude.

(2) As in (1), but superior forces = or > 0.025 sec if leftward magnitude is < 0.25 mv.

(3) Completely clockwise initial forces if the maximal QRS vector is to the left of 10°.

(4) If the loop is clockwise but the initial forces are inferior and to the right, then subsequent clockwise superior forces must be 0.25 sec in duration.

(5) If there is a short inferior leftward initial vector, then this is quickly reversed and followed by a superior clockwise loop = or > 0.025 sec in duration.

These criteria were derived on 100 patients with prior or present ECG evidence of inferior infarction and tested by comparing with VCGs of 315 normal subjects of all ages.

Starr et al. [9] analyzed the criteria of Young and Williams by testing these criteria in a group of normal individuals and in a group of individuals with clinical inferior infarction or angiographic evidence of inferior infarction. They found a false-positive incidence of 7% and a false-negative incidence of 12%. These authors proposed their own criteria and tested these criteria in a new group of patients. Their criteria are predicated on a clockwise initial loop in the frontal plane and include one of the following:

(1) time at which the QRS crosses the X axis = or > 0.025 sec and at a magnitude > 0.3 mv to the left,

(2) a maximal QRS vector to the left at 15°,

(3) maximal superior voltage = or > 0.1 mv and Q:R ratio in Y axis at least 1:5.

The difficulty in testing against a group of normal subjects is that conditions other than infarction may deform the QRS loop, and such patients would be excluded from the control group. On the other hand, any autopsy study eliminates consideration of healthy normal individuals from the control group. Understanding the genesis of the QRS loop and how it may be deformed allows interpretation of the vectorcardiogram as modified by clinical findings. We suggest that if a clockwise initial frontal plane QRS loop meets the following criteria--the 0.03 second vector above the null point; the LMSV > 0.4 mv; maximal QRS vector to the left of 10°--then one can be assured the patient has an inferior infarction. If the QRS loop is clockwise, if there is 0.025 sec of the initial vector above the X axis and LMSV is > 0.3 mv, and if there is no evidence of severe ventricular hypertrophy, the diagnosis of inferior infarct has a very high probability of being correct. If the QRS loop in the frontal plane is initially clockwise, if the 0.02 sec vector is inferior and the LMSV is < 0.16 mv, and if the maximal QRS vector is greater than 20°, then the diagnosis of inferior infarction is highly unlikely. Between these negative and positive criteria will be patients with and without infarction, and analysis of clinical data becomes important in the diagnosis. In this latter group will be a few normal patients, some patients with myocardial fibrosis and micro-infarction, patients with pulmonary embolism, and patients with left ventricular hypertrophy, particularly of the asymmetric type.

Posterior Infarction (figures 6 and 7)

In the absence of inferior wall infarction, it is difficult to diagnose true posterior infarction. Even though many would insist that the deformity of the QRS loop should be seen in the terminal forces, it is true that the posterior wall begins its activation process early and most of the criteria for diagnosis of this lesion are based on deformity of the initial forces of the QRS loop [2, 3, 10]. The loss of posterior forces allows the entire loop to move anteriorly. The criteria for the diagnosis include maximal anterior QRS voltage greater than 0.55 mv, the maximum horizontal QRS vector anterior to 20°, and the duration of the anterior forces greater than .05 seconds. In analysis of the terminal forces, we have found useful the criterion of a rather straight slow terminal segment directly posterior to the null point. The major causes for false-positive diagnoses of posterior infarction using these criteria are right ventricular hypertrophy and anterior displacement of the heart against the chest wall. This latter deformity is seen not only in the straight-back syndrome and pectus excavatum, but also in some normal individuals who happen to have somewhat diminished anterior-posterior thoracic diameters.

Mather and Levine [11] attempted to differentiate true posterior infarction from right ventricular hypertrophy by analyzing the vectorcardiograms of 360 patients with electrocardiograms suggestive of true posterior infarction or right ventricular hypertrophy. By autopsy or clinical evaluation, 85 of the patients were considered to have posterior infarction and 203 were considered to have right ventricular hypertrophy. Seventy-two patients were excluded because clinical differentiation could not be made. They then analyzed the VCG criteria that would differentiate the two groups and found the best differentiation could be made using two criteria: the direction of the half area vector in the horizontal plane, and the magnitude of the terminal rightward forces. If the terminal rightward QRS forces in the horizontal plane less than 1.0 mv and a half area QRS vector between 350° and 90° were used to identify posterior infarction, and terminal forces greater than 1.0 mv and QRS half area horizontal vector between 90° and 350° were used to identify right ventricular hypertrophy, then the patients were

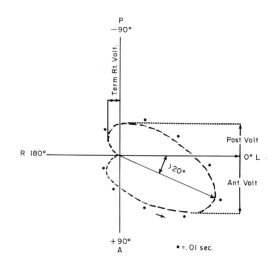

Fig. 6. Diagrammatic representation of the QRS_H loop in posterior infarction. Anterior voltage, posterior voltage, and terminal rightward voltage are shown. The left maximal vector is anterior to 20°.

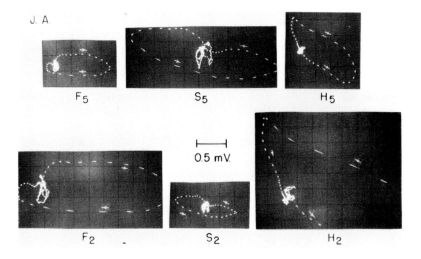

Fig. 7. Posterior infarction in addition to superior infarction meeting the following QRS_H criteria: anterior voltage > 0.55 mv, left maximum voltage anterior to 20°, terminal slow posterior forces less than 0.4 mv to the right, and the half area QRS_H vector between 350° and 90°.

correctly classified in 207 instances and incorrectly classified in 11 instances. In 70 instances these criteria were discordant--each indicating a different diagnosis. By adding the direction of the .04 sec vector to the criteria, classifying those in whom this vector was between 350° and 60° as posterior infarcts and those with this vector between 60° and 350° as right ventricular hypertrophy, then 41 of these 70 unclassified cases could be correctly classified.

Kini and Pipberger [12] analyzed the Frank lead orthogonal electrocardiogram in a group of 857 patients with myocardial infarction and selected 80 patients because the Q/R ratio in Z exceeded the upper limits of the 96th percentile range for normal subjects. They also analyzed the records of 843 patients with pulmonary emphysema and 121 patients with mitral stenosis. Sixty-three with emphysema and 8 with mitral stenosis were selected because they satisfied the above criteria. They ten tested Mather and Levine's criteria for usefulness in separating these groups, looked for significant differences between the scalar and planar vectorcardiograms in the two groups and also developed a classification of the groups by multivariate analysis. They were disappointed in the criteria of Mather and Levine in distinguishing the two groups and suggest that the difference may be in the high percentage of patients with emphysema in their own group. They give no figures for the results of the comparison. They found the most significant difference between the groups to be the large initial superior forces in the patients with posterior infarction. This is merely a reflection of their associated inferior infarction. If the Qy/Ry ratio exceeded 0.25 and the maximal T angle in the horizontal plane was between 90° and 180°, then 70% of posterior infarcts were identified with inclusion of only 15% of patients with right ventricular hypertrophy. If Q_Z was less than 0.04 sec, Rx/Sx was less than 1.0 and the maximal T_h angle was between 270° and 340°, then 55% of patients with RVH were identified, with only 13% of patients with posterior infarction included. For multivariate analysis, they used seven parameters and identified 78% of the posterior infarcts and 79% of the patients with right ventricular hypertrophy correctly, but they again used several y axis criteria.

Ha, Kraft and Stein [13] compared two groups of patients with anteriorly oriented QRS loops undergoing cardiac catheterization. They selected nine patients with evidence of occlusion of the coronary artery supply to the posterior wall and compared these vectorcardiograms to those of 138 patients with anterior oriented loops and no evidence of coronary disease or right ventricular hypertrophy. They added five healthy volunteers with anterior oriented loops to bring the normal group to 13 subjects. They examined the direction and magnitude of the horizontal plane 0.02, 0.03, 0.04, 0.05 and 0.06 sec vectors,

the half area vector and the maximal QRS vector. They also analyzed the magnitude of the terminal right vector, the maximum anterior and posterior vectors, the anterior accession time, the direction of rotation of QRS_h and T_h and the T_h angle. In the frontal and sagittal planes the 0.04 sec vector, the half area vector, the maximal QRS vector and direction of QRS and T were analyzed.

None of the criteria tested showed significant separation of the two groups. They do not comment on shape of the chest, placement of the heart in the thorax or A-P thoracic diameter in the normal group. By method of selection, it is not surprising that there was no differentiation between the two groups. It is interesting that none of the patients with posterior infarction satisfied ECG criteria for this diagnosis and no statement is made about this measurement in the normal subjects. It may be that the system of correcting resistances in the Frank lead system has pulled the loop anterior in patients with hearts close to the anterior chest wall. Inspection of the patient's chest and X-ray as well as the vectorcardiogram might have separated the two groups.

Review of the literature would suggest that it is not possible to diagnose posterior wall infarction unless lateral or inferior wall infarction co-exists. However, as a clinical tool the vectorcardiogram still has merit. The maximal QRS_h vector anterior to 20°, the Q_Z/R_Z ratio > 55/45, Q_Z > 0.55 mv and the duration of anterior forces > 0.05 sec all define an anteriorly displaced loop. If terminal rightward forces are less than 0.4 mv, if there is a straight slow terminal force behind the null point, if there is no evidence of pectus excavatum or narrow A-P diameter of the chest, then the diagnosis of posterobasal myocardial infarction is likely. If the loop is anterior, but the terminal rightward forces exceed 1.0 mv and there is clinical reason to suspect right ventricular hypertrophy, then this diagnosis becomes likely.

Lateral Wall Infarction (figure 8)

Initial rightward forces exceeding 0.16 mv and 0.022 seconds [6] even with normal rotation of the loop, suggests that there is either diminution in the mass of the lateral wall due to lateral wall infarction or exaggeration of the initial rightward and anterior forces of the septum as seen in left ventricular hypertrophy. The septal forces tend to be particularly large in aortic insufficiency and asymmetric septal hypertrophy. These criteria, therefore, would be useful for diagnosis of lateral myocardial infarction in patients who have no other evidence of left ventricular hypertrophy.

C.G.

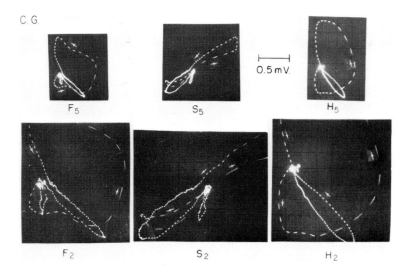

0.5 mV.

Fig. 8. Lateral wall infarction with initial anterior forces longer than 0.02 sec to the right and exceeding 0.16 mv to the right in the absence of left ventricular hypertrophy.

Myocardial Infarction in the Presence of Left Bundle Branch Block

The QRS deformity produced by left bundle branch block is best described in the horizontal plane, since the loop tends to lie close to the Z axis and is seen end on in the frontal plane [14, 15]. The initial forces are generated by the early activation of the septum around the base of the septal papillary muscle of the right ventricle and the right ventricular free wall. The septum is then activated in a right to left direction, giving a vector directed posteriorly and to the left. As the wave of activation reaches the anterior and posterior walls near the junction with the septum, the resultant vector moves posteriorly and left and the activation wave envelops the left ventricular cavity. The free wall of the left ventricle is activated last and slowly. Thus, the initial forces in left bundle branch block are the result of the early forces around the apex of the right ventricle and the right ventricular free wall, which produces a vector anterior and to the right. This is modified by the early depolarization of the septum in a right to left direction--a vector directed to the left and slightly posteriorly. The resultant vector is directed anteriorly and to the left, and persists for no more than .025 seconds. Then the forces of the left ventricular posterior wall and continued septal activation give a resultant vector directed posteriorly and slightly to the left. As the free wall of the left ventricle becomes activated, the resultant vector sweeps slowly back to the left along an irregular path to the null point.

The criteria for myocardial infarction in left bundle branch block, therefore, are different from the criteria in the presence of a normal QRS loop. Testing of these criteria, of course, is difficult because many of the patients with left bundle branch block have left ventricular hypertrophy, and the presence of myocardial infarction is not uncommon. Apical infarction, which would involve the apex of both ventricles, destroys the initial anterior forces and allows the loop to move directly posterior with initial anterior forces less than .01 msec. On the other hand, true posterior infarction allows the initial anterior forces to persist beyond 0.025 msec. With infarction of the septum, there is loss of the early leftward and posterior forces allowing the right ventricular forces to persist long enough to draw the loop anterior to the right and clockwise around the null point, giving the classic Q wave deformity in I, AVL, V_5 and V_6. Infarction of the lateral free wall allows the slowly progressing returning limb of the QRS loop to swing to the right of the efferent limb and return to the right of the null point, resulting in S waves in V_5 and V_6. Infarction of the lateral free wall allows the slowly progressing returning limb of the QRS loop to swing to the right of the efferent limb and return to the right of the null point, resulting in S waves in V_5 and V_6 and standard lead I. If the afferent limb crosses the X axis at a point greater than 0.5 mv to the right of the E point, the diagnosis of lateral free wall infarction is strengthened. These criteria do not distinguish inferior wall infarction from anterolateral infarction, but do distinguish

lateral free wall infarction from septal and posterobasal infarction. Using these criteria, the diagnosis
of infarction can be made in over 80% of patients with
left bundle branch block. However, the incidence of
false-positive diagnoses of infarction remains at the
35% level.

Left Ventricular Hypertrophy

The accuracy of the vectorcardiographic diagnosis of left ventricular hypertrophy (LVH) remains
less than satisfactory [16, 21]. Diagnostic criteria
for LVH are based on maximal QRS voltage, the angle
of the QRS vector, the T loop angle, and the QRS-T
angle. The more abnormal the VCG is by these criteria, the more certain is the diagnosis of LVH [17].
The vectorcardiographic diagnosis of LVH has been
tested against left ventricular pressures [18] and, in
young patients, against left ventricular weight and
thickness [19]. These measurements have been shown
to have prognostic implications in patients with suspected coronary artery disease [20]. However, a
common misdiagnosis in interpreting vectorcardiograms showing left ventricular hypertrophy is the
additional diagnosis of myocardial infarction, especially anteroseptal [22, 23]. This could have important implications in patients with aortic valve disease as well as coronary artery disease, especially
when aortic valve surgery is contemplated. To review and evaluate the diagnostic accuracy of the
Frank lead vectorcardiogram in LVH, we studied 45
patients with significant aortic valve disease, all of
whom were candidates for open heart surgery and
aortic valve replacement. There were 16 females
and 29 males. Left ventricular pressures were correlated with vectorcardiographic measurements using selected criteria for LVH as previously proposed
in the medical literature. Coronary arteriography
allowed scrutiny of the diagnosis of coronary artery
disease in the presence of LVH in these adult patients. Twenty-two patients had severe aortic stenosis; 13 patients had severe aortic regurgitation;
and 10 patients had mixed aortic valve lesions, i.e.,
stenosis and regurgitation. Mixed aortic valve lesions were defined by a peak to peak systolic gradient
less than 50 mmHg and severe aortic regurgitation
determined by an aortic root angiogram. Coronary
arteriograms were performed by standard techniques. Significant coronary obstruction was diagnosed when the vessel was narrowed by more than
60%. Special attention was given to the angle and the
magnitude (mv) of the 0.01, 0.02, and the 0.03 sec
vectors. Reversal of the inscription of the T loop in
any plane and high frequency notches on the QRS loop
were also examined for a potential relationship to
coronary artery disease.

Results

The data are presented in tables 2 and 3, and in
figures 9-11. R_X and R_Z of the orthogonal system
were added, and this was compared to the left maximal vector (LMV = $\sqrt{x^2+y^2+z^2}$). Figure 9 shows these
two values plotted against each other, and their correlation coefficients for the 45 patients in the three
groups. Fair correlation was demonstrated. The
QRS-T angle was abnormally widened in all cases.
Reversed T loop inscription was frequent, and varied
from 10% to 40% in the three groups. In the aortic
stenosis group, four of nine patients with reversed T
loops had significant coronary artery disease. In the
aortic regurgitation patients, no significant coronary
lesions were found, although five cases had reversed
T loops. High frequency notches were often present,
and varied between 46 and 60% in the three groups.
Coronary artery disease was present in 4 of 12 of the
aortic stenosis groups with notches, 1 of 6 of the
aortic regurgitation group, and 2 of the 6 mixed aortic
valve group, respectively. Significant coronary artery disease was present in 12 of the 45 patients (27%).

Figure 10 shows the distribution of the 0.02 sec
vector in the 22 patients with aortic stenosis. Of the
9 patients who had the 0.02 sec vector posterior to the
X axis in the horizontal plane, only 2 had significant
coronary artery disease. One of these 2 patients had
greater than three vessel coronary disease, while the
other had a lesion in the left anterior descending artery. The 0.02 sec vector posterior to the X axis in
the aortic regurgitation group predicted coronary
artery disease in 3 patients, but none actually had
significant coronary disease. The 0.02 sec vector
posterior incorrectly predicted 1 patient would have
coronary disease in the mixed aortic lesion group.
Five patients in this group had significant coronary
disease, but it was not predicted by the vectorcardiogram. Two of these 5 patients had greater than three
vessel disease, and 3 had single vessel disease. Two
of these latter 3 had left anterior descending obstruc-
tions. A comparison of the left maximal spatial vector and left ventricular peak pressures is shown in
figure 11. The correlation coefficient is positive
(r = 0.41) as shown. The correlation coefficients for
this comparison in the aortic regurgitation and mixed
aortic lesion groups were negative, -0.33 and -.073
respectively. Table 3 compares several studies to
our own with regard to the magnitude of the QRS vector in three planes, the QRS angle in two planes, and
the left maximal spatial vector when it is given.
There is a great range in the magnitude of the QRS
vectors in the three planes, although most of the patients had systolic overloaded left ventricles. There
is a large spread to the age range in these different
groups. Of these studies listed in table 3, only our
own consisted entirely of surgical candidates who had
coronary arteriograms as part of their evaluation for
aortic valve replacement.

Table 2

	Aortic Stenosis N = 22	Aortic Regurgitation N = 13	Mixed Aortic Valve Lesions N = 10
Age	56 years	43 years	56 years
Range	(37–72)	(25–63)	(36–72)
VCG Data			
Orthogonal $R_x + R_z$ (MV)	1.42	2.03	1.68
QRS–T angle			
H plane	166.5°	129.3°	93.9°
F plane	124.9°	91.5°	66.2°
Reversed T loop inscription cases	9/22 (41%)	5/13 (38%)	1/10 (10%)
High Frequency QRS Notches	12/22 (54%)	6.13 (46%)	6.10 (60%)
Hemodynamic Data			
Left Ventricular Pressure	228/18 mmHg	151/16	175/17
Peak to Peak Aortic Valve Gradient	104.9 mmHG		42 mmHg
Cardiac Index	2.5 L/min/M^2	2.6	2.6
Angiographic Coronary Artery Disease	5/22 (23%)	2/13 (15%)	5/10 (50%)

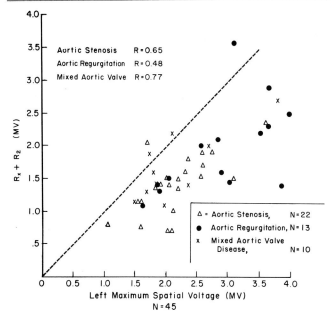

Aortic Stenosis   R = 0.65
Aortic Regurgitation R = 0.48
Mixed Aortic Valve   R = 0.77

△ = Aortic Stenosis,   N = 22
● = Aortic Regurgitation, N = 13
x = Mixed Aortic Valve
     Disease,   N = 10

Fig. 9. The measurement of R in X plus the R in Z is compared to left maximum spatial voltage calculated as $\sqrt{x^2 + y^2 + z^2}$ in patients with aortic stenosis, aortic insufficiency and mixed aortic stenosis and insufficiency.

Table 3

Authors	Type and # Patients	Magnitude of QRS Vector (MV)			QRS Angle		Left MSV (MV)
		H	F	S	H	LS	
Bristow[23]	41 Congenital and rheumatic aortic valve disease and hypertension (age mean 40 years)	3.29	2.95	2.32	$322^0 \pm 17 +$	$24^0 \pm 22$	
Murata[24]	63 Autopsied age av 60 years	1.50 ± 0.56	1.55 ± 0.65	1.23 ± 0.51	330^0		
Varriale[25]	50 Hypertension and aortic valve disease (average age 53 years)	2.61	2.28	1.90	320^0	+38	
Upshaw[26]	20 13 aortic valve disease 4 hypertension (average age 43 years)	1.82	1.68	1.49	322^0	$+27^0$	
Wallace[27]	24 Hypertension aortic valve disease (average age 51 years)	2.43 ± 0.82	2.15 ± 0.77	1.54 ± 0.61	332^0	$+35^0$	2.55 ± 0.80
Postell[28]	22 Aortic stenosis or coarctation of aorta (average age 34 years)		2.59 ± 0.54				2.70 ± 0.57
Abbott-Smith[29]	100 Hypertension aortic valve disease and mitral insufficiency (average age 47)	2.4	2.25				
This Study	45 Total						
	22 Aortic stenosis Average age 56 (37-72)	1.67	1.39	1.66	310^0	$+19.6^0$	2.20
	13 Aortic regurgitation Average age 43 (25-63)	2.5	2.0	2.3	313^0	$+14^0$	2.97
	10 Mixed aortic lesions Average age 56 (36-72)	1.59	1.59	1.43	318^0	+22.5	2.16

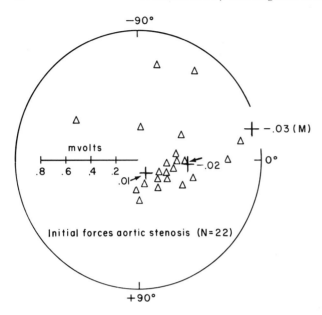

Fig. 10. Individual initial 0.02 sec vectors are plotted as △ in 22 patients with aortic stenosis. The mean .01, 02 and .03 sec vectors for the group are also plotted.

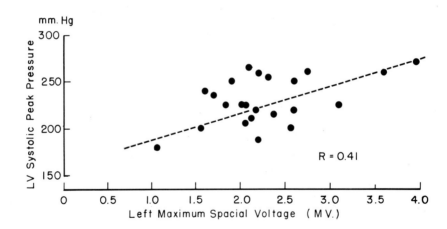

Fig. 11. Left ventricular peak systolic pressure is plotted against left maximum spatial voltage in patients with aortic stenosis.

Discussion

The addition of the R_X to R_Z was done to evaluate any relationship to the left maximal spatial vector ($\sqrt{x^2+y^2+z^2}$) which itself has good correlation with peak left ventricular pressures [18, 25]. The correlation was slightly different in each of the three groups for unexplained reasons (see figure 9). The correlation of the sum of R_X and R_Z to the peak left ventricular pressure for the three groups of patients was as follows: aortic stenosis r = 0.37, aortic regurgitation r = -0.85, and mixed aortic valve lesion r = -0.85. The correlation of peak left ventricular pressure and the left maximal spatial vector is much better in younger patients with aortic stenosis, i.e., r = 0.82 in the pediatric age group [30]. The correlation in our adult patients with aortic stenosis was half this value. Although a simpler calculation, the sum of R_X and R_Z cannot be recommended as a substitute for the left maximal spatial vector in these adult patients.

The abnormally widened QRS-T angle is a consistent finding in our study, as well as other studies of patients with LVH (see table 3). Reversal of the T loop inscription has been observed during ischemia induced by exercise [31]. In this study of patients with aortic valve disease, reversal of the T loop was not helpful in predicting coronary artery disease. Mashima et al. have suggested that the reversed T loop inscription is related to a wide QRS-T angle as well as the shape of the QRS loop [32]. This trend was also seen here. The average QRS-T angle in the horizontal plane in patients who received aortic prostheses and had a reversed inscription of the T loop was: aortic stenosis 205° (range 155-234), aortic regurgitation 194° (range 158-240), and mixed aortic valve disease 164°. When compared to the QRS-T angles in table 2, it can be seen that these values accounted for the wider QRS-T angles.

High frequency QRS notches were reasonably common in this group of patients with LVH. However, no additional information with regard to coronary disease was found from the notches. High frequency QRS notches probably have many causes, e.g., advancing age, ventricular hypertrophy, coronary artery disease, primary myocardial disease, etc. [33].

The diagnostic accuracy of conventional measurements of the Frank vectorcardiogram continue to be disappointing when used to predict left ventricular hypertrophy in the presence of valvular heart disease and coronary artery disease, and this is further complicated by advancing age.

References

[1] D. Durrer, R. T. van Dam, G. E. Freud, M. J. Janse, F. L. Meijler, and R. C. Arzbaecher, Total excitation of the isolated human heart, Circulation 41 (1970) 899.

[2] D. G. Hugenholtz, C. E. Forkner, and H. D. Levine, A clinical appraisal of the vectorcardiogram in myocardial infarction. II. The Frank system, Circulation 24 (1961) 825.

[3] R. M. Gunnar, R. J. Pietras, J. Blackaller, S. E. Dadmun, P. B. Szanto, J. R. Tobin, Jr., Correlation of vectorcardiographic criteria for myocardial infarction with autopsy findings, Circulation 35 (1967) 158.

[4] R. M. Gunnar, E. B. J. Winslow, G. I. Cabin, R. J. Pietras, J. Boswell, and P. B. Szanto, Autopsy correlation of vectorcardiographic criteria for the diagnosis of myocardial infarction. In: I. Hoffman (ed.), Proc. Long Island Jewish Hosp. Symposium, Vectorcardiography 2 (North-Holland, Amsterdam, 1971), p. 277.

[5] Y. Watanabe, K. Nishimima, H. Richman, and E. Simonson, Vectorcardiographic and electrocardiographic differentiation between cor pulmonale and anterior wall myocardial infarction, Am. Heart J. 84 (1972) 302.

[6] H. W. Draper, C. J. Peffer, F. W. Stallmann, D. Littman, and H. V. Pipberger, The corrected orthogonal electrocardiogram and vectorcardiogram in 510 normal men (Frank lead system), Circulation 30 (1964), 853.

[7] I. Hoffman, R. C. Taymor, and A. Gootnick, Vectorcardiographic residua of inferior infarction, Circulation 29 (1964) 562.

[8] E. Young and C. Willians, The frontal plane vectorcardiogram in old inferior myocardial infarction, Circulation 37 (1964) 604.

[9] J. W. Starr, G. S. Wagner, V. S. Behar, A. Walston, and J. C. Greenfield, Jr., Vectorcardiographic criteria for the diagnosis of inferior myocardial infarction, Circulation 49 (1974) 829.

[10] I. Hoffman and R. C. Taymor, Quantitative criteria for the diagnosis of dorsal infarction using the Frank vectorcardiogram, Am. Heart J. 70 (1965) 295.

[11] V. S. Mathur and H. D. Levine, Vectorcardiographic differentiation between right ventricular hypertrophy and posterobasal myocardial infarction, Circulation 42 (1970) 883.

[12] P. M. Kini and H. V. Pipberger, Criteria for electrocardiographic differentiation of right ventricular hypertrophy from true posterior myocardial infarction, Amer. J. Cardiol. 33 (1974) 608.

[13] D. Ha, D. I. Kraft, and P. D. Stein, The ante-
     riorly oriented horizontal vector loop: The
     problem of distinction between direct posterior
     myocardial infarction and normal variation,
     Am. Heart J. 88 (1974) 408.

[14] J. Neuman, J. R. Blackaller, J. R. Tobin, Jr.,
     P. B. Szanto, and R. M. Gunnar, The spatial
     vectorcardiogram in left bundle branch block,
     Amer. J. Cardiol. 16 (1965) 352.

[15] R. J. Pietras, E. B. J. Winslow, J. Boswell,
     P. B. Szanto, and R. M. Gunnar, The spatial
     vectorcardiogram in left bundle branch block.
     Correlation of autopsy findings with vectorcar-
     diogram. In: I. Hoffman (ed.), Proc. Long
     Island Jewish Hosp. Symposium, Vectorcar-
     diography 2 (North-Holland, Amsterdam, 1971),
     p. 277.

[16] E. Massie and T. J. Walsh, Clinical vector-
     cardiography and electrocardiography (Year
     Book Medical Publishers, Chicago, 1960).

[17] D. W. Romhilt and E. H. Estes, A point score
     system for electrocardiographic diagnosis of
     left ventricular hypertrophy, Am. Heart J. 75
     (1968) 752.

[18] P. G. Hugenholtz and R. Gamboa, Effect of
     chronically increased ventricular pressure on
     electrical forces of the heart, Circulation 30
     (1964) 511.

[19] P. G. Hugenholtz, R. C. Ellison, and O. S.
     Miettinen, Spatial voltages in the assessment
     of left ventricular hypertrophy, J. Electrocar-
     diol. 1 (1968) 77.

[20] W. B. Kannel, T. Gordon, W. P. Castelli, and
     J. R. Margolis, Electrocardiographic left ven-
     tricular hypertrophy and risk of coronary heart
     disease, Ann. Int. Med. 72 (1970) 813.

[21] E. Simonson, N. Tuna, N. Okamoto, and H.
     Toshima, Diagnostic accuracy of the vector-
     cardiogram and electrocardiogram, Amer. J.
     Cardiol. 17 (1966) 829.

[22] V. Beamer, M. Amidi, and J. Scheur, Vector-
     cardiographic findings simulating myocardial in
     aortic valve disease, J. Electrocardiol. 3
     (1970) 71.

[23] J. D. Bristow, G. A. Porter, and H. E.
     Griswold, Observations with the Frank system
     of vectorcardiography in left ventricular hyper-
     trophy, Am. Heart J. 62 (1961) 621.

[24] K. Murata, H. Kurihara, S. Hosoda, M. Ikeda,
     and M. Seki, Frank lead vectorcardiogram in
     left ventricular hypertrophy, Jap. Heart J. 5
     (1964) 543.

[25] P. Varriale, J. C. Alfenito, and R. J. Kennedy,
     The vectorcardiogram of left ventricular hyper-
     trophy, Circulation 33 (1966) 569.

[26] C. B. Upshaw, Simplified clinically applicable
     vectorcardiographic diagnosis of left ventricular
     hypertrophy, Am. Heart J. 74 (1967) 749.

[27] A. G. Wallace, B. W. McCall, and E. H. Estes,
     The vectorcardiogram in left ventricular hyper-
     trophy, Am. Heart J. 63 (1962) 466.

[28] W. N. Postell, R. L. Rainey, A. C. Witham,
     and J. H. Edmonds, Vectorcardiographic and
     electrocardiographic manifestations of increas-
     ing left ventricular pressure load, Am. Heart J.
     77 (1969) 33.

[29] C. W. Abbott-Smith and T. C. Chou, Vector-
     cardiographic criteria for the diagnosis of left
     ventricular hypertrophy, Am. Heart J. 79
     (1970) 361.

[30] R. C. Ellison and N. J. Restieaux, Vectorcar-
     diography in congenital heart disease (W. B.
     Saunders and Co., Philadelphia, 1972).

[31] J. H. Isaacs, M. Wilburne, H. Mills, R. Kuhn,
     S. L. Cole, and H. Stein, The ischemic T loop
     during and following exercise, J. Electrocar-
     diol. 1 (1968) 57.

[32] S. Mashima, F. Longtai, and F. Kokichi, The
     ventricular gradient and the vectorcardiographic
     T loop in left ventricular hypertrophy, J. Elec-
     trocardiol. 2 (1969) 55.

[33] N. C. Flowers, L. G. Horan, W. J. Tolleson,
     and J. R. Thomas, High frequency components
     in the orthogonal vectorcardiogram and in the
     scalar leads: Their basis, their significance,
     and their specificity. In: I. Hoffman (ed.),
     Proc. Long Island Jewish Hosp. Symposium,
     Vectorcardiography 2 (North-Holland, Amster-
     dam, 1971).

Vectorcardiography 3 I. Hoffman and R.I. Hamby eds.

VECTORCARDIOGRAPHIC DIAGNOSIS OF RIGHT VENTRICULAR HYPERTROPHY

IN THE PRESENCE OF RIGHT BUNDLE BRANCH BLOCK

Te-Chuan Chou, David Schwartz, and Samuel Kaplan

From the Division of Cardiology, Departments of Pediatrics and Medicine,
College of Medicine, University of Cincinnati, Cincinnati, Ohio

It is generally agreed that the diagnosis of right ventricular hypertrophy is difficult when right bundle branch block is present. A few electro and vectorcardiographic criteria have been proposed in the past; however, their reliability is still uncertain [1-6]. The purpose of this study is to define some simple vectorcardiographic criteria with acceptable sensitivity and specificity for the diagnosis of right ventricular hypertrophy in the presence of right bundle branch block. They are derived by examining two groups of patients. One group has both right bundle branch block and anatomical right ventricular hypertrophy and the other group has right bundle branch block but without right ventricular hypertrophy.

Material and Methods

Patients with tetralogy of Fallot or ventricular septal defect often develop right bundle branch block after surgical correction of the defect. The right bundle branch block has been attributed to injury to the proximal or distal branch of the right bundle during repair of the defect or right ventriculotomy [7, 8]. In these patients it is reasonable to assume that anatomical right ventricular hypertrophy is still present and mostly unaltered shortly after the surgical procedure. In the first group of patients in this study, which represents the group with right bundle branch block and right ventricular hypertrophy, the following requirements were met:

1. The patient had definite anatomical right ventricular hypertrophy supported by hemodynamic and operative findings.

2. The preoperative vectorcardiogram revealed either right ventricular hypertrophy or combined ventricular hypertrophy.

3. The postoperative vectorcardiogram was recorded within three weeks after surgery.

4. A prolongation of the QRS duration of more than 20 msec. had occurred after surgery with the appearance of a slowly inscribed terminal appendage directed rightward and anteriorly.

5. The patients who developed left anterior hemiblock in addition to right bundle branch block were excluded.

In the second group, which represents the group of patients with right bundle branch block but without right ventricular hypertrophy, the following subjects were included:

1. Patients whose electrocardiogram and vectorcardiogram were consistent with right bundle branch block. Their clinical examination revealed no other evidence of heart disease.

2. Patients whose right bundle branch block was the result of surgery, but without clinical or anatomical evidence to suggest right ventricular hypertrophy.

From the selected subjects the QRS loop in the transverse and frontal planes during right bundle branch block was examined. The loop was divided into two portions, namely the main body and the terminal appendage. The following measurements were made from the main body (figure 1):

1. The direction of inscription of the loop in the transverse plane.

2. The direction of the maximum QRS vector as projected in the transverse and frontal planes.

3. The maximum leftward and rightward forces projected on the X axis, R_x and S_x, and their ratio, R_x/S_x.

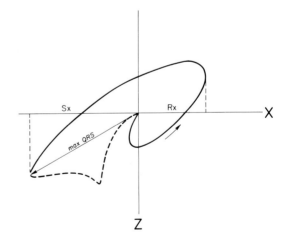

Fig. 1. Some of the measurements of the QRS loop used in this study.

Many other measurements were also made. Since they complicated the results without giving additional information, they are not included in this report.

Results

Group I: Right bundle branch block with right ventricular hypertrophy.

Thirty patients met the requirements for Group I. Twenty-two had tetralogy of Fallot, six had ventricular septal defect with pulmonary hypertension, and two had infundibular pulmonic stenosis. The age of the patients ranged from 1 1/2 to 15 years with an average age of 6.3 years. The postoperative tracings were obtained 4 to 21 days after surgery with a mean period of 10.5 days. The QRS duration before surgery varied from 52 to 84 msec. with an average of 70 msec. The QRS duration after the development of right bundle branch block was from 80 to 128 msec. The average increase was 39 msec. with a range of 22 to 58 msec.

The direction of inscription of the QRS loop in the transverse plane was clockwise in 13 patients, counterclockwise in 9, and a figure of eight pattern in 8. When this was compared with the preoperative records before the development of right bundle branch block, a change in the rotation had occurred in more than 50% of the cases.

The direction of the maximum QRS vector of the main body in the transverse and frontal projections is presented in figure 2. In 20 of the 30 subjects the maximum vector was directed rightward. All but 8 of the patients had a maximum vector directed to the right of 65 degrees in both planes, which is the upper limit of normal in the absence of conduction defect [9].

The magnitude of the maximum rightward QRS forces of the main body as projected on the X axis is illustrated in figure 3. The normal value for each age group in the absence of right bundle branch block as determined by Borun [10] is indicated by the horizontal line. Twelve of the 30 patients had abnormally large rightward forces (Sx). The ratio of the leftward to rightward QRS forces (Rx/Sx) was less than the lower normal limits for the various age groups [10] (0.92 for age 1-4; 0.67, age 5-9; 0.91, age 10-16) in 15 of the 30 cases.

Figures 4 and 5 are examples of right bundle branch block with right ventricular hypertrophy. Both patients had tetralogy of Fallot. The preoperative tracings are also shown.

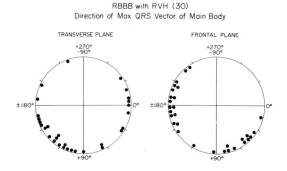

Fig. 2. The direction of the maximum QRS vector in the transverse and frontal planes in patients with right bundle branch block and right ventricular hypertrophy.

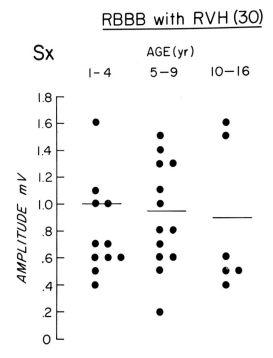

Fig. 3. The magnitude of the maximum rightward QRS forces as projected on the X axis (Sx) in patients with right bundle branch block and right ventricular hypertrophy.

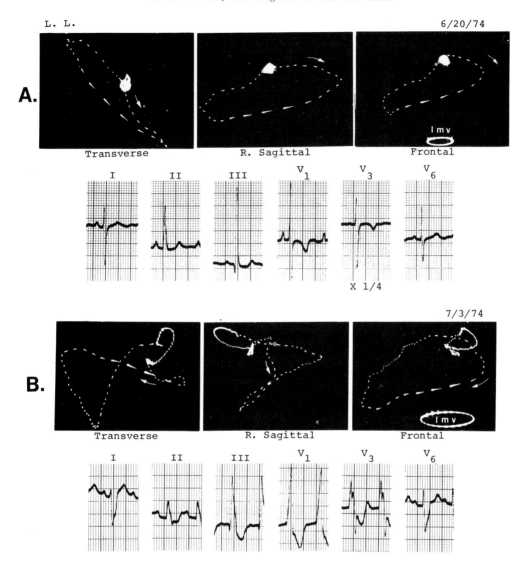

Fig. 4. The pre and postoperative vectorcardiograms and electrocardiograms of a 10-year-old girl with tetralogy of Fallot. The preoperative tracings (A) revealed right ventricular hypertrophy. The postoperative tracings (B) were recorded 8 days after surgery. They were consistent with right bundle branch block with a QRS duration of 128 msec. In the vectorcardiogram the main body of the QRS loop was displaced rightward. Except for the terminal slowing the frontal plane QRS loops before and after surgery were quite similar.

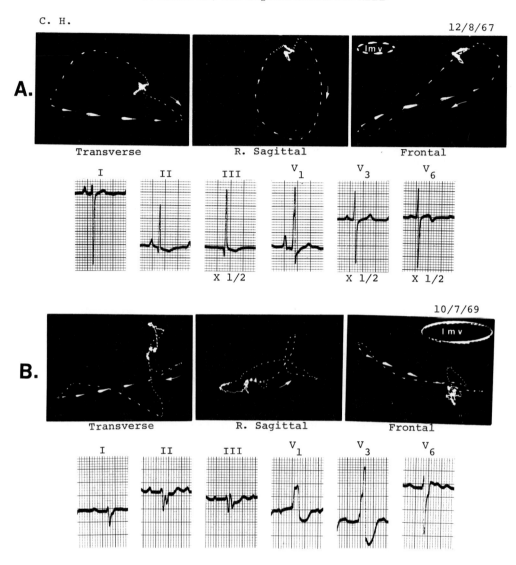

Fig. 5. Right bundle branch block with right ventricular hypertrophy in a 9-year-old boy with tetralogy of Fallot. The preoperative tracings (A) revealed typical findings of right ventricular hypertrophy. The postoperative records (B) were obtained 14 days after surgery. Although the QRS loop had decreased in amplitude, the majority of its main body was still located to the right of the isoelectric point.

Group II: Right bundle branch block without right ventricular hypertrophy.

Nine patients met the criteria for Group II. Two subjects had no evidence of heart disease other than the electrocardiographic finding of right bundle branch block. One of them had a history of rheumatic fever. The other seven patients had ventricular septal defect repairs six months to four years prior to the recording of the vectorcardiogram. Right bundle branch block developed during surgery. The electrocardiogram recorded before surgery revealed no right ventricular hypertrophy. Cardiac catheterization before surgery showed no pulmonary hypertension. Therefore, it is reasonable to assume that these patients did not have right ventricular hypertrophy in addition to right bundle branch block.

The age of the patients ranged from 6 to 18 years with an average age of 10. Both the vectorcardiogram and electrocardiogram were consistent with right bundle branch block. The total duration of the QRS loop varied from 100 to 132 msec. In the transverse plane the direction of inscription was counterclockwise in eight, but clockwise in one. The direction of the maximum QRS vector of the main body was less than 30° in the transverse plane in all of the patients. In the frontal projection it was superior to 50° in all (figure 6). The amplitude of the maximum rightward forces (Sx) was less than the upper normal limit for their age in the absence of block in all of the patients (figure 7). None of the nine patients had an Rx/Sx ratio under the normal limits.

Figures 8 and 9 illustrate the electro and vectorcardiographic findings in two of the patients in Group II.

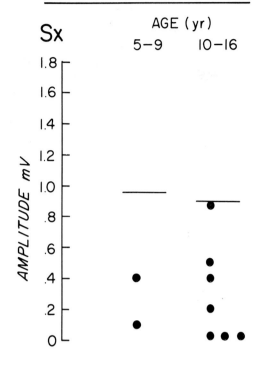

Fig. 7. The magnitude of the maximum rightward QRS forces as projected on the X axis (Sx) in patients with right bundle branch block but without right ventricular hypertrophy.

Summary

When the results of the two groups of patients were compared, it is apparent that using the main body of the QRS loop in patients with right ventricular hypertrophy certain information may be obtained which is helpful in the diagnosis of right ventricular hypertrophy. Using the direction of the maximum QRS vector, the maximum rightward QRS forces and the Rx/Sx ratio of the main body of the QRS loop, 25 of 30 patients with right ventricular hypertrophy were recognized. These same measurements resulted in no false positive diagnosis when they were applied to a group of individuals with right bundle branch block but without right ventricular hypertrophy.

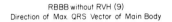
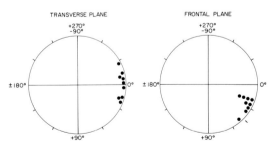

RBBB without RVH (9)
Direction of Max. QRS Vector of Main Body

TRANSVERSE PLANE   FRONTAL PLANE

Fig. 6. The direction of the maximum QRS vector in the transverse and frontal planes in patients with right bundle branch block but without right ventricular hypertrophy.

D. B.

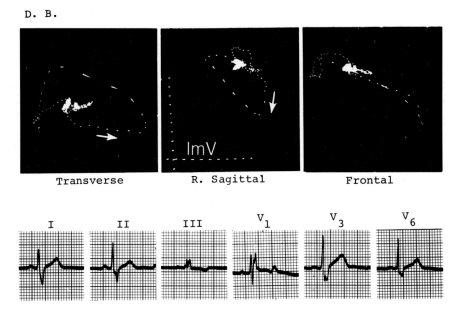

Fig. 8. Right bundle branch block in an 8-year-old girl with no clinical evidence of heart disease. Excluding the terminal appendage the amplitude of the rightward QRS forces in the vectorcardiogram was within the normal range.

Since both clockwise and counterclockwise loops may be seen in the transverse plane in patients with or without right ventricular hypertrophy and the direction of inscription may be changed as the result of the right bundle branch block, it is, therefore, not a reliable sign for the diagnosis of right ventricular hypertrophy.

It is to be emphasized that our results are obtained from patients with congenital heart disease in which the degree of right ventricular hypertrophy is usually severe. The use of the same method in the adult patient with acquired heart disease is still to be investigated. Since it is known that left posterior hemiblock may also result in abnormal rightward QRS forces, this abnormality should be considered in the differential diagnosis.

References

[1] R. W. Booth, T. C. Chou, and R. C. Scott, Electrocardiographic diagnosis of ventricular hypertrophy in the presence of right bundle-branch block, Circulation 18 (1958) 169.

[2] L. Scherlis and Y.C. Lee, Right bundle branch block following open heart surgery: Electrocardiographic and vectorcardiographic study, Am. J. Cardiol. 8 (1961) 780.

[3] L. Scherlis and Y.C. Lee, Transient right bundle branch block: An electrocardiographic and vectorcardiographic study, Am. J. Cardiol. 11 (1963) 173.

[4] I. D. Baydar, T. J. Walsh, and E. Massie, A vectorcardiographic study of right bundle branch block with the Frank lead system: Clinical correlation in ventricular hypertrophy and chronic pulmonary disease, Am. J. Cardiol. 15 (1965) 185.

[5] J. Wartak, Simplified vectorcardiography (J. B. Lippincott Co., Philadelphia, 1970), p. 108.

[6] R. C. Ellison and N. J. Restieaux, Vectorcardiography in congenital heart disease (W. B. Saunders Company, Philadelphia, 1972), p. 128.

[7] J. L. Titus, G. W. Daugherty, J. W. Kirklin, and J. E. Edwards, Lesions of the atrioventricular conduction system after repair of ventricular septal defect: Relation to heart block, Circulation 28 (1963) 82.

[8] E. Krongrad, S. E. Hefler, F. O. Bowman Jr., J. R. Malm, and B. F. Hoffman, Further observations on the etiology of the right bundle branch block pattern following right ventriculotomy, Circulation 50 (1974) 1105.

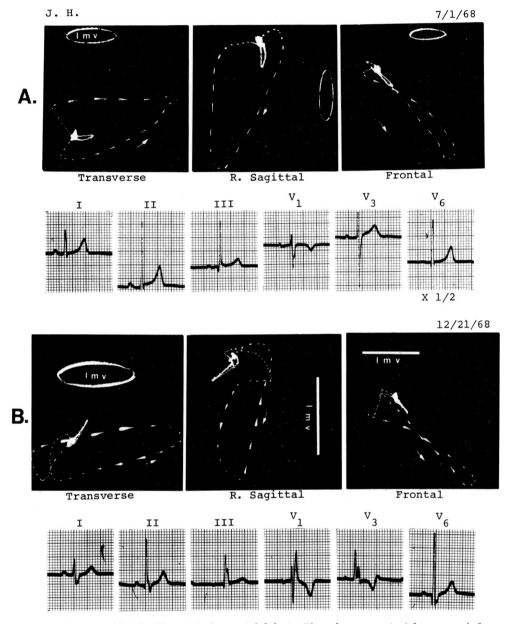

Fig. 9. An 11-year-old girl with ventricular septal defect. The pulmonary arterial pressure before surgery was normal. The preoperative tracings (A) were consistent with left ventricular hypertrophy. The postoperative tracings (B) taken about 6 months after repair of the septal defect showed right bundle branch block. The main body of the QRS loop revealed no abnormal rightward forces.

[9] G. H. Khoury and R. S. Fowler, Normal Frank vectorcardiogram in infancy and childhood, Brit. Heart J. 29 (1967) 563.

[10] E. F. Borun, S. O. Sapin, and S. J. Goldberg, Scalar amplitude measurements of data recorded with cube and Frank leads from normal children, Circulation 39 (1969) 859.

Vectorcardiography 3 I. Hoffman and R.I. Hamby eds.

DIRECT POSTERIOR MYOCARDIAL INFARCTION

A Problem in Differential Diagnosis

Richard J. Kennedy, Joseph C. Alfenito, and Melvin S. Schwartz

From the Department of Medicine, St. Vincent's Hospital
and Medical Center, New York, New York

In most standard texts and in several papers the electrocardiographic (ECG) and vectorcardiographic (VCG) criteria of posterior myocardial infarction are so deceptively simple that one would expect the diagnosis to be made with assurance [1, 2, 3, 4]. Actually, however, this type of infarct often can not be differentiated from other conditions that may mimic it, such as right ventricular hypertrophy (RVH) and a group of normals who present with anteriorly oriented QRS loops on VCG and its ECG counterpart the early rightward transition (ERT). This second group has been largely neglected in the differential diagnosis of posterior infarction (PMI) and an important unanswered question remains, can this normal variant with increased anterior forces be differentiated from PMI?

True or direct posterior myocardial infarction rarely occurs in the absence of inferior or lateral involvement. Because of this over 98% of infarcts analyzed here as in previous studies, were complicated by involvement of the inferior or lateral wall. These combined infarcts were judged to be representative of direct posterior infarction on the premise that the combined infarcts did not affect the altered forces due to the posterior infarct.

Methods

A total of 170 subjects, divided into four groups were included in the study. The number of cases, sex and age range in each group is shown in table 1.

Table 1

Total cases, sex distribution and age range in four groups studied by Frank VCG system

Group	No. Cases			Age Range
Normal	47	M	25	16–80
		F	22	16–87
Early Transition	22	M	13	39–82
		F	9	36–70
R.V.H.	47	M	25	4–67
		F	22	8–68
Posterior Infarct	54	M	52	39–78
		F	2	50–55

The VCG was recorded by the Frank system with the electrodes at the level of the 4th intercostal space with the patient in the supine position [5]. The recording equipment consisted of a Tetronic amplifier and oscilloscope. Horizontal (H), right sagittal (S) and frontal (F) loops were photographed directly from the oscilloscopic screen on Polaroid film. The loops were interrupted 400 times per second, each dash representing 0.0025 sec. The standard calibration was 0.1mV equivalent to 1.0 cm. Twelve lead electrocardiograms as well as the X, Y and Z leads were recorded on the same day as the VCG.

The following characteristics of the H and S plane QRS loops were measured (figure 1).

1. Maximum anterior voltage (MAV) on the Z axis ($90^\circ - 270^\circ$).
2. Maximum posterior voltage (MPV) on the Z axis.
3. Anterior duration (AD). The total duration of the loop in seconds anterior to the X axis in the H plane and the Y axis in the S plane.
4. Posterior duration (PD). The total duration of the loop in seconds posterior to the X axis in the H plane and the Y axis in the S plane.
5. Anterior accession time (AAT). The time in seconds from the onset of the QRS loop to the peak anterior voltage on the X axis in the H plane and the Y axis in the S plane.
6. The angle of the 0.04 second vector.

Other parameters were measured in the H and S planes but proved to be of no diagnostic value. These included the 0.01, 0.02, 0.03 sec. vectors, maximum T voltage, T angle and T length/width ratio. The maximum or 1/2 area QRS vector gave information similar to the 0.04 sec. vector.

The primary aim of the study was to attempt to identify diagnostic criteria for posterior wall infarction (PMI). It soon became evident that it was necessary to differentiate the following conditions that may mimic this infarct.

1. Some normal QRS loops.
2. Anteriorly oriented vector loops defined as those in which the maximum QRS vector or the half area vector is anterior to the X axis in the H plane [6]. The ECG counterpart of this is the early

rightward transition (ERT) with an R/S complex in V_1 or V_2 in which the R voltage is greater than the S without a preceding Q wave. None of the patients in this group had either historical or objective evidence of heart disease.

3. Right ventricular hypertrophy (RVH) with dominant anterior loops. This group included patients with RVH of various etiologies including rheumatic mitral disease, emphysema and congenital lesions.

The above three groups were compared with the infarct group, 98% of which had combined posteroinferior infarction. These patients fell into two subgroups, one with a history of past myocardial infarction and the other with acute infarction characterized by typical chest pain, ECG changes consistent with posterior infarction as well as serial enzyme rises. In this latter group VCG and ECG were performed two to four weeks after the acute stage.

The six parameters listed were measured and compared in each of the four groups in the H and S planes. In the attempt to differentiate the groups cut-off points for each parameter were established. These were derived by normal equivalent deviate analysis (NED analysis) or probit analysis, a form of normal curve analysis by which the distribution pattern for a given parameter can be represented by a straight line if the distribution of values is bell shaped. This method was chosen in preference to the percentage of criteria method which has been used in small groups of patients [6, 9]. Probit analysis clearly demonstrates the overlap or percent of error between groups and helps to identify those parameters which are significant. One of its chief values is that it allows projection from small samples to large population groups.

Results

Although the age distribution was broad for each group, no significant correlation for age was found in any parameter in either H or S planes.

Vector angles up to 0.04 sec., T voltages, angles and length/width ratios were not diagnostic determinants.

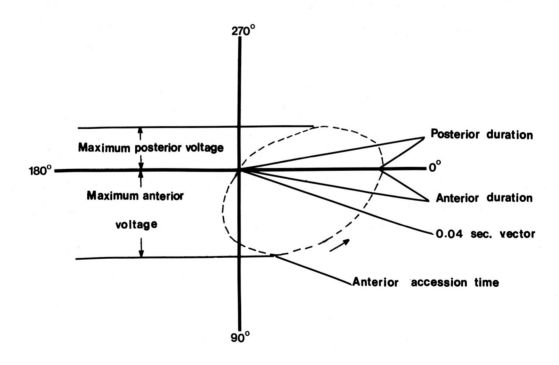

Fig. 1. Diagram (prototype) of horizontal plane anterior QRS loop showing the six characteristics measured.

Table 2

MAV (mV)

	Lit. Norms.	Normals		ERT		S.V.H. RVH		PMI
		M	F	M	F	M	F	M
No.	11	26	20	13	9	25	22	52
H.P.								
M.	.268	.258	.200	.334	.279	.339	.508	.401
S.D.	.164	.179	.159	.124	.174	.216	.472	.161
S.P.								
M.	.283	.243	.217	.339	.253	.333	.436	.414
S.D.	.165	.135	.168	.127	.162	.242	.440	.206
Corr.	.964	.916	.857	.899	.838	.565	.981	.673
Coeff.	p < .001	p < .001	p < .001	p > .001	.1 > p > .001	.01 > p > .001	p > .001	p < .001

MAV (HP)

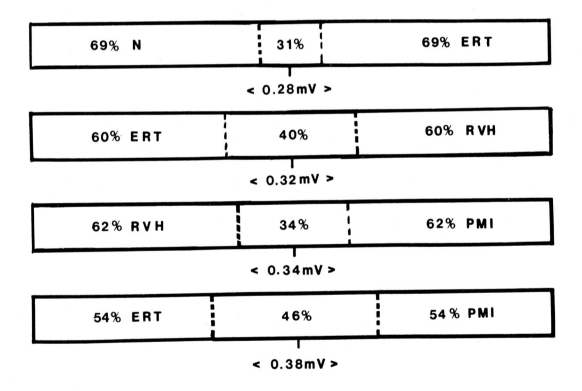

Fig. 2. In this and in the following figures, the percent in the center of the bars represents the percent of error. See text for details.

The correlation between the H and S plane measurements was good so that measurements for both planes are shown only for MAV (table 2). Probit analyses of these measurements are shown in figures 2 and 2a. In this parameter a difference exists only between normals and the other three groups. A noticeable difference is present between the cut-off points between the groups.

Table 3 is the data on MPV. There is a corresponding decrease in the cut-off points in voltage compared to the anterior voltage but the percentage of error in the four groups is unacceptable (figure 3).

Measurements of anterior duration are listed in table 4. The separation between RVH and both PMI and ERT is good with only 1% error. The 42% error between PMI and ERT is unacceptable (figure 4).

Data for PD are listed in table 5 and in figure 5.

The data for AAT are contained in the next table, table 6. The result of analysis is shown in figure 6. ERT is differentiated from RVH with 1% error and PMI from RVH by 1%. Again the error is 40% in attempting to differentiate ERT and PMI.

MAV (SP)

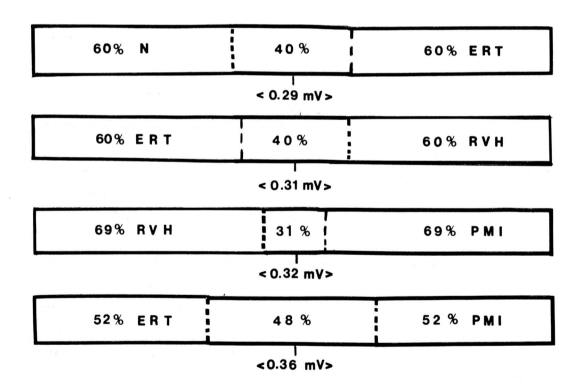

Fig. 2a. For this and other figures, see text for details.

Table 3

MPV (mV)

| | Lit. Norms. | S.V.H. | | | | | | |
| | | Normals | | ERT | | RVH | | PMI |
		M	F	M	F	M	F	M
No.	11	26	20	13	9	25	22	52
H.P.								
M.	.640	.527	.356	.238	.092	.337	.332	.170
S.D.	.274	.315	.229	.195	.119	.188	.240	.144
S.P.								
M.	.716	.564	.415	.209	.097	.298	.255	.194
S.D.	.243	.321	.251	.194	.120	.185	.216	.163
Corr.	.933	.896	.569	.455	.920	.824	.934	.924
Coeff.	p < .001 < p	.001	.01 > p > .001	p > .1	p < .001	p < .001	p < .001	p < .001

MPV (H P)

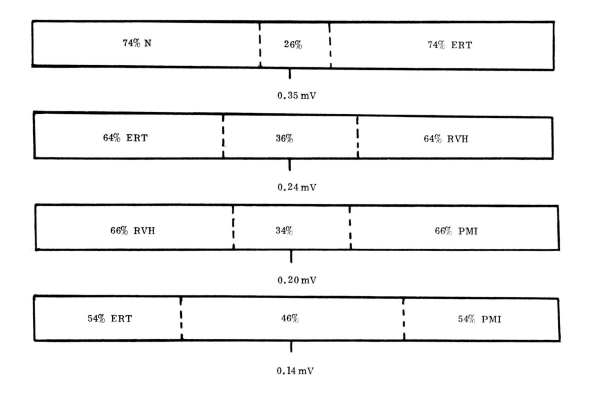

Fig. 3.

Table 4

AD (sec)

	Lit. Norms.	Normals		S.V.H.				PMI
				ERT		RVH		
		M	F	M	F	M	F	M
No.	11	26	20	13	9	25	22	52
H.P.								
M.	.030	.039	.035	.050	.057	.0410	.052	.059
S.D.	.008	.011	.009	.007	.026	.009	.020	.030
S.P.								
M.	.030	.038	.036	.054	.0278	.042	.052	.056
S.D.	.010	.013	.010	.017	.0064	.010	.021	.017
Corr.	.436	.852	.726	-0.491	-0.643	.533	.932	-0.288
Coeff.	$p > .1$	$p > .001$	$p < .001$	$.1 > p > .05$	$.1 > p > .05$	$.01 > p > .001$	$p < .001$	$.05 > p > .02$

A D (H P)

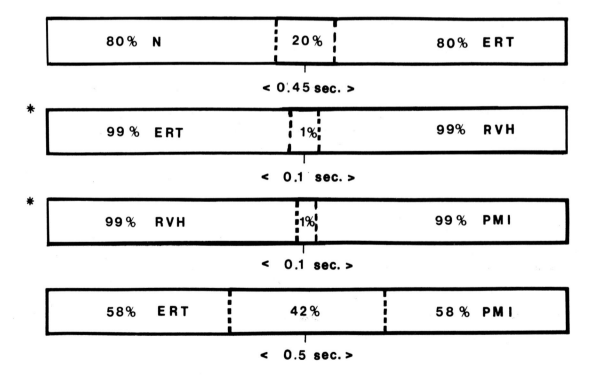

Fig. 4.

Table 5

PD (sec)

| | Lit. Norms. | Normals | | ERT | | RVH | | PMI |
		M	F	M	F	M	F	M
No.	11	26	20	13	9	25	22	52
H.P.								
M.	.036	.053	.053	.037	.133	.087	.043	.035
S.D.	.015	.013	.014	.017	.325	.121	.018	.0199
S.P.								
M.	.041	.058	.054	.041	.085	.077	.043	.034
S.D.	.014	.015	.015	.018	.172	.131	.017	.020
Corr.	.964	.825	.786	.927	.995	.270	.932	.705
Coeff.	p < .001	p < .001	p < .001	p < .001	p < .001	p > .1	p < .001	p < .001

PD (HP)

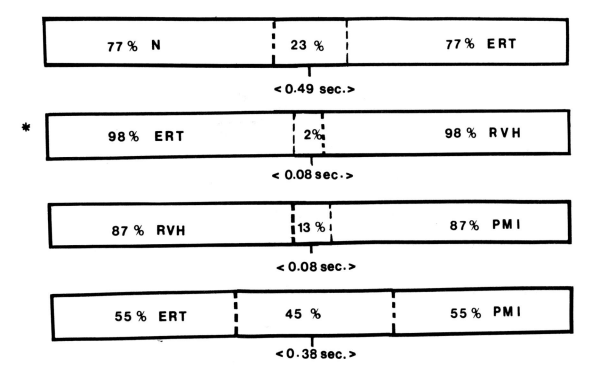

Fig. 5.

Table 6

AAT (sec)

	Lit. Norms.	Normals		S.V.H.				PMI
				ERT		RVH		
		M	F	M	F	M	F	M
No.	11	26	20	13	9	25	22	52
H.P.								
M.	.018	.026	.023	.035	.069	.028	.036	.049
S.D.	.005	.008	.007	.012	.096	.008	.014	.057
S.P.								
M.	.019	.026	.025	.034	.032	.030	.033	.034
S.D.	.007	.006	.008	.011	.014	.013	.011	.012
Corr.	.475	.371	.525	.735	-0.745	.253	.791	-0.437
Coeff.	p > .1	.1 > p > .05	.02 > p > .01	.01 > p > .001	.05 > p > .01	p > .1	p < .001	.01 > p > .001

A A T (H P)

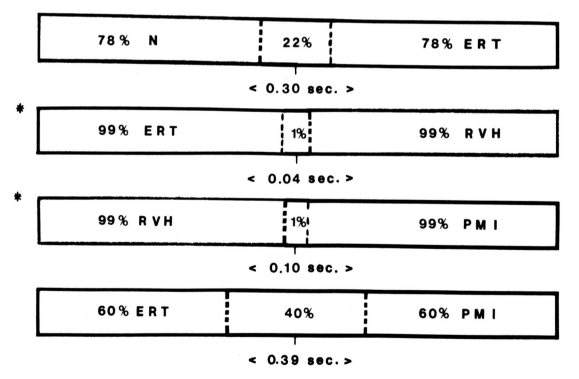

Fig. 6.

Discussion

Definite criteria have been published, with which the present study is in agreement, separating PMI from RVH [6, 7]. The problem remaining is can the anteriorly oriented QRS loop or ERT be differentiated from PMI? Anterior loops are not uncommon and in the absence of combined inferior or lateral infarction present a diagnostic challenge in the absence of a typical history of infarction and serial enzyme changes. Ha, Kraft and Stein are the only investigators to our knowledge who have attempted to answer this question [8]. They compared the VCG findings in nine patients with complete occlusion of either the dominant right coronary artery, its posterior branch or the left circumflex artery with 13 patients with anteriorly oriented QRS loops who had no evidence of coronary artery disease. Both groups fulfilled the combination of criteria for PMI used by McConahay and associates [9] which was based on the criteria of Hoffman and associates [10] and of Chou and Helm [11]. They concluded that the VCG of PMI can not be differentiated from the anteriorly oriented loop of normal individuals. Although pathology was documented by angiocardiography their series was small consisting of 9 infarcts and 13 normals with anterior loops. They calculated the incidence of criteria on a percentage basis. We questioned whether such calculations were valid for such a small series. In this study, the data on 54 patients with posterior infarction and 22 with anterior loops were analyzed by probit analysis. Although the MAD and MAV in this series were greater and the MPD and MPV less than in theirs and in the series of Toutouzas and associates [12] our standard deviation was greater and we have to conclude from probit analysis that our findings are entirely consistent with those of Ha, Kraft and Stein. The VCG and ECG of patients with posterior myocardial infarction usually can not be differentiated from those of normal patients with anteriorly oriented QRS loops or early rightward transition unless there is clear evidence of associated inferior or lateral infarction or one has a prior VCG or ECG for comparison.

References

[1] D. Littman, Textbook of electrocardiography (Harper and Row, New York, 1962).

[2] B. S. Lipman and E. Massie, Clinical scalar electrocardiography (Yearbook Pub., Chicago, 6th ed.).

[3] J. K. Perloff, The recognition of strictly posterior myocardial infarction by conventional scalar electrocardiography, Circulation 30 (1964) 706.

[4] T. Winsor, Primer of vectorcardiography (Lea and Febiger, Philadelphia, 1972).

[5] E. Frank, An accurate clinically practical system for spatial vectorcardiography, Am. Heart J. 70 (1956) 365.

[6] V. S. Mathur and H. D. Levine, Vectorcardiographic differentiation between right ventricular hypertrophy and posterobasal myocardial infarction, Circulation 42 (1970) 883.

[7] M. P. Kini and H. V. Pipberger, Criteria for differentiation of right ventricular hypertrophy from true posterior myocardial infarction, Am. J. Cardiol. 33 (1974) 608.

[8] D. Ha, D. I. Kraft, and P. D. Stein, The anteriorly oriented horizontal vector loop, Am. Heart J. 88 (1974) 408.

[9] D. R. McCanahay, B. D. McCallister, F. J. Hallerman, and R. E. Smith, Comparative quantitative analysis of the electrocardiogram and the vectorcardiogram: Correlations with the coronary arteriogram, Circulation 42 (1970) 245.

[10] I. Hoffman, R. C. Taymor, M. H. Morris, and D. Kittell, Quantitative criteria for the diagnosis of dorsal infarction using the Frank vectorcardiogram, Am. Heart J. 70 (1965) 295.

[11] T. C. Chou and R. A. Helm, Clinical vectorcardiography (Grune and Stratton, New York, 1967).

[12] A. K. Toutouzas, P. Papadopoulos, and D. Augoustakis, Anterior QRS forces in posterolateral infarction, Brit. Heart J. 35 (1973) 1245.

[13] D. J. Finney, Probit analysis (Cambridge Press, Boston, 3rd ed., 1971).

Vectorcardiography 3 I. Hoffman and R.I. Hamby eds.
© 1976 North-Holland Publishing Company - Amsterdam

THE FRANK VECTORCARDIOGRAM IN SUBJECTS WITH

TRIPLE VESSEL CORONARY ARTERY DISEASE

Alberto Benchimol, Charles L. Harris, and Kenneth B. Desser

From the Institute for Cardiovascular Diseases, Good Samaritan Hospital,
1033 East McDowell Road, Phoenix, Arizona 85006

Several studies have demonstrated insensitivity of the resting 12 lead electrocardiogram for predicting the extent of underlying coronary artery disease [1-9]. We recently reported that 29% of subjects with angiographically demonstrable triple vessel coronary artery disease had normal QRS complexes on their resting electrocardiograms [9]. Furthermore, 17 of 106 patients with a similar degree of occlusive disease had completely normal scalar tracings. In an effort to improve the sensitivity of non-invasive methods for diagnosis, Frank vectorcardiograms obtained in this population were reviewed and compared with findings on the resting electrocardiograms. We report here the results of such study.

Material and Method

All selective coronary cineangiograms done at this institution between January 1970 and November 1971 were reviewed. A total of 583 angiograms were performed and 229 demonstrated coronary artery disease. Of all subjects with this latter diagnosis, 106 had significant triple vessel involvement; the study group was comprised of these 106. "Significant" triple-vessel coronary artery disease is defined here as at least a 50% obstruction of the luminal diameter of the anterior descending, left circumflex and right coronary arteries. There were 94 men and 12 women whose ages ranged from 39 to 70 with a mean of 54 years. Details regarding the technique for recording electrocardiograms and performance of coronary cineangiography have been previously described [9].

Frank vectorcardiograms were available for study in 98 of the 106 patients with triple vessel coronary artery disease. Vectorcardiograms in the three plane projections were recorded in the supine position using the Frank lead system [10]. The fourth intercostal space was used for placement of the chest electrodes as suggested by Langner et al. [11] for the supine position. The vectorcardiograms were recorded in a DR-8 Electronics for Medicine light beam oscilloscopic photographic recorder using a vectorcardiographic channel (Model VET-6). Still and

timed [12, 13] vectorcardiograms (running loops) were taken in the frontal, left sagittal and horizontal planes. The still loops were magnified in order to provide optimal analysis of the initial components of the QRS loop; this degree of magnification averaged from 50 to 80 mm. for 0.25 mv. The loops were interrupted at intervals of 2 msec. and the direction of rotation was indicated by a comet with the "tail" pointing in the direction of inscription. Further information regarding our recording method has recently been described in detail [14].

These vectorcardiograms were examined for disturbances of intraventricular conduction, maximal QRS deflection vectors, QRS loop voltage, and abnormalities of the OJ vector and T loop. The direction, rotation and amplitude of the initial 10, 20, 30 and 40 millisecond QRS vectors were carefully noted. All vectorcardiograms were interpreted by three experienced cardiologists. Electrovectorcardiographic diagnoses of myocardial infarction were made on the basis of widely accepted standard criteria [8, 14, 15].

Results

Seventeen of 106 patients (16%) with significant triple vessel coronary artery disease had normal resting electrocardiograms. Vectorcardiograms from 14 of these 17 subjects were available for review. Seven of the 14 (50%) vectorcardiograms were compatible with myocardial ischemia (1) or transmural myocardial infarction [6]. The distribution and extent of coronary arterial disease in these 7 subjects along with their vectorcardiographic findings are listed in table 1. In no case did the vectorcardiogram reveal an anterior wall myocardial infarction in the presence of a completely normal electrocardiogram. All infarctions detected in such cases were inferior, lateral or posterior in location (figures 1 and 2). Vectorcardiograms and electrocardiograms in the remaining seven patients were within normal limits. Fourteen other patients (13%) manifested normal QRS complexes on their electrocardiograms but had S-T segment and T wave changes thought to be secondary to digitalis, ischemia or of a nonspecific nature. In three of these latter cases, the vectorcardiogram was diagnostic of either inferior or posterior wall infarction (figure 3).

Supported, in part, by the Nichols and Sigsworth Memorial Funds.

Table 1

Results of coronary cineangiography and Frank vectorcardiogram
in seven subjects with normal resting electrocardiograms

Patient	Age	Sex	Percent Coronary Artery Obstruction			Vectorcardiographic Diagnosis
			RCA	LAD	LCA	
G.G.	49	M	60	70	80	Inf. Lat. Post. Myo. Infar.
J.B.	50	M	80	80	90	Inf. Lat. Myo. Infar.
H.D.	48	M	70	100	70	Inf. Post. Myo. Infar.
J.P.	50	M	90	80	60	Post. Myo. Infar.
T.A.	49	M	90	90	50	Ischemia
C.B.	51	M	70	80	80	Post. Myo. Infar.
E.W.	52	M	80	60	70	Post. Myo. Infar.

RCA = Right Coronary Artery   Inf. = Inferior Wall
LAD = Left Anterior Descending Coronary Artery   Lat. = Lateral Wall
LCA = Left Circumflex Coronary Artery   Post. = Posterior Wall
Myo. Infar. = Myocardial Infarction

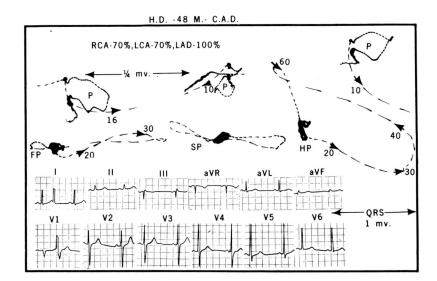

Fig. 1. Frank vectorcardiogram and scalar electrocardiogram in a 48 year old man with triple
vessel coronary artery disease. The resting electrocardiogram is normal. The vectorcardiogram
demonstrates superior displacement of the frontal plane (FP) 24 to 40 msec. QRS vectors, diagnostic
of inferior wall myocardial infarction. The initial 40 msec. QRS vectors are directed anteriorly in
the horizontal plane (HP), indicating posterior wall myocardial infarction. In addition, at least 40%
of the QRS loop area is anterior to the X axis. The degree of coronary arterial obstruction is indicated.

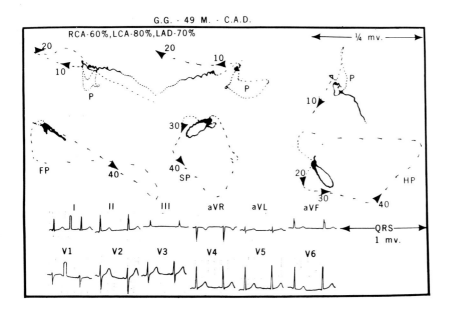

G.G. - 49 M. - C.A.D.

RCA-60%, LCA-80%, LAD-70%

Fig. 2. Frank vectorcardiogram and scalar electrocardiogram in a 49 year old man with triple vessel coronary artery disease. The electrocardiogram is within normal limits. Initial 20 to 30 msec. QRS vectors are oriented superiorly and to the right, indicating inferolateral wall myocardial infarction. The initial 42 msec. QRS vectors are displaced anteriorly in the horizontal plane, diagnostic of posterior wall myocardial infarction. Note that greater than 50% of the QRS loop area is directed anterior to the X axis in the horizontal plane (HP). The degree of coronary arterial obstruction is indicated.

Fig. 3. Selective coronary cineangiograms, Frank vectorcardiogram and scalar electrocardiogram in a 65 year old man with triple vessel coronary artery disease. Coronary arteriograms demonstrate multiple occlusive lesions (arrows) of coronary vessels. The Frank vectorcardiogram demonstrates abnormal S-T and T vectors suggesting myocardial ischemia. Horizontal plane (HP) initial 40 msec. QRS vectors are directed anteriorly, diagnostic of posterior wall infarction. The electrocardiogram shows diffuse S-T segment and T wave changes compatible with myocardial ischemia but no signs of posterior wall myocardial infarction. Note the inverted P waves in scalar leads II, III and aVF and the superiorly directed P loops in the frontal (FP) and sagittal (SP) planes. These P loop abnormalities indicate an A-V junctional or low atrial rhythm.

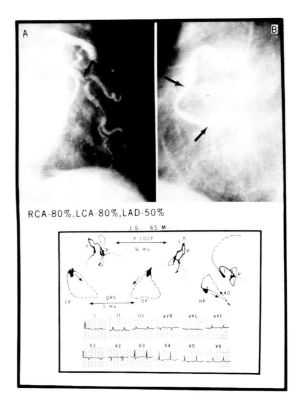

RCA-80%, LCA-80%, LAD-50%

J.S. - 65 M.

A sub-group of seven patients had electrocardiographic QRS complexes which were of normal duration, without diagnostic Q waves of infarction. The
scalar abnormalities in this group were based on abnormal frontal plane QRS axis, low voltage or ventricular hypertrophy. Four of these subjects (57%)
had vectorcardiographic findings compatible with
transmural myocardial infarction; the anatomic sites
of infarction were: posterior--2, inferior--1, and
lateral--1 (figures 4-5).

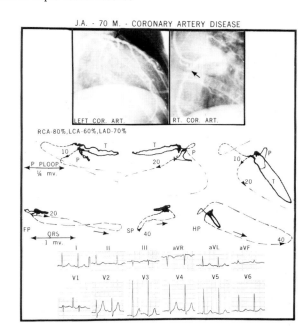

Fig. 4. Selective coronary cineangiograms,
Frank vectorcardiogram and scalar electrocardiogram in a 70 year old man with triple vessel coronary
artery disease. Angiograms show multiple obstructive lesions of all three major coronary arteries.
Sagittal and horizontal plane vectorcardiograms demonstrate major QRS loop area anterior to the X and Y
axis with the initial 52 msec. vectors displaced in the
same direction, these findings indicating posterior
wall myocardial infarction.

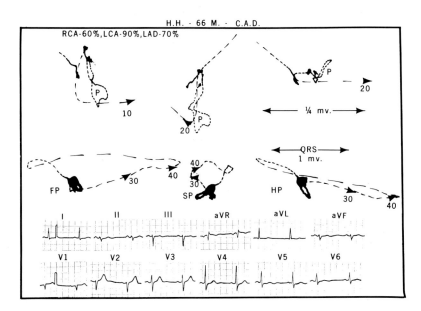

Fig. 5. Frank vectorcardiogram and scalar electrocardiogram in a 66 year old man with triple vessel
coronary artery disease. The vectorcardiogram shows evidence of left anterior hemiblock. The horizontal
plane initial 52 msec. QRS vectors are oriented in an anterior direction, diagnostic of posterior wall myocardial
infarction. The electrocardiogram demonstrates left anterior hemiblock and non-specific abnormalities of the
S-T segments and T waves. There are no electrocardiographic signs of posterior wall infarction.

Frank vectorcardiograms were performed in 59 of 64 subjects with Q waves of infarction on their electrocardiograms. Abnormal QRS vectors diagnostic of myocardial infarction corresponded to the Q waves of infarction for each anatomic site in all cases. The vectorcardiogram, however, detected infarction at locations which were not predicted by the electrocardiogram in 9 of 59 (15%) patients. In 6 cases, the vectorcardiogram demonstrated evidence of posterior wall myocardial infarction when there were no criteria for this diagnosis on the scalar tracing. The other locations of infarction noted on the vectorcardiogram were inferior wall, inferolateral wall and anterolateral wall respectively.

Discussion

Various investigations have been performed in order to correlate the electrocardiogram and vectorcardiogram with post-mortem cardiac findings, or in the case of living subjects, coronary angiograms [1–9]. Burch et al. [6] examined necropsied heart specimens and found that the vectorcardiogram favorably supplemented the electrocardiogram, specifically improving the diagnosis of smaller myocardial infarcts. Gunnar et al. [7] demonstrated high sensitivity of the vectorcardiogram for detecting autopsy proven myocardial infarctions. The vectorcardiogram was predictive of infarction in 92% of 53 hearts and correctly localized the infarcts in 74%. McConahay et al. [8] correlated the electrocardiogram and vectorcardiogram with findings on coronary cineangiography and left ventriculography in 210 subjects presenting with chest pain. Their study concluded that the vectorcardiogram was superior to the electrocardiogram for the diagnosis of transmural myocardial infarction and was more sensitive for revealing multiple infarction sites.

The study described here differed from these other investigations in that it concentrated on electro-vectorcardiographic manifestations in a population with angiographically proven triple vessel coronary artery disease. The fact that normal resting electrocardiograms were present in 17 of 106 subjects afflicted with such a severe degree of coronary artery disease implies that in the individual case, the electrocardiogram is decidedly unreliable for adequate non-invasive screening programs. The actual percentage of normal electrocardiograms in subjects so affected is probably higher, since the vast majority of our cases underwent coronary arteriography for symptoms referable to the cardiovascular system. Clearly, the prognostic implications of so unfavorable a detection rate require that more sensitive techniques be utilized. Our data indicate that the Frank vectorcardiogram reduced by 50 percent the number of false-negative diagnoses as ascertained by examination of the electrocardiogram. Furthermore, infarction patterns were noted on the vectorcardiogram in four of seven patients who had no Q waves of infarction but other QRS abnormalities on the scalar tracings.

It was noteworthy that in the majority of studied cases, the vectorcardiogram detected infarctions of the inferior and posterior walls in absence of diagnostic changes on the electrocardiogram. Interesting as these data may be, they are not surprising and are consistent with the acknowledged superiority of the vectorcardiogram for the recognition of infarctions at these respective anatomic sites [14, 16–20].

A greater sensitivity of the Frank vectorcardiogram for the diagnosis of myocardial infarction in subjects with angiographically documented coronary artery disease can be ascribed to the theoretical and practical advantages of a corrected orthogonal lead system and high fidelity recordings of high frequency components of the QRS vector loop [14]. Previous study has demonstrated that electrocardiograms diagnostic of myocardial infarction can revert to a normal state in at least 20% of cases [21]. It is possible that the vectorcardiogram reveals definitive changes in a significant portion of this patient group. It is our impression that the vectorcardiogram rarely reverts to normal after indicating changes of myocardial infarction and further research in this area is warranted.

Exercise electrocardiography might have resulted in diagnostic S-T segment changes in some of the 17 subjects described here with normal resting electrocardiograms and triple vessel coronary artery disease. There are, however, a few points worthy of consideration in this context. Firstly, for the purposes of diagnosis alone the exercise electrocardiogram would not appear to enhance non-invasive capabilities when definite vectorcardiographic evidence of myocardial infarction is present in subjects with angina pectoris and normal resting electrocardiograms. Secondly, it is possible that initial QRS vector changes diagnostic of myocardial infarction represent more conclusive evidence of underlying coronary artery disease when compared with ischemic S-T segment responses to stress testing. Thirdly, post-exercise or stress Frank orthogonal lead changes or O-J vector loop displacement analysis may be superior to electrocardiographic monitoring under similar conditions in patients with normal resting electrocardiograms and vectorcardiograms. [22].

Our results indicate that the Frank vectorcardiogram should play an integral role in the routine non-invasive evaluation of subjects with possible coronary artery disease, and particularly when there is

a normal QRS complex on the resting 12 lead electrocardiogram.

Summary

Frank vectorcardiograms were obtained in 98
patients with angiographically demonstrable triple
vessel coronary artery disease. Fourteen subjects
with this degree of obstructive disease had normal
resting 12 lead scalar electrocardiograms. Seven of
these 14 patients (50%) had Frank vectorcardiograms
diagnostic of myocardial infarction (6/7) or myocardial ischemia (1/7). All such detected infarctions
were inferior, lateral or posterior in location. Three
of 14 other patients with normal electrocardiographic
QRS complexes and abnormal S-T segments or T
waves had vectorcardiographic evidence of infarction.
A sub-group of 7 subjects with abnormal scalar QRS
complexes, not diagnostic of myocardial infarction,
had vector evidence of the latter diagnosis in 4/7
(57%). Nine of 59 patients (15%) with definite scalar
Q waves of infarction had vectorcardiographic signs
of infarction at other sites which were not predicted
by the electrocardiogram.

It is concluded that (1) the vectorcardiogram is
a more sensitive technique for the detection of myocardial infarction in patients with triple vessel coronary artery disease, and (2) vectorcardiography
should be routinely applied for the non-invasive evaluation of patients with suspect chest pain, particularly when the scalar electrocardiogram appears
normal.

Acknowledgements

We wish to acknowledge the technical assistance
of Carole Crevier, Jeanette R. Goff, Carol Graves,
R.N., Bettie Jo Massey, Nancy Moffatt, R.N., and
Sydney Peebles.

References

[1] M. A. Martinez-Rios, B. C. Bruto Da Costa,
     F. A. Cecena-Seldner, and G. G. Gensini,
     Normal electrocardiogram in the presence of
     severe coronary artery disease, Am. J. Car-
     diol. 25 (1970) 320.
[2] H. G. Kemp, H. Evans, W. C. Elliott, and
     R. Gorlin, Diagnostic accuracy of selective
     coronary cinearteriography, Circulation 36
     (1967) 526.
[3] R. B. Allison, F. L. Rodriquez, E. A.
     Higgins, Jr., J. P. Leddy, W. H. Abelman,
     L. B. Ellis, and S. L. Robbins, Clinicopatho-
     logic correlations in coronary atherosclerosis.

Four hundred thirty patients studied with post-
     mortem coronary angiography, Circulation 27
     (1963) 170.
[4] W. Likoff, H. Kasparian, B. L. Segal, P.
     Novack, and S. Lehman, Clinical correlation of
     coronary arteriography, Am. J. Cardiol. 16
     (1965) 159.
[5] A. Saltups, B. D. McCallister, F. J.
     Hallerman, R. B. Wallace, R. E. Smith, and
     R. L. Frye, Left ventricular hemodynamics in
     patients with coronary artery disease and in
     normal subjects, Am. J. Med. 50 (1971) 8.
[6] G. E. Burch, L. G. Horan, J. Ziskind, and
     J. A. Cronvich, A correlative study of post-
     mortem, electrocardiographic and spatial vec-
     torcardiographic data in myocardial infarction,
     Circulation 18 (1958) 325.
[7] R. M. Gunnar, R. J. Pietras, J. Blackaller,
     S. E. Dadmun, P. B. Szanto, and J. R. Tobin,
     Jr., Correlation of vectorcardiographic crite-
     ria for myocardial infarction with autopsy find-
     ings, Circulation 35 (1967), 158.
[8] D. R. McConahay, B. D. McCallister, F. J.
     Hallerman, and R. E. Smith, Comparative
     quantitative analysis of the electrocardiogram
     and the vectorcardiogram. Correlation with
     the coronary arteriogram, Circulation 42 (1970)
     245.
[9] A. Benchimol, C. L. Harris, K. B. Desser,
     B. T. Kwee, and S. D. Promisloff, Resting
     electrocardiogram in major coronary artery
     disease, J.A.M.A. 224 (1973) 1489.
[10] E. Frank, An accurate, clinically practical
     system for spatial vectorcardiography, Circu-
     lation 13 (1956) 739.
[11] P. H. Langner, Jr., R. H. Okada, S. Moore,
     and H. L. Fies, Comparison of four orthogonal
     systems of vectorcardiography, Circulation 17
     (1958) 46.
[12] R. H. Selvester, L. J. Haywood, and D. E.
     Griggs, The timed vectorcardiogram: a useful
     clinical tool. (As applied to the study of 1,500
     subjects), Dis. Chest 47 (1965) 170.
[13] A. Benchimol and A. Pedraza, The timed vec-
     torcardiogram in the diagnosis of cardiac ar-
     rhythmias, J. Electrocardiol. 2 (1969) 363.
[14] A. Benchimol, Vectorcardiography (The Wil-
     liams & Wilkins Company, Baltimore, 1973).
[15] P. G. Hugenholtz, C. E. Forkner, Jr., and
     H. D. Levine, Clinical appraisal of the vector-
     cardiogram in myocardial infarction. II. The
     Frank system, Circulation 24 (1961) 825.
[16] A. Benchimol and E. C. Barreto, Serial vec-
     torcardiograms with the Frank system in pa-
     tients with acute inferior wall myocardial
     infarction, J. Electrocardiol. 2 (1969) 159.
[17] E. Young, H. D. Levine, P. S. Vokonas,
     H. G. Kemp, and R. A. Williams, The frontal
     plane electrocardiogram in old inferior myo-

cardial infarction. II. Mid-to-late QRS changes, Circulation 42 (1970) 1143.

[18] A. Benchimol and K. B. Desser, The electro-vectorcardiographic diagnosis of posterior wall myocardial infarction, Cardiovasc. Clin. 5 (1974) 183.

[19] P. Toutouzas, P. Hubner, G. Sainani, and J. Shillingford, Value of vectorcardiogram in diagnosis of posterior and inferior myocardial infarctions, Brit. Heart J. 31 (1969) 629.

[20] W. Gray, M. Corbin, J. King, and M. Dunn, Diagnostic value of vectorcardiogram in strictly posterior infarction, Brit. Heart J. 34 (1972) 1163.

[21] C. J. Burns-Cox, The occurrence of a normal electrocardiogram after myocardial infarction, Am. Heart J. 75 (1968) 572.

[22] W. Gray and H. H. Bell, Vectorcardiographic T loop analysis in ischemic heart disease, Brit. Heart J. 33 (1971) 917.

Vectorcardiography 3 I. Hoffman and R.I. Hamby eds.
© 1976 North-Holland Publishing Company - Amsterdam

VENTRICULAR DYSFUNCTION IN INFERIOR INFARCTION:

HEMODYNAMIC AND VCG STUDIES

Jawahar Mehta, Irwin Hoffman, Joseph Hilsenrath, and Robert I. Hamby

From the Department of Medicine, Division of Cardiology, Long Island
Jewish/Hillside Medical Center, New Hyde Park, New York and Queens
Hospital Center Affiliation, Jamaica, New York, Health Sciences
Center, State University of New York, Stony Brook, New York

Left ventricular function as measured by left ventriculography and hemodynamics is more frequently impaired when the electrocardiogram indicates anterior wall myocardial infarction than is the case with inferior infarction patterns [1-6]. Indeed, in a study of 264 patients [1], it was concluded that anterior or anterior plus inferior infarction patterns correlated with poor left ventricular function because these two groups share anterior wall damage. When the "isolated" inferior infarction group was closely examined, it became evident that although the mean values for ejection fraction and end-diastolic volume were normal, a large scatter was evident with many values clearly falling in the abnormal range. It was also observed that 25% of the patients in this group had unexpected asynergy of the anterior or apical wall of the left ventricle.

A study was therefore designed to determine if the patients with electrocardiographic evidence of "isolated" inferior infarction, but with poor left ventricular ejection also demonstrated dysfunction of the anterior wall on left ventricular angiography and further, if such dysfunction was detectable with vectorcardiography.

Materials and Methods

We compared a group of 26 patients with isolated transmural inferior myocardial infarction patterns on electrocardiogram and who had abnormal ejection fractions, with another group of 26 patients with similar inferior wall infarctions but with normal left ventricular ejection fractions. These 52 patients were selected from a group of 435 with chest pain who underwent coronary arteriography and left ventricular angiography at the Long Island Jewish-Hillside Medical Center. Twelve lead electrocardiograms were performed with a Marquette Series 3000 machine operated at a paper speed of 25 mm/second and standardization adjusted to 1 cm./mv. Tracings demonstrating anterior, posterior or lateral wall infarction, left or right bundle branch block, left anterior or posterior hemiblock, left or right ventricular hypertrophy or artificial cardiac pacing were excluded from the study.

All patients had a chest x-ray interpreted by a radiologist to define the presence or absence of cardiomegaly. Frank vectorcardiograms were available on 35 patients, which were interpreted according to accepted criteria [7, 8, 9]. Vectorcardiograms were recorded using a Hewlett Packard/Sanborn vector amplifier and Visoscope Model No. 569A. Loops were photographed using Polaroid high speed film. The usual magnification employed was 1 mv = 5 cm.

Left ventricular angiograms were obtained in the right anterior oblique projection by injecting 0.50 to 0.75 ml/kg of 75% sodium meglumine diatrozoate through either the retrograde or trans-septal catheter. Cineangiograms were taken with a 35 mm camera at a rate of 60 frames per second. After the completion of the left ventricular injection, selective coronary angiograms were performed in multiple projections using methods described by Sones and Shirey [10] or Judkins [11]. The pattern of left ventricular contraction was determined by superimposition of the end-diastolic and end-systolic silhouettes as defined by Herman et al. [12]. Left ventricular volumes were obtained by using a modification of the area length method [13] and the regression equation derived by Hermann and Bartle [14]. By this method the ejection fraction was determined in each patient. Significant disease of a coronary artery was assumed if the lumen was occluded 50% or more [15]. Obstruction in each of the three main coronary arteries and the left main coronary artery was graded 0-6 depending on the severity of obstruction as defined by Bruschke et al. [15]. ECG-VCG and angiographic data were analyzed by separate observers.

Results

Twenty-six patients with inferior infarction patterns (ECG) and poor ejection fractions (Group A) were compared with 26 patients with similar inferior infarction patterns and good ejection fractions (Group B). There were 25 males and one female in each group. The mean age for the two groups was identical (52 ± 7 years in Group A and 52 ± 5 years in Group B). Cardiomegaly was present in 8 patients in Group A, whereas none of the patients in Group B had any evidence of cardiac enlargement.

Table 1

Left ventricular contractile pattern in isolated inferior infarction

	Range	Ejection Fraction % Mean ± 1 S.D.	Asynergy			
			Inferior	Anterior	Apical	Generalized Hypokinesia
Group A (E.F. < 50%) n = 26	16-49	39 ± 9.59	23	10	7	2
Group B (E.F. > 50%) n = 26	51-75	62 ± 6.58	17	3	2	0

E.F. - Ejection Fraction

n = number

Left ventricular contractile patterns and coronary disease. -- Table 1 lists the left ventricular contractile patterns in the two groups. Sixty-three percent of the patients with poor ejection fractions associated with inferior infarction (Group A) had evidence of asynergy of the anterior and/or apical wall of the left ventricle in addition to the expected infero-posterior asynergy. Two patients had generalized hypokinesia.

Twenty-three of the 26 patients had the expected asynergy of the inferior wall. In comparison, fewer patients in Group B had involvement beyond the infero-posterior wall (Anterior 3 and apical 2). One patient in Group A had moderate mitral insufficiency as well. The mean ejection fraction in the two groups were 39±9.59% and 62±6.58% respectively.

Mean coronary scores for each artery in the two groups were calculated. The severity of right coronary artery disease was identical in both groups, whereas Group A manifested greater involvement of the circumflex (3.50±1.72 vs 2.10±1.74) and left anterior descending (3.96±1.48 vs 2.78±1.50) arteries. The number of vessels involved with significant disease was different in the two groups (table 2). The frequency of triple vessel disease in Group A was 65% (17 of 26 patients) compared to only 32% (8 patients) in Group B. Single vessel disease (right coronary or dominant circumflex artery) was present in only one patient of Group A but in nine of Group B. One patient in Group B had no significant disease in any of the coronary arteries, yet had evidence of inferior infarction on the electrocardiogram.

Table 2

Results of coronary arteriography in isolated inferior infarction

	Number of Vessels Involved			
	None	Single	Double	Triple
E.F. < 50% n = 26	0	1	8	17
E.F. > 50% n = 26	1	9	8	8

E.F. - Ejection Fraction

Vectorcardiographic correlations. --Vectorcardiograms were available in 18 patients in Group A and 17 patients in Group B. These were correlated with the catheterization data. The results of vectorcardiographic interpretation are shown in tables 3A and 3B. All patients showed evidence of inferior infarction confirming the electrocardiograms. Vectorcardiographic evidence of posterior wall (dorsal) infarction was present in three patients in each group. All six manifested asynergy of the infero-dorsal wall of the left ventricle as seen on the left ventricular angiograms. Evidence of anterior infarction was found in five patients in Group A (28%) but in only one

Table 3A

ECG-VCG, Arteriographic and ventriculographic correlations

Group A No.	ECG	VCG	Coronary Artery Dis. LAD	RCA	Cx	Asynergy Inferior	Anterior	Apical	E.F. (%)
1.	IMI	IMI+AMI	+	+	+	+	0	+	44
2.	IMI	IMI+AMI	+	+	+	+	+	0	45
3.	IMI	IMI+AMI+LAHB	+	+	+	+	+	0	49
4.	IMI	IMI+AMI	+	+	+	+	+	0	43
5.	IMI	IMI+AMI	+	+	+	0	+	+	32
6.	IMI	IMI	+	+	+	0	0	+	47
7.	IMI	IMI	+	+	+	+	0	0	46
8.	IMI	IMI	0	+	0	+	0	0	48
9.	IMI	IMI	+	+	+	+	0	+	43
10.	IMI	IMI+LVH	+	+	+	+	0	+	22
11.	IMI	IMI	+	+	+	+	+	0	16
12.	IMI	IMI	+	+	0	+	0	0	47
13.	IMI	IMI	+	+	+	+	+	0	43
14.	IMI	IMI+DMI	+	+	+	+	+	0	26
15.	IMI	IMI+DMI+LVH	+	+	0	+	0	0	38
16.	IMI	IMI-LVH	+	+	0	+	0	+	38
17.	IMI	IMI+DMI	+	0	+	+	0	0	45
18.	IMI	IMI	+	+	+	+	0	0	46

ECG - Electrocardiogram
VCG - Vectorcardiogram
LAD - Left anterior descending artery
RCA - Right coronary artery
Cx - Circumflex artery

E.F. - Ejection fraction
IMI - Inferior wall myocardial infarction
DMI - Dorsal wall myocardial infarction
AMI - Anterior wall myocardial infarction
LVH - Left ventricular hypertrophy

Table 3B

Group B No.	ECG	VCG	Coronary Artery Dis. LAD	RCA	Cx	Asynergy Inferior	Anterior	Apical	E.F. (%)
1.	IMI	IMI+DMI	+	+	0	+	0	0	64
2.	IMI	IMI	+	+	+	+	0	0	64
3.	IMI	IMI	+	+	+	+	0	+	53
4.	IMI	IMI	+	+	0	+	0	0	51
5.	IMI	IMI	0	+	0	+	0	0	60
6.	IMI	IMI	0	0	0	+	0	0	75
7.	IMI	IMI	0	+	0	+	0	0	66
8.	IMI	IMI+LVH	+	+	0	+	0	0	63
9.	IMI	IMI+DMI	0	+	0	+	0	0	66
10.	IMI	IMI	+	+	+	+	0	0	60
11.	IMI	IMI+AMI	+	+	0	+	+	0	52
12.	IMI	IMI	+	+	+	+	0	0	52
13.	IMI	IMI	0	+	0	+	0	0	65
14.	IMI	IMI+DMI	0	+	0	+	0	0	62
15.	IMI	IMI	+	0	+	0	0	0	66
16.	IMI	IMI	0	+	0	+	0	0	59
17.	IMI	IMI	+	+	+	+	0	0	75

Symbols are the same as in table 3A.

patient of Group B (6%). These six patients all had anterior and/or apical asynergy by left ventriculography. The vectorcardiograms also revealed left anterior hemiblock in one patient and left ventricular hypertrophy in three patients in Group A. In contrast left ventricular hypertrophy was present in only one patient in Group B and none had left anterior hemiblock. These results are summarized in table 4. Typical examples of patients in Groups A and B are shown in figures 1-4.

Table 4

Summary of VCG findings in 35 patients with inferior infarction

	IMI	AMI	DMI	LVH	LAHB
E.F. < 50% n = 18	18	5	3	3	1
E.F. > 50% n = 17	17	1	3	1	0

IMI - Inferior myocardial infarction
AMI - Anterior myocardial infarction
DMI - Dorsal myocardial infarction
LVH - Left ventricular hypertrophy
LAHB - Left anterior hemiblock
n - number of patients

Discussion

The classic vectorcardiographic abnormality in anterior wall myocardial infarction consists of a posterior horizontal loop with clockwise rotation and very small or absent anterior initial QRS forces [7, 8]. This picture has recently been correlated with extensive anterior wall asynergy [16]. The present study addresses itself to more subtle VCG residuals of anterior wall disease which are insufficient in themselves to eliminate precordial unipolar R waves or to change the major rotation of the horizontal QRS loop.

In this study, all the 35 frontal plane vectorcardiograms exhibited leftward QRS loops with clockwise movement and with the 30 msec. vector superior to the X axis, meeting accepted criteria for inferior wall myocardial infarction. The VCG criteria that we accepted as evidence for anterior wall myocardial infarction are summarized in figure 5 (adapted from Van Herpen et al. [9] and reproduced with permission).

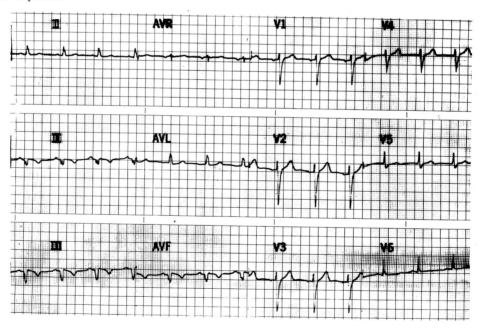

Fig. 1. 12 lead ECG typical of inferior infarction. Ejection fraction normal (Pt. I.G., 47, male), Group B.

I.G. 47 year old male.

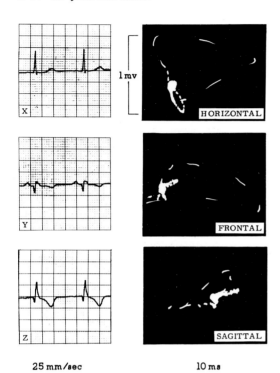

1 mv

X

Y

Z

25 mm/sec   10 ms

Fig. 2. VCG corresponding to Fig. 1.
Note normal anterior forces in lead Z
and in horizontal QRS loop.

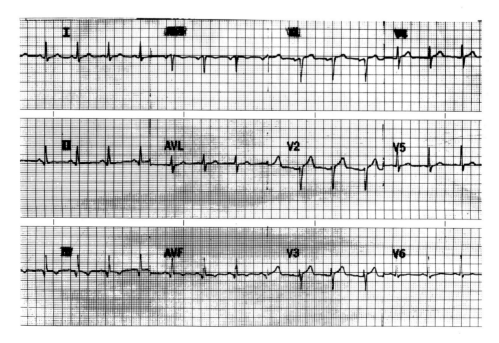

Fig. 3. 12 lead ECG typical of inferior infarction. Ejection fraction abnormally low. (Pt. J.K., 43, male) Group A.

J.K. 43 year old male.

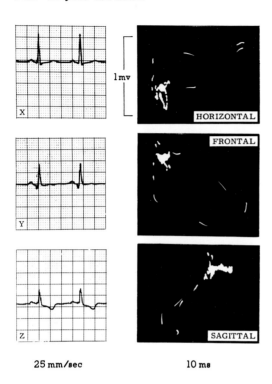

25 mm/sec   10 ms

Fig. 4. VCG corresponding to Fig. 3. Note absent anterior QRS forces in lead Z and posterior early "bite" in horizontal QRS loop indicating anterior infarction.

In 5 of 18 patients with unequivocal ECG evidence of inferior infarction and poor ejection fractions, one or more of these criteria were satisfied. In 4 of the 5 cases, anterior asynergy was observed and in the fifth, apical asynergy was present. Three additional patients in this group had anterior and 4 had apical asynergy, but none of these 7 satisfied criteria for anterior wall infarction by VCG. Thus, of all 12 patients with inferior infarction, poor ejection fraction and anterior asynergy, VCG correctly identified 5 (42%).

In addition to detection of unsuspected anterior infarction, vectorcardiography proved of additional value, in the poor ejection fraction group, in the diagnosis of dorsal wall infarction in three, left ventricular hypertrophy in three, and left anterior hemiblock in one patient.

In sharp contrast stand the 17 patients with inferior wall infarction and normal ejection fractions.

Only two had anterior or apical asynergy, and only one of these met VCG criteria for anterior myocardial infarction. It seems clear from these results that a poor ejection fraction in inferior wall myocardial infarction has a high correlation with anterior and/or apical left ventricular dysfunction and that about 40% of such cases can be correctly identified on the basis of VCG criteria for anterior wall myocardial infarction.

Marked differences were observed in the severity and extent of coronary obstruction between the abnormal ejection fraction Group (A) and normal ejection fraction group (B). Triple vessel disease was twice as common in Group A. In contrast, single vessel disease was found in only one of 26 patients in Group A (47%) whereas in Group B, a single vessel lesion was observed in 9 of 26 patients.

It is generally recognized that patients with isolated inferior infarctions have better ventricular function than those with anterior wall pathology [1, 3, 6]. However, our study strongly suggests that the scalar ECG is not entirely reliable in identifying isolated inferior infarction. When vectorcardiography is done in these patients, as a supplementary study, the diagnosis of occult anterior wall infarction is of great significance. An explanation for the increased sensitivity of the VCG in this situation is presented in figure 6. Left ventricular hypertrophy, dorsal wall infarction and left anterior hemiblock may also be revealed and are clues to more extensive myocardial damage, more extensive coronary disease and poor left ventricular emptying. Thus vectorcardiography, in addition to improving the accuracy of diagnosis of myocardial damage as reported by Burch et al. [17] and Gunnar et al. [18], may also prove valuable in the prediction of ventricular function.

Summary

Twenty-six patients with electrocardiographic evidence of localized inferior myocardial infarction and poor ejection fraction (less than 50%) were compared with 26 patients with similar ECGs, but with normal ejection fraction (over 50%). The poor ejection fraction group had significantly more frequent and more severe disease in left anterior descending artery and a higher incidence of triple coronary obstruction than the normal ejection fraction group. The poor ejection fraction group had a significantly greater incidence of ventricular asynergy in the anterior and apical segments of left ventricle. Vectorcardiography was available in 35 of the 52 patients studied, and frequently supplied diagnostic information not available in the scalar electrocardiograms. Of 18 patients with scalar ECG patterns of isolated inferior wall infarction and poor ejection fractions,

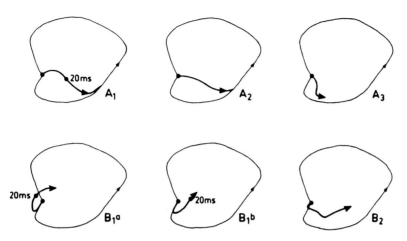

Fig. 5. Criteria for antero-septal infarction

(A1) Initial part of the vector loop takes a leftward and posterior course. In isolated antero-septal infarction, the 20 msec. vector should return to a point anterior of E.

(A2) The initial part, although anterior of E, recedes to the left. This may result in a flat concavity.

(A3) Circumscript concavity from the right and anterior during the initial 15 msec.

Criteria for strictly anterior infarction

(B1) Following the forward septal activity, the centrifugal part of the loop turns immediately to posterior, the 20 msec. vector has a posterior direction. This is manifested in two ways in the horizontal projection. (B1a)--The centrifugal part runs a clockwise course behind the point E. (B1b)--The centrifugal part follows a counterclockwise course in front of E.

(B2) A concavity from anterior occurring after 15 to 30 msec.

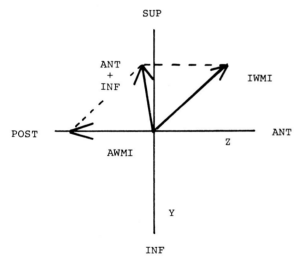

Fig. 6. The resultant of the anterior infarct vector (AWMI) and the inferior infarct vector (IWMI) is directed markedly superiorly (ANT + INF), almost perpendicular to the Z axis. If the precordial V leads are left or superior to the E point, initial R waves will result. The corrected Frank Z lead registers a posterior deflection.

vectorcardiography identified 5 cases with anterior infarction, 3 with left ventricular hypertrophy and one with left anterior hemiblock. Vectorcardiography is a valuable supplementary tool in the clinical assessment of patients with apparently isolated inferior infarction. When extensive coronary and poor ventricular function exist, vectorcardiographic clues may be expected in about half the patients.

References

[1] R. E. Hamby, I. Hoffman, J. Hilsenrath et al., Clinical, hemodynamic and angiographic aspects of inferior and anterior myocardial infarctions in patients with angina pectoris, Am. J. Cardiol. 34 (1974) 513-19.

[2] K. Chatterjee, M. Sacoor, G. C. Sutton et al., Angiographic assessment of left ventricular function in patients with ischemic heart disease without clinical heart failure, Gr. Heart J. 33 (1971) 559-64.

[3] B. J. Field, R. O. Russell, Jr., J. T. Dowling et al., Regional left ventricular performance in the year following myocardial infarction, Circulation 46 (1972) 679-89.

[4]   J. W. Linhart, F. J. Hildner, S. S. Barold, et al. , Myocardial function in patients with coronary artery disease, Am. J. Cardiol. 23 (1969) 379-85.

[5]   R. R. Williams, P. F. Cohen, P. S. Vokonas, et al. , Electrocardiographic, arteriographic and ventriculographic correlations in transmural myocardial infarction, Am. J. Cardiol. 31 (1973) 595-99.

[6]   R. O. Russell, Jr. , D. Hunt, C. E. Rackley et al. , Left ventricular hemodynamics in anterior and inferior myocardial infarction, Am. J. Cardiol. 32 (1973) 8-16.

[7]   T. Chou and R. A. Helm, Clinical vectorcardiography (Grune and Stratton, New York and London, 1967).

[8]   E. Massie and T. J. Walsh, Clinical vectorcardiography and electrocardiographic (Yearbook Publishers, Chicago, 1960), pp. 268-316.

[9]   G. Van Herpen, A. V. G. Bruschke, and A. W. Hansen, The correlations between the coronary arteriogram and other diagnostic parameters. Proc. Long Island Jewish Hosp. Symposium Vectorcardiography 2 (North-Holland, Amsterdam, 1971), pp. 352-61.

[10] F. M. Sones, Jr. , and E. K. Shirey, Cinecoronary arteriography, Mod. Concepts Cardiovasc. Dis. 31 (1962) 735-38.

[11] M. P. Judkins, Percutaneous transfemoral selective coronary arteriography, Radiolog. CII. North Am. 6 (1968) 467-92.

[12] M. V. Herman, R. A. Heinle, M. D. Klein et al. , Localized disorders in myocardial contractions. Asynergy and its role in congestive heart failure, New Engl. J. Med. 277 (1967) 222-32.

[13] H. T. Dodge, H. Sandler, D. W. Ballew et al. , The use of biplane angiocardiography for the measurement of left ventricular volume in man, Am. Heart J. 60 (1960) 762-76.

[14] H. J. Hermann and S. H. Bartle, Left ventricular volumes by angiocardiography; comparison of methods and simplification of technique, Cardiovasc. Research 2 (1968) 404-14.

[15] A. V. G. Bruschke, The diagnostic significance of the coronary arteriogram. A study of its value in relation to other diagnostic methods (Utrecht, Kremink en orn N.V., 1970).

[16] E. Young, P. F. Cohn, R. Gorlin, et al. , Vectorcardiographic diagnosis and electrocardiographic correlation in left ventricular asynergy due to coronary artery disease, Circulation 51 (1975) 467-76.

[17] G. E. Burch, L. G. Horan, J. Ziskind et al. , A correlative study of postmorten electrocardiographic and spatial vectorcardiographic data in myocardial infarction, Circulation 18 (1958) 325-40.

[18] R. M. Gunnar, R. Pietras, J. Blackaller, et al. , Correlation of vectorcardiographic criteria for myocardial infarction with autopsy findings, Circulation 35 (1967) 158-71.

SECTION 2.
VECTORCARDIOGRAPHY OF THE P AND T WAVES

Vectorcardiography 3 I. Hoffman and R.I. Hamby eds.
© 1976 North-Holland Publishing Company - Amsterdam

AN OVERVIEW OF P AND T LOOPS

J. A. Abildskov

From the Cardiovascular Research and Training Institute and Cardiology
Division, Department of Internal Medicine, University of Utah,
College of Medicine, Salt Lake City, Utah 84132

The P and T loops of the vectorcardiogram and
their counterparts in other displays of electrocardiographic data almost certainly contain significant medical information that has not yet been usefully identified. At present, the major utility of P waves is related to identification of the cardiac rhythm and involves their presence and temporal relation to the
ventricular complex. The form of P waves and loops
has utility in the recognition of atrial enlargement,
cardiac pacemaker site and intra-atrial conduction
disorders. In current use, the form of ST-T waves
and loops has major medical significance but this is
mainly a consequence of the high incidence of abnormalities rather than the specificity of ST-T abnormalities. Improved definition of the physiologic basis of
P and T waves and loops and extended correlations
between these deflections and the presence, severity
and course of both organic disease and functional
states offer excellent possibilities for improvement in
the range and precision of clinical electrocardiography.

The other papers in this section on vectorcardiography of the P and T loops will present the
current state of information as to the physiologic
basis of the T wave and loop and the value of P loops
in recognizing and differentiating atrial enlargement
and intra-atrial conduction defects. This "overview"
will not repeat specific information to be included in
those communications but will have the theme of possibilities for increased clinical utility of P and T
waves and loops. The material has been organized
into three sections. One of these concerns information furnished by the combination of T waves and T
loops which is not provided by either display alone.
The second section considers possible prognostic use
of P and T waves and loops and the third section concerns possibilities for increased diagnostic specificity of these deflections.

Supported, in part, by Program Project Grant
#HL 13480, Contract NHLI 72-2988 from the National
Institutes of Health, and the Richard A. and Nora
Eccles Harrison Fund for Electrocardiographic Re-
search.

T Waves and T Loops

Since the symposium particularly concerns
vectorcardiograms and this section specifically includes consideration of the T loop, the merit of that
display in relation to scalar electrocardiographic
leads will be considered. It should be clearly recognized that the same cardiac phenomena are responsible for T waves and T loops. The identical cardiac
events which determine features of T loops displayed
as Lissajou figures also determine those of the T deflection in vectorcardiograms displayed in terms of
polar coordinates. Likewise, the same cardiac
states responsible for T waves in a single electrocardiographic lead determine the body surface potential pattern based on hundreds of electrodes. The
cardiac origin of deflections in these and other displays does not differ, but the displays differ in the
completeness with which that origin is reflected.

The T wave of scalar electrocardiographic
leads and the T loop of the vectorcardiogram provide
an excellent example of different displays furnishing
complementary information. One of the most important features of the normal electrocardiogram is that
polarity of the major QRS deflection and of T waves
is usually the same in an individual lead. This feature led to one of the most important insights into the
physiologic basis of the electrocardiogram, namely
that the sequence of ventricular repolarization differed from that of excitation. The clinically significant consequences of the observation that normal QRS
and T deflections had the same polarity and the insight into the mechanisms of this finding, were studies which established discordant QRS and T deflections to have value in the recognition of heart disease.

An equally important observation and insight as
to its mechanism was that the normal T loops are
usually inscribed in the same direction as QRS loops
in a particular plane projection. One of the earliest
publications employing the term "vectorcardiogram"
noted that the similar inscription direction of QRS and
T loops required substantial similarities of the normal ventricular excitation and recovery orders [1].
Scalar electrocardiographic leads furnish evidence
that normal excitation and recovery must differ but
vectorcardiograms provide equally persuasive evidence that the two processes must have features in

common [2,3]. Deviations from the normal differences
in excitation and recovery patterns as reflected in T
waves of abnormal polarity have been extremely useful in diagnostic electrocardiography. Deviations
from the normal similarities of the two processes
recognizable from the T loop have not been as fully
explored for their diagnostic value although pertinent
studies have been conducted and strongly suggest substantial diagnostic value [4-13].

Prognostic Electrocardiography and Vectorcardiography

Cardiac arrhythmias, particularly ventricular
fibrillation, are the most frequent mechanism by which
death occurs in the United States. The cause of death
is usually considered to be the underlying disease process and this is most often ischemic heart disease
and particularly the manifestation of acute myocardial
infarction. It is well established that mortality in this
condition can be modified by the prevention or man-
agement of the frequently associated arrhythmias.
These facts form the background for a major and
largely new area of possible utility for the electrocardiogram and vectorcardiogram. The general area
referred to is that of prognosis and, more specifically, the area is that of evaluating susceptibility of the
heart to arrhythmias prior to their actual ocurrence.
It should be emphasized that a possible rather than an
established area of utility is being discussed.

There are a number of electrophysiologic states
with established relations to arrhythmia susceptibility
and at the same time are known to be determinants of
electrocardiographic and vectorcardiographic waveform. One of these is the degree of inequality of repolarization. In the case of the atria, inequalities of
recovery time produced by vagal stimulation have
striking influence on the ease with which atrial fibrilla-
tion can be induced and sustained [14-16]. The same
agency alters P waveform and suggests at least the
possibility of recognizing an atrial state of greater
than normal susceptibility to fibrillation. In the same
sense, vulnerability to ventricular fibrillation has been
established to have a close relation to disparities in
the time of recovery of ventricular excitability [17-23].
These disparities must be reflected in the time course
of repolarization and this is also the organ level determinant of ST-T wave and loop form [24-28].

Some correlations which suggest T waveform
might have utility in recognizing ventricular states
vulnerable to arrhythmias already exist. The high incidence of arrhythmias in the early phases of acute
myocardial infarction is at least roughly correlated
with a period of high peaked T waves in the body surface electrocardiogram. The magnitude of ST segment displacement has also been shown to have

prognostic significance in patients with acute myocardial infarction [29]. At present these relations
are not firmly enough established and the optimum
electrocardiographic and vectorcardiographic parameters for their recognition have not been well enough
defined for useful application to prognosis in individual cases. As part of this overview of P and T waves
and loops however, the possibility of recognizing cardiac states of altered arrhythmia susceptibility prior
to the occurrence of these events, and with the expec-
tation that arrhythmia ausceptibility by appropriate
therapy is possible, can be cited as one of the most
promising areas for electrocardiographic and vectorcardiographic research.

Diagnostic Specificity

Finally in this overview of P and T loops and
waves, the need for and possibility of improved specificity in the recognition of cardiac states responsible
for abnormalities of these components of the electrocardiogram and vectorcardiogram will be reviewed.
At present, there is an unfortunately widespread practice of equating abnormalities of the ST-T deflection
with ischemic heart disease [30]. Increasing interest
in and dependence on exercise testing for the diagnosis
of ischemic heart disease has resulted in the practice
becoming even more widespread. While the number
and significance of diagnostic errors based on assum-
ing ST-T abnormalities to be the result of ischemic
cardiac disease is unknown, the fact that such errors
occur is certain. Drug effects, particularly those of
digitalis on the ST-T deflection, are well known and
recognized in the evaluation of ST-T abnormalities.
They are usually recognized, however, by discarding
the diagnostic utility of electrocardiographic findings
in patients with such drug effects. Less often considered are the possible influences of the autonomic
nervous system, particularly the direct influences of
the sympathetic system on ventricular repolarization.
These are powerful influences in experimental prepa-
rations and their occurrence in clinical conditions in
association with neurologic disease suggests they
should be given greater account in the evaluation of
ST-T deflections [31-44]. The role of this mechanism
in determining normal ventricular repolarization and
the form of the normal ST-T deflection, its role in
stress induced alterations of electrocardiographic and
vectorcardiographic form and the possibility of separating these effects and those of drugs and other
agencies from those of organic disease as well as the
more precise definition of specific disease entities
themselves are important goals for future studies of
ST-T waves and loops.

Summary

The P and T components of the electrocardio-gram and vectorcardiogram offer substantial poten-tialities for increasing the range and precision of cardiac evaluation on the basis of the heart's electri-cal state. These have been illustrated by examples of the complementary information furnished by T waves and T loops. Specifically, T waves in single scalar leads reflect differences in the normal sequence of excitation and recovery while T loops indicate sub-stantial similarity of these processes. The full diag-nostic utility of deviation from the similarity of these processes by means of the T loop has not yet been achieved.

In a second illustration of the possible improve-ment of cardiac evaluation by examination of electri-cal activity, the common electrophysiologic origin of abnormalities of P and T loops and waves and states susceptible to arrhythmias was cited. This furnishes a basis for possible identification of hearts susceptible to arrhythmias prior to the occurrence of such events.

Finally, the need for increased specificity in the evaluation of abnormalities of P and T waves and loops was stated and documented by examples of var-ied mechanisms capable of producing the abnormali-ties.

All of the examples given in this overview and others which could be cited represent possibilities for improved evaluation of the heart by examination of its electrical activity. All will require improved defini-tion of the physiologic basis of P and T waves, loops and other displays of cardiac electrical activity. All will also require experimental and most importantly, documentation of their utility in actual clinical prac-tice.

References

[1] F. N. Wilson and F. D. Johnston, The vector-cardiogram, Am. Heart J. 16 (1938) 14.
[2] S. Mashima and K. Fukushima, The ventricular gradient and vectorcardiographic T loop in left ventricular hypertrophy, J. Electrocardiol. 2 (1969) 55.
[3] J. A. Abildskov, K. Millar, M. J. Burgess, and L. Green, Characteristics of ventricular recov-ery as defined by the vectorcardiographic T loop, Am. J. Cardiol. 28 (1971) 670.
[4] N. Kimura, The vectorcardiogram, Jap. Circ. J. 13 (1949) 312.
[5] C. E. Forkner, P. G. Hugenholtz, and H. D. Levine, The vectorcardiogram in normal young adults, Am. Heart J. 62 (1961) 237.

[6] W. J. Wajszizuk and G. E. Burch, Analysis of the TsE loop in normal subjects of different ages, Am. J. Cardiol. 10 (1962) 505.
[7] K. Harumi, S. Mashima, C. Sato, Y. Yanai, and H. Ueda, A study on the direction of the vectorcardiographic T loop in left and right ventricular hypertrophy, Jap. Heart J. 4 (1963) 586.
[8] T. Chou, R. A. Helm, and R. Lach, The sig-nificance of a wide TsE loop, Circulation 30 (1964) 400.
[9] M. J. Burgess, J. A. Abildskov, and K. Millar, The relation of ventricular recovery boundary geometry to T loop form. In: I. Hoffman, R. I. Hamby, and E. Glassman (eds.), Vectorcar-diography-2 (North-Holland, Amsterdam, 1971) p. 664.
[10] K. Harumi, An analysis of the T loop by a theoretic model. In: I. Hoffman, R. E. Hamby, and E. Glassman (eds.), Vectorcardiography-2 (North-Holland, Amsterdam, 1971), p. 656.
[11] H. Ueda, M. Murayama, K. Harumi, C. Sato, and S. Murao, Spatial T wave changes produced by exercise in health and disease, Jap. Heart J. 8 (1967) 83.
[12] J. H. Isaacs, H. Mills, and S. Cole, The post exercise T loop. In: I. Hoffman, R. E. Hamby, and E. Glassman (eds.), Vectorcardiography-2 (North-Holland, Amsterdam, 1971), p. 670.
[13] I. Hoffman, R. Taymor, and I. Kittell, T loop rotation in ischemic heart disease. In: I. Hoff-man, and R. C. Taymor (eds.), Vectorcardiog-raphy 1965 (North-Holland, Amsterdam, 1966), p. 181.
[14] G. K. Moe and J. A. Abildskov, Atrial fibrilla-tion as a self sustaining arrhythmia independent of focal discharge, Am. Heart J. 58 (1959) 59.
[15] R. Alessi, M. Nusynowitz, J. A. Abildskov, and G. K. Moe, Non-uniform distribution of vagal effects on the atrial refractory period, Am. J. Physiol. 194 (1958) 406.
[16] G. K. Moe, W. C. Rheinboldt, and J. A. Abildskov, A computer model of atrial fibrilla-tion, Am. Heart J. 67 (1964) 200.
[17] J. A. Abildskov, The atrial complex of the electrocardiogram, Am. Heart J. 57 (1959) 930.
[18] J. Han and G. K. Moe, Non-uniform recovery of excitability in ventricular muscle, Circ. Res. 14 (1964) 44.
[19] J. Han, P. D. Garcia de Jalon, and G. K. Moe, Adrenergic effects on ventricular vulnerability, Circ. Res. 14 (1964) 516.
[20] J. Han, P. D. Garcia de Jalon, and G. K. Moe, Fibrillation threshold of premature ventricular responses, Circ. Res. 18 (1966) 18.
[21] J. Han, D. Millet, B. Chizzonitti, and G. K. Moe, Temporal dispersion of recovery of excit-ability in atrium and ventricle as a function of heart rate, Am Heart J. 71 (1966) 481.

[22] J. Han, J. DeTraglia, D. Millet, and G. K. Moe, Incidence of ectopic beats as a function of basic rate in the ventricle, Am. Heart J. 72 (1966) 632.

[23] J. Han, A. M. Malozzi, and C. Lyons, Ventricular vulnerability to paired-pulse stimulation during acute coronary occlusion, Am. Heart J. 73 (1967) 79.

[24] K. Harumi, M. J. Burgess, and J. A. Abildskov, A theoretic model of the T wave, Circulation 34 (1966) 657.

[25] M. J. Burgess, K. Harumi, and J. A. Abildskov, Application of a theoretic T wave model to experimentally induced T wave abnormalities, Circulation 34 (1966) 669.

[26] R. T. Van Dam and D. Durrer, Experimental study on the intramural distribution of the excitability cycle and on the form of the epicardial T wave in the dog heart in situ, Am. Heart J. 61 (1961) 537.

[27] J. A. Abildskov, M. J. Burgess, K. Millar, R. Wyatt, and G. Baule, The primary T wave--A new electrocardiographic waveform, Am. Heart J. 81 (1971) 242.

[28] G. Autenrieth, B. Surawicz, and C. S. Kuo, Sequence of repolarization on the ventricular surface in the dog, Am. Heart J. 89 (1975) 463.

[29] R. Zalter and K. Sadik, Prognostic significance of the magnitude of ST segment shift in myocardial infarction, Circulation 24 (1961) 1075.

[30] J. A. Abildskov, Nonspecificity of ST-T changes. In: A. N. Brest (ed.), Cardiovascular Clinics (F. A. Davis Co., Philadelphia, 1973), p. 170.

[31] G. E. Burch, R. Meyers, and J. A. Abildskov, A new electrocardiographic pattern observed in cerebrovascular accidents, Circulation 9 (1954) 719.

[32] E. Byer, R. Ashman, and L. A. Toth, Electrocardiograms with large upright T waves and long Q-T intervals, Am. Heart J. 33 (1947) 796.

[33] G. E. Burch, R. S. Sohal, S. C. Sun, and H. L. Colcolough, Effects of experimental intracranial hemorrhage on the myocardium of mice. Am. Heart J. 77 (1969) 427.

[34] G. E. Burch, S. C. Sun, H. L. Colcolough, N. P. DePasquale, and R. S. Sohal, Acute myocardial lesions following experimentally induced intracranial hemorrhage in mice: A histological and histochemical study, Arch. Pathol. 84 (1967) 517.

[35] R. C. R. Connor, Heart damage associated with intracranial lesions, Brit. Med. J. 3 (1968) 29.

[36] A. O. Fleisch, Zur klinischen Bedeutung der 2-gipfligen T-Welle im Ruhe-und Belastungs elektrokardiogramm, Cardiologia 44 (1964) 177.

[37] J. H. Greenhoot and D. D. Reichenbach, Cardiac injury and subarachnoid hemorrhage: A clinical, pathological and physiologic correlation, J. Neurosurg. 30 (1969) 521.

[38] S. Hayashi, J. Watanabe, S. Miyagawa, S. Tamakuma, and H. Nagaki, Studies of electrocardiographic patterns in cases with neurosurgical lesions, Jap. Heart J. 2 (1961) 92.

[39] C. Hersch, Electrocardiographic changes in head injuries, Circulation 28 (1961) 853.

[40] P. G. Hugenholtz, Electrocardiographic changes typical for central nervous system disease after right radical neck dissection, Am. Heart J. 74 (1967) 438.

[41] G. C. J. Kortiweg, J. Th. F. Boeles, and J. T. TenCate, Influence of stimulation of some subcortical areas on the electrocardiogram, J. Neurophysiol. 20 (1957) 100.

[42] P. Koskelo, S. Punsar, and W. Sipila, Subendocardial haemorrhage and ECG changes in intracranial bleeding, Brit. Med. J. 1 (1964) 1479.

[43] K. Millar and J. A. Abildskov, Notched T waves in young persons with central nervous system lesions, Circulation 37 (1968) 597.

[44] F. Yanowitz, J. B. Preston, and J. A. Abildskov, Functional distribution of right and left stellate innervation to the ventricles: Production of neurogenic electrocardiographic changes by unilateral alteration of sympathetic tone, Circ. Res. 18 (1966) 416.

Vectorcardiography 3 I. Hoffman and R.I. Hamby eds.
© 1976 North-Holland Publishing Company - Amsterdam

SEQUENCE OF NORMAL VENTRICULAR RECOVERY AND ITS RELATION TO T WAVEFORM

Mary Jo Burgess

From the Cardiovascular Research and Training Institute and Cardiology
Division, Department of Internal Medicine, University of Utah,
College of Medicine, Salt Lake City, Utah

Diagnostic electrocardiography and vectorcardiography have the aim of determining from data recorded on the body surface, the cardiac electrical events responsible for recorded waveforms. Since there is no unique solution to this problem, the accuracy of diagnosis is dependent on limiting the number of possible solutions on the basis of additional electrophysiologic data concerning both normal and abnormal cardiac states. The work of Scher [1] concerning normal canine ventricular activation sequence and, more recently, the work of Durrer's group [2] concerning human activation sequence has been extremely helpful in explaining normal QRS waveform and predicting QRS abnormalities associated with loss of cardiac tissue or ventricular conduction defects. Many models relating activation sequence to QRS waveform have been developed on the basis of those studies and applied to ECG diagnosis. Interpretation of the ST segment and T of the ECG however is still based mainly on empiric correlations. Published data concerning ventricular recovery properties are much less detailed than that concerning ventricular activation sequence. This is partly due to the fact that recovery is an extremely labile process and it is difficult to maintain stable states for study, and partly due to the fact that unlike activation, recovery properties cannot be directly assessed from electrograms. Ventricular recovery is a relatively long process and the most frequently used method of assessing it is with measurements of refractory periods. This measurement provides information concerning only one point in the recovery process, namely the earliest time at which the ventricle can be re-excited by a low intensity, 1 1/2 to 2 times threshold, stimulus. The duration of the refractory period is dependent on both the duration of the transmembrane action potential, and the slope of its downstroke. Therefore, refractory periods at various sites can be compared to each other only if the form of action potential downstrokes is the same. In addition, since refractory period measurements are independent of activation sequence, information concerning time of recovery at one site relative to time of recovery at other sites can only be obtained by taking activation sequence as well as refractory periods into consideration. Data concerning the normal sequence of ventricular recovery are still relatively limited. Interestingly, several reports about recovery sequence appeared after rather than before

development of models relating ventricular action potential duration and form to T wave configuration. Additional information concerning ventricular recovery properties in normal and abnormal states, and the development of clinically practical models for analyzing T waveform should provide further improvement in the diagnostic utility of the ECG.

Models Relating Recovery Properties to T Waveform

One of the earliest models of the T wave was that reported by MacLeod in 1938 [3]. The model was based on the graded stages of activity recorded from frog atria from which an ECG was graphically derived. Later Churney [4] and Hecht [5] reported models of T waveform based on the form of the downstroke of limited numbers of ventricular transmembrane action potentials. A more complete model of the relationship of ventricular action potential form to the T wave was reported by Harumi in 1966 [6]. In that model, the downstroke of the transmembrane action potential was considered to be related to the T wave of the body surface ECG in the same way the upstroke of the action potential is related to the QRS. The downstroke of the action potential was divided into 54 time units and the difference in height of the downstroke from the beginning to the end of each time unit was considered to represent moment by moment changes in potential in recovering tissue. Action potentials with various durations were assigned to areas of the ventricles on the basis of van Dam and Durrer's [7] measurements of the intramural distribution of ventricular refractory periods which was the only information concerning normal ventricular recovery sequence available at the time. Moment by moment differences in potential in areas of the ventricles with action potentials of different duration were estimated from the difference in height of action potentials in adjacent areas and magnitude and direction of repolarization vectors were assigned as illustrated in figure 1. Three muscle strips activated from left to right are shown. The action potentials assigned to the strips along with the ECG that would be recorded from a horizontal ECG lead with the negative electrodes on the left are diagrammed. In part A, the action potentials in the entire muscle strip have the same configuration and duration. With this assignment of action potentials, the T polarity is opposite that of the QRS because area 1 of the muscle strip is relatively negative with respect to area 2 during

Supported, in part, by Program Project Grant #HL 13480 and Research Grant #HL 12611 from the National Institutes of Health.

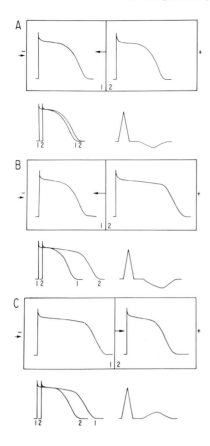

Fig. 1. Diagrams of three muscle strips which are
activated from left to right. The orientations of recovery vectors at the boundaries of areas 1 and 2 are
indicated. The temporal relationships of action potential upstrokes and downstrokes and ECGs from a
horizontal lead are shown beneath each muscle strip.
In part A, the action potentials in areas 1 and 2 have
the same configuration and the QRS and T have equal
areas and opposite polarities. In part B, the action
potentials in area 2 are longer than those in area 1.
The QRS and T have opposite polarities, but the T
area is larger than the QRS area. In part C, the action potentials in area 1 are longer than those in area
2 and the QRS and T have the same polarity.

cases the order of action potential upstrokes is the
same as the order in which downstrokes are completed. However, with the assignment of action potentials shown in part B, the QRS and T areas are not
equal. The T area is greater than the QRS because
the difference in time of completion of the downstrokes is greater than the difference in timing of the
upstrokes. In part C, a longer action potential has
been assigned to area 1 than to area 2. With this assignment of action potentials the order of completion
of action potential downstrokes is opposite the order
of onset of the upstrokes. Area 1 is relatively negative with respect to area 2 during both activation and
recovery and the QRS and T therefore have the same
polarity. As shown in these diagrams, repolarization vectors between areas with different recovery
properties are directed towards the area in which the
action potential is completed first. The magnitude of
repolarization vectors is determined by two additional
factors. The first is the magnitude of the difference
in the time course of recovery in the two areas and
the other is the degree to which the boundary between
the two areas is expressed in a vectorcardiographic
lead. The latter factor can be represented by the
length of the line necessary to close the boundary between areas with different recovery properties [8].
With this model of the T wave it is possible to predict
the changes in T waveform associated with localized
areas of altered recovery properties [9, 10] in the
same way that alteration in QRS form associated with
localized destructive lesions can be predicted. Even
with the limited data now available concerning recovery properties, the model has been useful in predicting T waveform for animals with experimentally induced alterations of recovery properties, and T waveform to be expected in association with acute ischemia
and hypertrophy [10, 11]. As additional information
concerning normal and abnormal ventricular recovery
properties is reported, more detailed descriptions of
the relation of these properties to ST and T waveform
will be possible.

Ventricular Recovery Properties

As early as 1934 Wilson recognized that normal
ventricular recovery properties were not uniform.
In his paper on the ventricular gradient concept [12]
he stated that the sum of the QRS and T areas of the
electrocardiogram was a measure of local variations
in the duration of the excited state. In the late 1950s
and early 1960s Pipberger [13] and Haas [14] estimated ventricular recovery properties from electrograms recorded from multiple ventricular sites.
Pipberger's study concluded that recovery properties
at the base of the left ventricle were shorter than
those at the apex and the study of Haas et al. came to
the opposite conclusion. An attempt to quantitate the
magnitude of differences in recovery properties was

activation and relatively positive with respect to area
2 during recovery. The QRS and T have equal areas
because the configuration of the action potentials is
the same. In part B, a longer action potential has
been assigned to area 2 than to area 1. With this assignment of action potentials the QRS and T have opposite polarities, as they did in part A, because in both

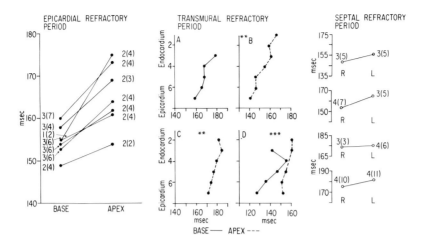

Fig. 2. Graphs summarizing the distribution of normal canine ventricular refractory periods. Data shown are averages and the numbers next to data points indicate the number of sites and number of measurements included in the averages. Epicardial refractory periods are graphed in the left panel. In all seven dogs, refractory periods at the base were shorter than those at the apex. The middle panel shows that there is progressive shortening of refractory periods from endocardium to epicardium at both base and apex. The asterisks represent refractory periods at an epicardial reference site and are an indication of the stability of the preparation. The panel on the right shows that refractory periods on the right side of the septum are shorter than those on the left side of the septum.

not made in either study. The longer duration of endocardial than epicardial recovery properties was suspected because of the normal upright polarity of T waves before studies of the distribution of ventricular refractory periods were actually carried out. Later, in acute dog experiments Reynolds and van der Ark [15] found that when endocardial refractory periods were longer than epicardial refractory periods, T waves recorded from an epicardial electrode were upright, and when endocardial refractory periods were shorter than epicardial refractory periods the T waves were negative. In that study epicardial refractory periods were longer than those on the endocardium at almost all sites tested. These findings were probably due to cooling of the epicardium and consequent prolongation of epicardial surface refractory periods. In 1961 van Dam and Durrer [7] reported their findings on the intramural distribution of refractory periods at a site in mid-anterolateral portion of the left ventricle. They found that endocardial refractory periods were longest, epicardial refractory periods were intermediate in duration and the shortest refractory periods were in the middle layers of the ventricle. The study supported the longer endocardial than epicardial refractory periods that had previously been inferred on the basis of T polarity. It was findings of this study that were used to assign action potential durations in reports concerning derivation of T waves of normal dogs [6] and the T waves of dogs with experimentally induced abnormalities of

recovery properties [9]. A more detailed description of normal canine refractory periods was reported from our laboratories in 1972 [16]. Graphs summarizing findings of that study are shown in figure 2. Functional refractory periods were measured at the apex and base of the left ventricle, intramurally from the endocardium to epicardium at the left ventricular base and apex, and at several sites in the interventricular septum. Refractory periods were progressively shorter from endocardium to epicardium. Apical refractory periods were longer than those at the base, in both the free wall of the left ventricle and in the interventricular septum, and refractory periods on the left side of the septum were longer than those on the right. The findings indicated that ventricular recovery properties were inversely related to activation order. Areas of the ventricles activated early had long refractory periods and areas of the ventricles activated late had short refractory periods. In a study employing suction electrodes, Autenreith et al. [17] have recently confirmed the shorter basal than apical recovery properties on the epicardial surface of the canine ventricle.

Refractory period measurements provide information about intrinsic recovery properties but unless they are related to ventricular activation sequence, the time course of recovery in one area with respect to other areas cannot be inferred from them. Studies of the relationship of activation sequence, refractory period duration and ventricular recovery sequence have recently been conducted by Abildskov [18]. In that study maps of epicardial recovery order closely resembled epicardial activation sequence maps with areas activated early recovering early, and areas activated late recovering late. On the endocardium, however, the relationship of recovery sequence to activation sequence was less consistent. Although apical endocardial sites were activated earlier than basal endocardial sites, some basal sites recovered earlier and some later than apical sites.

Relation of Ventricular Recovery Properties to T Waveform

The ECG manifestations of ventricular recovery have some features similar to the ECG manifestations of ventricular activation and other features that are unlike the ECG manifestations of activation. The ECG effects of boundaries of potential difference during both activation and recovery can be considered in terms of the magnitude of the potential difference across them and the length of the line necessary to close the boundary. During activation only a relatively limited number of boundaries of potential difference exist at any one time, and the magnitude of potential differences across each activation boundary is equal. Because of the long duration of ventricular repolarization it is a much more diffuse process. During a major portion of the recovery process multiple boundaries of potential differences which are distributed throughout both ventricles exist. In addition to this complexity, magnitudes of potential differences across recovery boundaries are not equal to each other because of the inhomogeneity of action potential durations in various portions of the ventricles. In spite of the complexities concerning the recovery process and the limited data available about the distribution of normal and abnormal recovery properties, a more critical approach to interpreting the significance of T wave configuration of clinical electrocardiograms is now possible. Positive T waves in normal electrocardiograms are probably due to the endocardial to epicardial gradient of ventricular refractory periods, with endocardium recovering later than epicardium. The clockwise inscription of both QRS and T loops implies that some features of ventricular recovery properties repeat features of activation sequence, and the apex to base distribution of endocardial recovery properties may be the responsible factor. In the presence of localized abnormalities of ventricular recovery the T vector can be expected to be directed more toward the abnormal area if its recovery times are shortened, and can be expected to be directed away from the abnormal area if its recovery times are prolonged. As further information is obtained concerning ventricular recovery properties in both normal and abnormal conditions, the diagnostic utility of the ECG should be further enhanced.

References

[1] A. Scher and A. Young, Ventricular depolarization and the genesis of QRS, Ann. N.Y. Acad. Sci. 65 (1957) 168.

[2] D. Durrer, R. Th. vanDam, G. E. Freud, M. J. Janse, F. L. Meijler, and R. C. Arzebacher, Total excitation of the isolated human heart, Circulation 41 (1970) 899.

[3] A. S. MacLeod, The electrocardiogram of cardiac muscle, an analysis which explains the regression or T deflection, Am. Heart J. 15 (1938) 165.

[4] L. Churney, R. Ashman, and E. Byer, Electrogram of turtle heart immersed in a volume conductor, Am. J. Physiol. 154 (1948) 241.

[5] H. Hecht, Some observations and theories concerning the electrical behavior of heart muscle, Am. J. Med. 30 (1961) 720.

[6] K. Harumi, M. J. Burgess, and J. A. Abildskov, A theoretic model of the T wave, Circulation 34 (1966) 657.

[7] R. Th. Van Dam and D. Durrer, Experimental study on the intramural distribution of the excitability cycle and on the form of the epicardial T wave in the dog heart in situ, Am. Heart J. 61 (1961) 537.

[8] J. A. Abildskov, M. S. Barnes, and B. L. Hisey, Studies of normal and ectopic atrial excitation, Am. Heart J. 52 (1956) 496.

[9] M. J. Burgess, K. Harumi, and J. A. Abildskov, Application of a theoretic T wave model to experimentally induced T wave abnormalities, Circulation 34 (1966) 669.

[10] W. J. Mandel, M. J. Burgess, J. Neville, and J. A. Abildskov, Analysis of T wave abnormalities associated with myocardial infarction using a theoretic model, Circulation 38 (1968) 178.

[11] P. S. Thiry, R. M. Rosenberg, and J. A. Abbot, A mechanism for the electrocardiogram response to left ventricular hypertrophy, Circ. Res. 36 (1975) 92.

[12] F. N. Wilson, A. G. MacLeod, P. S. Barker, and F. D. Johnston, The determination and significance of the areas of ventricular deflections of the electrocardiogram, Am. Heart J. 10 (1934) 46.

[13] H. Pipberger, L. Schwartz, R. Massumi, and M. Prinzmetal, Studies on the nature of the repolarization process. XIX Studies on the mechanism of ventricular activity, Am. Heart J. 53 (1957) 100.

[14] H. G. Haas, Ein beitrag zur theorie des ventrikelgradienten, Cardiologia 36 (1960) 321.

[15] E. W. Reynolds, Jr. and C. R. VanderArk, An experimental study of the origin of T waves based on determinations of effective refractory period from epicardial and endocardial aspects of the ventricle, Circ. Res. 7 (1959) 943.

[16] M. J. Burgess, L. S. Green, K. Millar, R. Wyatt, and J. A. Abildskov, The sequence of normal ventricular recovery, Am. Heart J. 84 (1972) 660.

[17] G. Autenreith, B. Surawicz, and C. S. Kuo, Sequence of repolarization on the ventricular surface in the dog, Am. Heart J. 89 (1975) 463.

[18] J. A. Abildskov, The sequence of normal recovery of excitability in the dog heart, Circulation (in press).

Vectorcardiography 3 I. Hoffman and R.I. Hamby eds.

RELATIONSHIP OF TRANSMEMBRANE ACTION POTENTIAL

FORM TO THE T WAVE AND T LOOP

Chien-Suu Kuo and Borys Surawicz

From the Cardiovascular Division, Department of Medicine,
University of Kentucky Medical Center,
Lexington, Kentucky 40506

Introduction

During each cardiac cycle, each myocardial cell undergoes a rapid reversal of its transmembrane potential from intracellular negative to positive. This event is followed by slow repolarization which restores the negative intracellular potential. Depolarization lasts less than two milliseconds and repolarization several hundred milliseconds. These electrical activities of ventricular myocardial cells correspond to the QRS complex and T wave in the surface electrocardiogram.

Since the process of repolarization represents reversal of depolarization, uniform duration and speed of repolarization would be expected to produce a T wave of an opposite polarity to the QRS but equal in area to the QRS complex. However, in man and in many of the experimental animals used in the study of the T wave, the QRS and T wave polarities are concordant. This is due to nonuniform repolarization in the normal heart. Experimental studies in dogs have elucidated some of the following causes of this nonuniformity: (1) the refractory periods in the subepicardial layers of the ventricular wall are longer than those in the subendocardial layers [17], (2) the refractory periods as well as the action potential durations are longer at the apex than at the base of the ventricles [1,4], and also longer on the left side than on the right side of the interventricular septum [4].

Harumi and co-workers developed a theoretical model of the T wave in dog [3,10]. Using this model, a T wave similar to the recorded T wave can be computed when the following parameters are known: (1) sequence of depolarization, (2) durations of action potentials in different parts of the ventricle, and (3) shape of the ventricular action potential. This indicates that the combination of these three factors determines the polarity and the shape of the T wave.

The T wave abnormalities can be divided into primary and secondary as shown in table 1 [16]. Secondary T wave abnormalities are due to changes in the sequence of depolarization with normal ventricular action potentials and primary T wave abnormalities are due to changes in the shape and/or the duration of the ventricular action potentials while the depolarization sequence is normal. Undoubtedly some T wave abnormalities are due to various combinations of primary and secondary T wave abnormalities.

Relation between the Shape
of Action Potential and
the T Wave

A typical ventricular action potential and the corresponding electrocardiogram are shown diagrammatically in figure 1. Phase 0 is the rapid depolarization corresponding to the QRS complex.

Table 1

Classification of T wave abnormalities

Sequence of Depolarization	Shape and Duration of Ventricular AP	Sequence of Repolarization	Type of Abnormality
Abnormal	Normal	Abnormal	Secondary
Normal	Uniformly abnormal	Normal	Primary
Normal	Nonuniformly abnormal	Abnormal	Primary

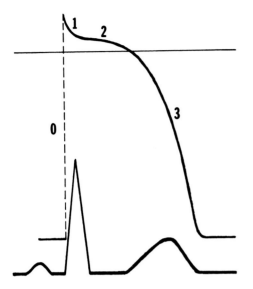

Fig. 1. Correlation between ventricular transmembrane action potential and surface electrocardiogram. The horizontal line indicates zero potential for transmembrane action potential. Positive potential is above and negative potential below the zero potential line. The numbers denote different phases of the action potential. See text.

This phase is followed by short phase 1, a notch, slow repolarization phase 2 or plateau, and phase 3-- a more rapid terminal repolarization. Phase 2 corresponds to the ST segment and phase 3 to the T wave. A general relation between the action potential and the electrocardiogram was stated by one of us (B.S.) as follows [16]:

1) The end of ventricular action potential coincides approximately with the end of the T wave; shortening of all action potentials is accompanied by corresponding shortening of the Q-T interval, while lengthening of all or some action potentials is accompanied by the prolongation of the Q-T interval.

2) Prolonged plateau is associated with a lengthening of the ST segment and a shortened plateau with a shortening of the ST segment.

3) Increased slope of phase 2 which tends to abolish the plateau is associated with disappearance of the isoelectric portion of the ST segment and with deviation of the ST segment from the baseline.

4) An increase in the slope of phase 3 is associated with a narrow and peaked T wave.

5) A more uniform repolarization slope approaching a straight line is associated with a decrease of T wave amplitude.

6) Prolongation of the terminal portion of repolarization is associated with an increase of U wave amplitude.

These relations hold only when the changes in action potentials are uniform in all ventricular fibers. Some clinical examples are shown diagrammatically in figure 2.

Nonuniform Changes of Ventricular Repolarization

The effects of nonuniform repolarization have been studied by us recently in anesthetized, open-chested dogs [2]. The electrocardiogram was recorded with orthogonal leads, and the monophasic action potentials from the surface of the ventricles with suction electrodes. Isoproterenol (ISP) in doses ranging from 0.06 μg to 4 μg was infused rapidly into: (1) pulmonary artery (PA), (2) left circumflex coronary artery (LCA), (3) the first major branch of LCA (LCA branch) and (4) right coronary artery (RCA). Figure 3 shows the ISP-perfused regions as dotted areas. Isoproterenol shortened the total duration of action potential due to shortening of phase 2. The ISP-induced shortening of monophasic action potentials in these four groups was similar and averaged from 12-18 msec while the QRS was not changed (figure 4). The average changes in T wave amplitude in each group are shown in figure 3. Positive values indicate upright T waves and negative values inverted T waves. These studies showed that:

1) Shortening the monophasic action potential by 12-18 msec in a localized area comprising 8% of total ventricular myocardium was sufficient to change the T wave amplitude.

2) Within the same region of the ventricle perfusion of a larger mass of myocardium with ISP produced a greater increase in T wave amplitude.

3) Perfusion of the entire heart with ISP caused lesser T wave change than perfusion of one region in the left ventricle. This can be explained by cancellation.

4) Injection of ISP into RCA produced changes in T wave polarity opposite to those produced by ISP injection into LCA. However, the magnitude of change was smaller even though the perfused ventricular myocardial mass was larger than that affected by injection into branch of LCA. This may be due to differences in the location of the perfused myocardial mass, or in the thickness of ventricular wall of the two perfused areas. This study shows that when the change in action potentials is not uniform, the T wave change is influenced by the mass of myocardium affected by this change, and the

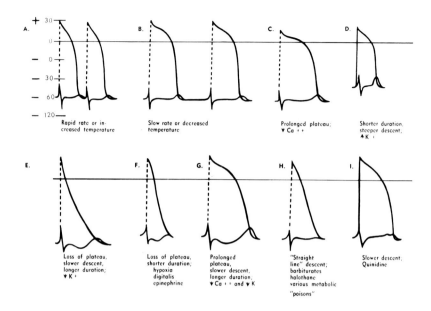

Fig. 2. Diagrammatic presentation of the relation between the ventricular transmembrane action potential and the electrocardiogram. Sections A through I show the effect of various factors which alter the duration and velocity of the repolarization. The scale on the top left represents amplitude in millivolts. The upstroke of the action potential is represented by an interrupted line except in D and I where the upstroke is drawn as a solid line to indicate the decreased velocity of depolarization produced by hyperpotassemia and quinidine.

anatomical location of this mass. This study also demonstrates the clinically well known high sensitivity and low specificity of T wave abnormalities.

Vectorcardiographic T Loop

The high sensitivity and the low specificity of T wave abnormalities underscores the difficulty in separating various T wave abnormalities by the available methods. More specific but no less sensitive methods of analysis of electrocardiographic repolarization abnormalities need to be developed. Vectorcardiography is a major alternate way of expressing electrical activity. During the past decade several investigators studied the vectorcardiographic T loop [8,9,11,12,13, 14,15], particularly in patients with ischemic heart disease. Vectorcardiography may have certain advantages over the ECG because it can record: (1) the sense of rotation, (2) the speed of inscription, and (3) the form of the T loop expressed by Chou et al. [6] as length-width ratio (L/W ratio).

The studied characteristics of the T loop have included: (1) direction of maximal vector in frontal, horizontal and right saggital planes, (2) magnitude of the maximal vector in each plane, (3) L/W ratio,

(4) rotation of the T loop in each plane, (5) speed of inscription, and (6) QRS-T angle. The normal T loop [5,11] in adults is a long ellipse with L/W ratio of > 2.6 (average 7.16 ± 4.18). The amplitude of the maximal vector ranges from 0.2 to 0.75 mV (mean 0.5 mV in frontal and horizontal planes, and 0.4 mV in the right saggital plane). The normal T wave loop is directed to the left, anteriorly and inferiorly. In the horizontal plane the rotation is characteristically counterclockwise, occasionally not definable because of a very narrow loop, and rarely clockwise; in the right saggital plane, clockwise and very rarely counterclockwise with a narrow loop; in the frontal plane either clockwise or counterclockwise. As a rule, the inscription of the efferent loop is slower than that of the afferent loop. The QRS-T angle shows marked variation in horizontal and right saggital planes but is usually less than 28° in the frontal plane. The spatial QRS-T angle ranges from 26° to 134°.

In left ventricular hypertrophy [12,13], the T loop shifts rightward, inferiorly and either anteriorly, or posteriorly; the spatial QRS-T angle increases; the T loop becomes wider and therefore the L/W ratio decreases (3.37-4.21). The rotation in the frontal plane is frequently counterclockwise. In the

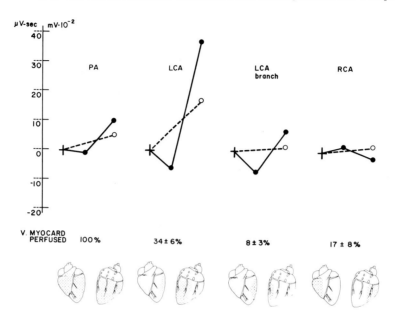

Fig. 3. Effect of isoproterenol (ISP) on T wave amplitude in 10^{-2} mV (solid line) and T wave area in $\mu \bar{V}$ sec (broken line) in four groups of experiments in dogs. The points represent average change from control values. In each panel the proximal solid dot represents the T amplitude at the center of QT interval and the distal dot the amplitude at the apex of the T wave. The lower part shows the percent of the ventricular myocardial mass perfused with ISP. The ISP-perfused area of the ventricles is indicated by the dotted area in the diagram under each number. In each panel the anterior surface of the heart is shown on the left and the posterior surface on the right. The abbreviations are: PA = pulmonary artery, LCA = left circumflex coronary artery, LCA branch = left circumflex coronary artery branch and RCA = right coronary artery.

horizontal plane the rotation is clockwise in approximately one third of all patients. In 75% of patients with clockwise horizontal T loops, the T loop is located within the 90° - 180° quadrant although only 40% of T loops located within this quadrant have clockwise rotation. Left bundle branch block produces similar changes in T loops as left ventricular hypertrophy. In right ventricular hypertrophy the T loop vector shifts posteriorly but maintains the leftward orientation; it becomes wider and the L/W ratio decreases [9]; the rotation in the horizontal plane is frequently clockwise and in the right saggital plane counterclockwise. The T loop changes in right bundle branch block [14] are also similar to those in right ventricular hypertrophy. These observations indicate that T wave abnormalities frequently shift the direction of maximal T vectors, increase the QRS-T angles, change the rotation, and increase the width of the T loops.

The shift of the T loop vector can be readily recognized as change in T wave polarity in the scalar electrocardiogram. We have already stated previously that this is a sensitive but nonspecific indicator

of repolarization abnormalities. The changes in rotation and in L/W ratio are not readily derived from the scalar electrocardiogram. Several investigators studied the diagnostic usefulness of these vectorcardiographic parameters, particularly in patients with ischemic heart disease. Chou et al. [6] reported that L/W ratio <2.6 occurred in 2.5% of normal subjects and in 17% of patients with various cardiac abnormalities, predominantly myocardial infarction or ischemia. De Ambroggi, Sachero and Riva [8] reported similar findings. In their study 34% of 50 patients with ischemic heart disease had a wide T loop with L/W ratio of <2.6. Ischemic heart disease is a frequent but not the sole cause of wide T loops. In patients with QRS abnormalities due to left ventricular hypertrophy (LVH) or intraventricular conduction disturbance (IVCD), the incidence of wide T loops was similar in the presence or absence of ischemic heart disease (LVH group 46% vs. 55%, and IVCD group 39% vs. 25%) [11]. A wide T loop therefore appears to have low specificity in identifying T abnormalities caused by myocardial ischemia.

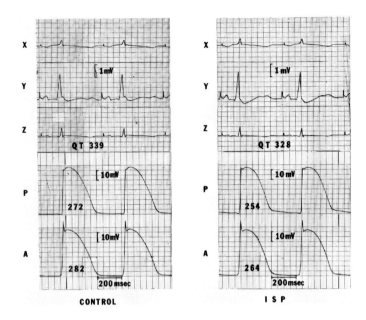

Fig. 4. Effect of isoproterenol (ISP) on electrocardiogram and ventricular monophasic action potentials (MAP) in dogs. A and P indicate MAP's from the anterior and the posterior surfaces of the left ventricle respectively. ECG and MAP's were recorded simultaneously. The durations of QT interval and MAP are shown in milliseconds. The heart rate was kept constant by atrial pacing. ISP (3 μ g) was administered via pulmonary artery. ISP shortened MAP by 18 msec in both P and A. Note the increases in T wave amplitude, shortening of the QT interval and no change of the QRS complex.

Smithline, Hamby, Hilsenrath and Hoffman [15] analyzed the clinical significance of a clockwise horizontal T loop in a group of patients with arteriosclerotic, rheumatic valvular, primary myocardial and congenital heart disease. They found that coronary artery disease or myocardial "ischemia" was frequently associated with other types of heart disease, and suggested that this association was responsible for the abnormal clockwise horizontal T loop when the expected rotation was counterclockwise, e.g. in LVH. Others [11,13] found that in patients with electrocardiographic pattern of LVH or IVCD the incidence of a clockwise horizontal T loop was similar in the presence and in the absence of ischemic heart disease (LVH group 27% vs 33%, and LVCD group 30% vs 38%, presence, or absence of ischemic heart disease, respectively). Mashima and Fu [12] reported that direction of rotation in the horizontal T loop was dependent on the QRS-T angle. Murato et al. [13] found

that the rotation of T loop in the horizontal plane was almost always clockwise if the maximal T vector was directed to the right more than 130°.

The above review of literature suggests that abnormal T loop rotation is not specific for myocardial ischemia. Our studies support this conclusion. Three pertinent examples from our studies are shown in figures 5, 6 and 7. The patient whose ECG is shown in figure 5 was a 66 year old woman with nontransmural infarction. ECG (control panel) shows deep, symmetrical T wave inversion, prolonged QT interval, and normal QRS complex. The enlarged T loop (control panel, upper) is directed rightward, posteriorly, and superiorly, and its rotation is clockwise in the horizontal plane. The inscription of a T loop is uniform in speed. Figure 6 shows an ECG and enlarged T loop of a 41 year old woman with delirium tremens and Wernicke syndrome but no heart disease.

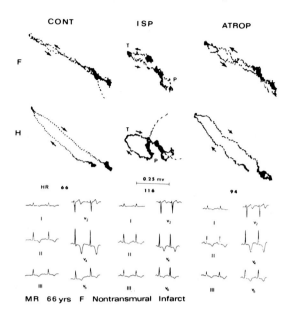

Fig. 5. ECG and enlarged T loop in horizontal (H) and frontal (F) planes in a patient with nontransmural myocardial infarction. The effects of isoproterenol (8 μ g i.v.) and atropine (0.8 mg i.v.) are shown in the middle (ISP) and right (ATROP) panels. ISP increased the heart rate, decreased the T wave amplitude and the magnitude of maximal T vector but did not change the polarity of T wave or the T loop vector. Atropine increased the heart rate but did not change the T wave, or the T loop.

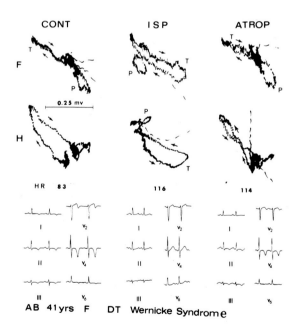

Fig. 6. ECG and enlarged T loop in horizontal (H) and frontal (F) planes in a patient with delirium tremens and Wernicke syndrome. The effects of isoproterenol (4 μ g i.v.) and atropine (0.8 mg i.v.) are shown in the middle (ISP) and right (ATROP) panels. ISP increased the heart rate and "normalized" the abnormal T wave and T loop. Atropine induced a similar increase in heart rate but did not "normalize" the T wave or the T loop.

The T wave and T loop show identical abnormalities as those in figure 5 although in this patient the T changes were transient, and probably "functional" and neurogenic (CVA pattern).

The enlarged T loop shown in figure 7 was recorded from a healthy 24 year old medical student with a normal ECG. The T loop (control panel) is located anteriorly, inferiorly and to the left. The loop is narrow and has a slow efferent and a fast afferent loop; the rotation is normal. When isoproterenol was administered intravenously, the heart rate was increased, QRS did not change, the T loop became wide, uniform in the speed of inscription, and the rotation in the horizontal plane became clockwise. These T loop changes were transient and regressed within 5 minutes. These findings show no distinct differences between functional abnormalities of repolarization in normal persons, and abnormal T waves in patients with organic heart disease. It appears therefore that the advantages of T loop records showing the sense of rotation, the form and the speed of inscription have not contributed to increased diagnostic accuracy or to increased specificity in detection of changes due to myocardial ischemia, or organic heart disease.

Pharmacologic Tests

Several pharmacologic tests have been used for the diagnosis of various types of T wave abnormalities. We found the isoproterenol test particularly helpful for such purposes [7]. In our study, intravenous administration of isoproterenol (1-9 ʋg) increased the amplitude of upright T waves in normal subjects, did not reverse the secondary T wave abnormalities, or the primary T wave abnormalities in patients with myocardial infarction and pericarditis but reversed more than 90% of primary T wave abnormalities due to various other causes (figures 5,6).

Summary

T wave abnormalities can be classified as primary and secondary. In the primary T wave abnormalities, the sequence of depolarization is normal while the shape and/or the duration of ventricular action potentials is abnormal. In the secondary T wave abnormalities, the sequence of depolarization is abnormal while the ventricular action potentials are normal. In the primary T wave abnormalities, the ventricular action potentials may be uniformly abnormal,

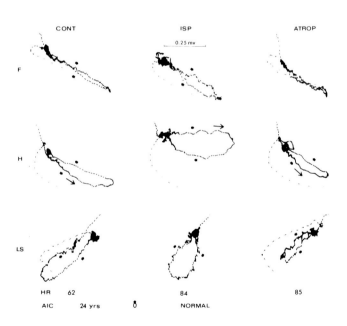

Fig. 7. Enlarged T loops in frontal (F), horizontal (H) and left saggital (LS) planes in a normal subject. CONT: control, ISP: after intravenous administration of isoproterenol (6 ʋg), ATROP: after intravenous administration of atropine (0.8 mg). Heart rates (HR) are shown on the bottom of each panel. See text.

without changes in sequence of repolarization, e.g. due to effect of electrolytes or drugs. When the abnormalities in the ventricular action potential are not uniform, the T wave is influenced by the anatomical location and the distribution of myocardial mass generating the abnormal action potentials. The T wave is a sensitive but a non-specific indicator of repolarization abnormalities. Review of literature and personal studies suggest that analysis of the T loop does not increase diagnostic specificity of T wave changes. The differences in the response to isoproterenol are helpful in differentiating abnormal T waves due to ischemia or pericarditis from similar abnormal T waves due to other causes.

References

[1]   G. Autenrieth, B. Surawicz, and C. S. Kuo, Sequence of repolarization on the ventricular surface in the dog, Am. Heart J. 89 (1975) 463-469.

[2]   G. Autenrieth, B. Surawicz, C. S. Kuo, and M. Arita, Primary T wave abnormalities caused by uniform and regional shortening of ventricular monophasic action potential in dog, Circulation 51 (1975) 668-676.

[3]   M. J. Burgess, K. Harumi, and J. A. Abildskov, Application of a theoretic T wave model to experimentally induced T wave abnormalities, Circulation 34 (1966) 660.

[4]   M. J. Burgess, L. S. Green, K. Millar, R. Wyatt, and J. A. Abildskov, The sequence of normal ventricular recovery, Am. Heart J. 84 (1972) 660-669.

[5]   T. Chou, R. A. Helm, and S. Kaplan, Clinical vectorcardiography (Grune & Stratton, New York, 1974).

[6]   T. Chou, R. A. Helm, and R. Lach, The significance of a wide TsE loop, Circulation 30 (1964) 400-405.

[7]   F. S. Daoud, B. Surawicz, and L. Gettes, Effect of Isoproterenol on the abnormal T wave, Amer. J. Cardiol. 30 (1972) 810-819.

[8]   L. De Ambroggi, A. Sachero, and D. Riva, The T vector loop in ischemic heart disease, Cardiologia 53 (1968) 351-364.

[9]   R. I. Hamby, I. Hoffman, and E. Glassman, The T loop in right ventricular hypertrophy, Dis. Chest 55 (1969) 105-109.

[10] K. Harumi, M. J. Burgess, and J. A. Abildskov, A theoretical model of the T wave, Circulation 34 (1966) 657-668.

[11] I. Hoffman, R. Taymor, and I. Kittell, T loop rotation in ischemic heart disease. In: I. Hoffman (ed.), Proc. Long Island Jewish Hosp. Symposium, Vectorcardiography 1965 (North-Holland, Amsterdam, 1966), p. 182.

[12] S. Mashima, L. Fu, and K. Fukushima, The ventricular gradient and the vectorcardiographic T loop in left ventricular hypertrophy, J. Electrocardiol. 2 (1969) 55-62.

[13] K. Murata, H. Kurihara, S. Matsushita, M. Ikeda, and M. Seki, Significance of T loop change in vectorcardiographic diagnosis of left ventricular hypertrophy, Am. Heart J. 73 (1967) 49-54.

[14] S. Rubler, I. Hoffman, W. D. Franklin, and R. C. Taymor, The T loop in right bundle branch block: A vectorcardiographic study of 82 cases, Am. Heart J. 76 (1968) 217-226.

[15] F. Smithline, R. I. Hamby, J. Hilsenrath, and I. Hoffman, The clockwise horizontal plane T loop: A study of 73 patients, J. Electrocardiol. 7 (1974) 43-56.

[16] B. Surawicz, The pathogenesis and clinical significance of primary T-wave abnormalities. In: Advances in electrocardiography (Grune & Stratton, 1972), p. 377.

[17] R. T. Van Dam and D. Durrer, Experimental study on the intramural distribution of the excitability cycle and on the form of the epicardial T wave in dog heart in situ, Am. Heart J 61 (1961), 537.

Vectorcardiography 3 I. Hoffman and R.I. Hamby eds.
© 1976 North-Holland Publishing Company - Amsterdam

VECTORCARDIOGRAPHIC DIAGNOSIS OF ATRIAL HYPERTROPHY

Alberto Benchimol, Kenneth B. Desser, Stephen Tio, and Bettie Jo Massey

From the Institute for Cardiovascular Diseases, Good Samaritan Hospital,
1033 East McDowell Road, Phoenix, Arizona 85006

The limitations of standard electrocardiography for the diagnosis of atrial hypertrophy are well known and particularly so for the recognition of left atrial hypertrophy, where an intra-atrial conduction defect can mimic left atrial enlargement. Routine unmagnified still loop vectorcardiography is similarly of little value for the study of atrial depolarization. The analysis of atrial vectors by high magnification of the P loop, in combination with timed vectorcardiography has proven very useful for the non-invasive evaluation of atrial disease [1-4].

The purpose of this paper is to describe the vectorcardiographic features of right and left atrial hypertrophy utilizing the Frank lead system.

MATERIAL AND METHOD

One hundred and four patients were studied and divided into three groups.

Group I--Normal Subjects: Fifty-two normal subjects comprised the control group. Twenty-one male and 31 female subjects whose ages ranged from 3 to 70 with a mean of 28 years had no laboratory evidence of heart disease. These patients were studied because of the presence of atypical chest pain or functional systolic murmurs which were originally attributed to organic heart disease.

Group II--Left Atrial Hypertrophy: Twenty-eight patients with left atrial hypertrophy secondary to various forms of acquired heart disease were studied. There were 16 men and 12 women whose ages ranged from 15 to 64 with a mean of 43 years. The distribution of cardiac abnormalities was as follows: 8--mitral stenosis, 4--aortic valvular stenosis, 4--combined aortic stenosis and insufficiency, 3--isolated aortic regurgitation, 2--coronary artery disease and 7--combined valvular lesions.

Group III--Right Atrial Hypertrophy: Seventeen male and 7 female subjects whose ages ranged from 2 to 56 with a mean of 15 years were studied. Eight had Tetralogy of Fallot, 5 atrial septal defect, 3 pulmonary valvular stenosis, 2 ventricular septal defect and 6 had right heart disease of varied etiology.

Supported, in part, by the Nichols and Sigsworth Memorial Funds.

All diagnoses were established on the basis of complete right and left heart catheterization, indicator dilution curves, blood oxygen saturation data and selective cineangiocardiography. In the older subjects, selective coronary arteriography was routinely performed. The diagnosis of atrial hypertrophy was supported by chamber enlargement on atriography and abnormal elevation of the mean right or left atrial and pulmonary arterial "wedge" pressures.

Vectorcardiograms in the three plane projections were recorded in the supine position using the Frank reference system [5]. The fourth intercostal space was used for chest electrode placement as suggested by Langner et al. [6] for the supine position. All vectorcardiograms were recorded on a DR-8 Electronics for Medicine oscilloscopic photographic recorder using a model VT-6 vectorcardiographic channel. Still loops and timed vectorcardiograms [1-4] were obtained in the frontal, left sagittal and horizontal planes. The still loops were magnified and by using a gating system, only the portion of the cardiac cycle encompassing the P loop was displayed and recorded. This degree of magnification averaged 5 cm. for 0.25 mv. The vector loops were interrupted at intervals of 2 msec. and the direction of rotation was indicated by a tear-drop shaped inscription with the thin portion representing its leading point. The frequency response of the amplifier was 0.1 to 500 Hertz. Optional filtering was occasionally utilized at 25, 50 and 500 Hertz. The amplifier noise was 0.003 mv. peak-to-peak over the spectrum of 0.1 per 1500 Hertz.

The following P loop measurements were made on all vectorcardiograms: (1) direction of 10, 20, 30, 40, 50, 60, 70 and 80 msec. vectors in all three planes and of the maximal deflection vector (maximal distance from the E point), (2) rotation of the P loop, (3) magnitude in mv. of the maximal anterior and of the maximal posterior deflection vectors of the P loop as defined by maximal anterior and posterior distances of these vectors from the E point in the horizontal plane and (4) ratio of the magnitude of maximal posterior/anterior vectors in the horizontal plane; in four cases this latter measurement could not be made. Twelve lead scalar electrocardiograms were obtained in all subjects.

RESULTS

Group I--52 Normal Subjects: The direction of the 20, 40, 60 or 80 msec. vectors and of the maximal deflection vectors of the P loop are shown in figures 1, 2 and 3 for all three planes. It can be seen that the initial 20 msec. vector is oriented inferiorly, anteriorly and to the left in most cases; the 40 msec. vector, inferiorly to the left and anteriorly or posteriorly; and the 60 msec. vector inferiorly, posteriorly and to the left. The maximal deflection vector of the P loop is usually directed inferiorly, posteriorly and to the left.

The rotation of the P loop was predominantly counterclockwise in the frontal plane, counterclockwise in the sagittal plane and counterclockwise in the horizontal plane. A figure-of-eight rotation was observed on the horizontal plane vectorcardiograms of 17/52 subjects. The magnitude of the maximal anterior and posterior deflection vectors and the posterior/anterior vector ratios in normal subjects are shown in figures 4-6.

Group II--28 Cases--Left Atrial Hypertrophy: The direction of the 20, 40, 60 msec. vectors and of the maximal deflection vectors of the P loop in the frontal, left sagittal and horizontal planes is shown in figures 7-9. The magnitude of the anterior and posterior deflection vectors and the posterior/anterior ratios are shown in figures 4-6. There was no significant difference between the mean values for the

maximal anterior deflection vectors in Groups I and II (Group I = 0.04 ± 0.02 mv., Group II = 0.04 ± 0.01 mv., P > 0.03, figure 4). There was a highly significant difference between the mean values for the maximal posterior deflection vectors in the normal subjects (Group I) and those patients with left atrial hypertrophy (Group II), (Group I = 0.06 ± 0.02 mv., Group II = 0.13 ± 0.03 mv., P < 0.001, figure 5). The maximal posterior deflection vector was significantly increased above 0.09 mv. in all but 3 cases with left atrial hypertrophy. There was a statistically significant difference between the mean posterior/anterior vector ratios in Groups I and II (Group I = 1.60 ± 0.93, Group II = 3.72 ± 1.93, P < 0.001, figure 6). Despite the presence of scatter overlap, the posterior/anterior vector ratio was greater than 2 in all but 4 patients with left atrial hypertrophy. A representative example of the vectorcardiographic findings in a patient with left atrial hypertrophy is shown in figure 10.

The rotation of the P loop was predominantly counterclockwise in the frontal plane, counterclockwise in the sagittal plane and figure-of-eight in the horizontal plane. A figure-of-eight rotation of the P loop was quite common in the horizontal plane of patients with left atrial hypertrophy. All P loops had a duration exceeding 0.1 second.

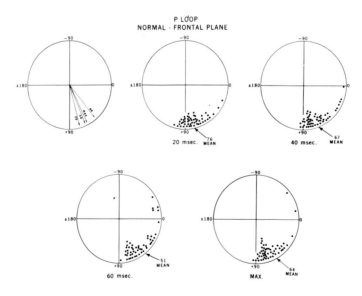

Fig. 1. Direction of the 20, 40, 60 msec. vectors and of the maximal deflection vector of the P loop in the frontal plane in normal subjects.

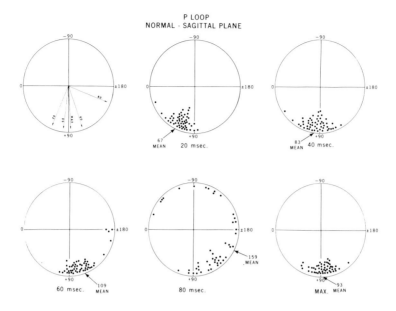

Fig. 2. Direction of the 20, 40, 60, 80 msec. vectors and of
the maximal deflection vectors of the P loop in the left sagittal plane
in normal subjects.

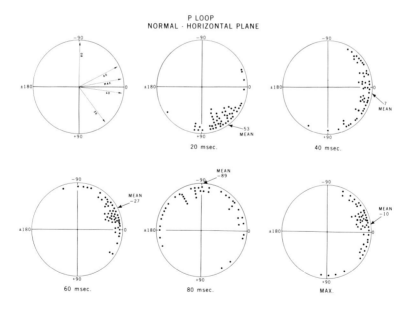

Fig. 3. Direction of the 20, 40, 60, 80 msec. vectors and of
the maximal deflection vector of the P loop in the horizontal plane in
normal subjects.

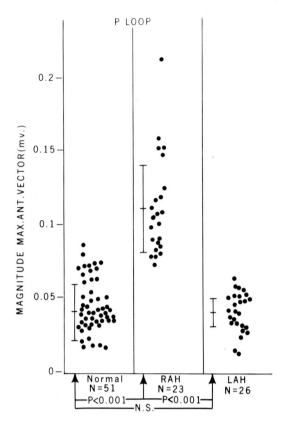

Fig. 4. Magnitude of the maximal anterior vectors of the P loop in the horizontal plane in normal subjects, right atrial hypertrophy (RAH) and left atrial hypertrophy (LAH). The mean value ($\pm$ 1 standard deviation) for each group is properly indicated. Note the significant difference between the mean values for right atrial hypertrophy and left atrial hypertrophy or normal subjects.

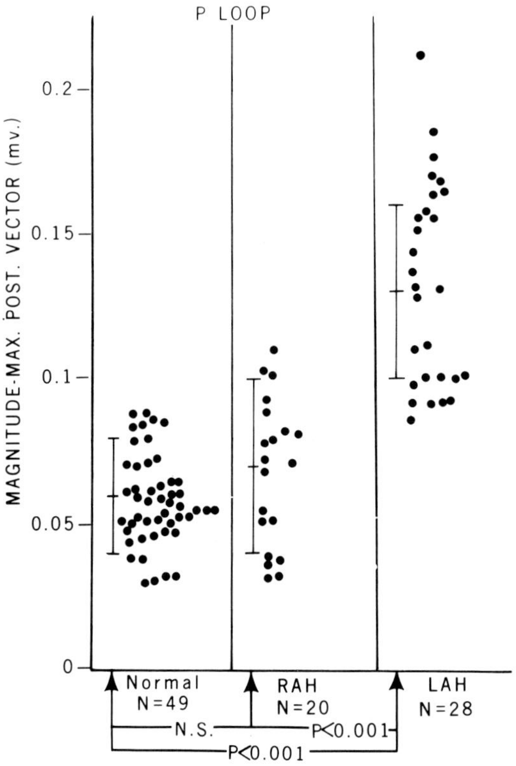

Fig. 5. Magnitude of the maximal posterior deflection vector of the P loop in normal subjects, right atrial hypertrophy (RAH) and left atrial hypertrophy (LAH). The mean value ($\pm$ 1 standard deviation) for each group is properly indicated. Note the significant differences between mean values for right atrial hypertrophy and left atrial hypertrophy.

Group III--24 cases--Right Atrial Hypertrophy: The direction of the 20, 40, 60 and of the maximal deflection vectors of the P loop in the three planes are shown in figures 11, 12 and 13.

The direction of the 20, 40, 60 msec. vectors and of the maximal deflection vector of the P loop in the frontal plane was essentially the same as that seen in normal subjects. In the left sagittal plane, the 40 msec. vector and the maximal deflection vectors were different from normals or patients with left atrial hypertrophy in that they were usually oriented anteriorly and inferiorly in the group with right atrial hypertrophy as compared to the patients with left atrial

hypertrophy. In the horizontal plane, an important sign of right atrial hypertrophy was the anterior orientation of the maximal deflection vector (figure 13).

The distribution of the maximal anterior and posterior deflection vectors and the posterior/anterior vector ratios are shown in figures 4-6. There was a significant difference between the mean values for the magnitude of anterior vector deflection in Group III and Groups I and II (Group I = 0.04 ± 0.02 mv., Group III = 0.11 ± 0.03 mv., $P < 0.001$). The majority of subjects with right atrial hypertrophy manifested a maximal anterior vector which was

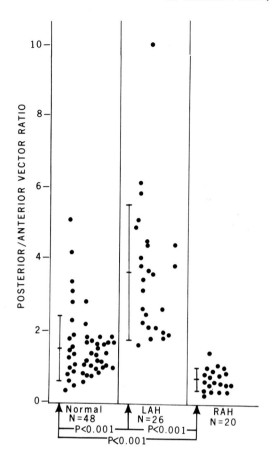

Fig. 6. Ratio of the magnitude of the posterior and anterior vectors in normal subjects, left atrial hypertrophy (LAH) and right atrial hypertrophy (RAH). The mean value ($\pm$ standard deviation) for each group is properly indicated. Note the significant difference between the mean values for all three groups.

greater than 0.09 mv. in the presence of a normal posterior deflection vector. As a result of these relationships, the posterior/anterior vector ratios were less than 1 in the vast majority of subjects with right atrial hypertrophy. There was a significant difference between the mean posterior/anterior vector ratios in normal subjects (1.60 $\pm$ 0.93) and patients with right atrial hypertrophy (0.70 $\pm$ 0.31, P < 0.001). A typical example of a P loop indicating right atrial hypertrophy is shown in figure 14.

The rotation of the P loop was predominantly counterclockwise in the frontal plane, counterclockwise in the sagittal plane and counterclockwise in the horizontal plane. A figure-of-eight rotation was extremely rare in patients with right atrial hypertrophy in contradistinction to what was noted in patients with left atrial hypertrophy as described above. When present, clockwise rotation of the P loop in the horizontal plane was virtually diagnostic of right atrial hypertrophy. All P loops had a duration of less than 0.1 second.

Of all the P loop measurements, the posterior/anterior vector magnitude ratio in the horizontal plane provided the best diagnostic separation among the three groups studied.

DISCUSSION

Owing to its close anatomical relationship to the sino-atrial node, the right atrium depolarizes before the left atrium by approximately 30 to 50 msec. [1]. The right atrial depolarization sequence results in initial vectorial forces which are directed anteriorly, inferiorly and to the right or slightly to the left. Subsequently, the left atrium depolarizes and this process is responsible for vectorial forces which are directed posteriorly and to the left. Thus it follows that the initial anterior and terminal posterior components of the P loop are due to depolarization of the right and left atria respectively.

Atrial enlargement can occur without an appreciable increase in vector forces [7]. Indeed, the small magnitude of P loop forces in relation to those of the QRS complex combined with a low degree of recording magnification renders the accurate diagnosis of atrial hypertrophy quite difficult when utilizing conventional electrocardiography [8].

The above comments apply in equal degree to standard still loop vectorcardiographic recording. Without the benefit of high fidelity amplification and magnification the initial and terminal components of the P loop are not uncommonly "blurred" in the O-E points or obscured by the early and late components of the QRS loop. Furthermore, P loop duration is difficult to measure even on magnified still P loops. The gating system utilized in our laboratory, in combination with timed vectorcardiography, permits highly accurate assessment of the atrial depolarization sequence [1-4].

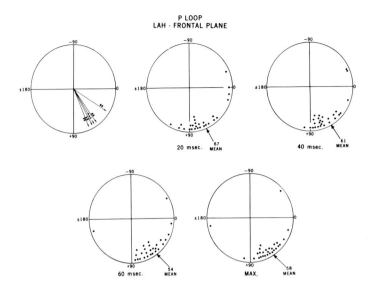

Fig. 7. Direction of the 20, 40, 60, 80 msec. vectors
and of the maximal deflection vector of the P loop in the
frontal plane in patients with left atrial hypertrophy.

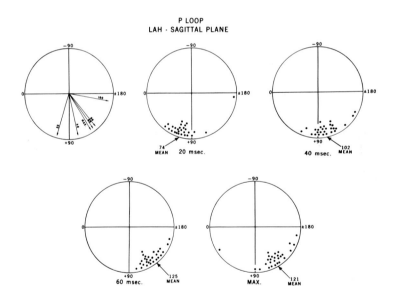

Fig. 8. Direction of the 20, 40, 60 msec. vectors
and of maximal deflection vector of the P loop in the
left sagittal plane in patients with left atrial hypertrophy.

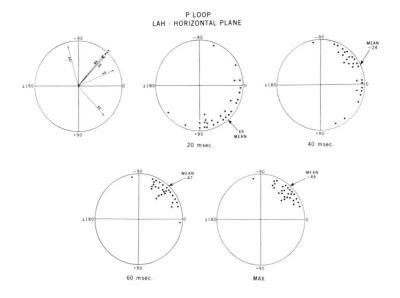

Fig. 9. Direction of the 20, 40, 60 msec. vectors and of the maximal deflection vector of the P loop in the horizontal plane in patients with left atrial hypertrophy.

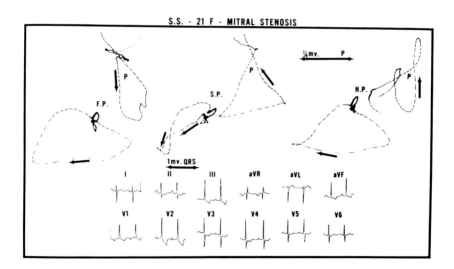

Fig. 10. Vectorcardiogram and electrocardiogram in a patient with typical signs of right and left atrial hypertrophy secondary to mitral stenosis. Note the major anterior and posterior P loop deflections in the horizontal plane.

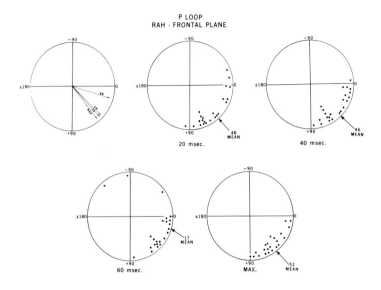

Fig. 11. Direction of the 20, 40, 60 msec. vectors and of the maximal deflection vector of the P loop in the frontal plane in patients with right atrial hypertrophy.

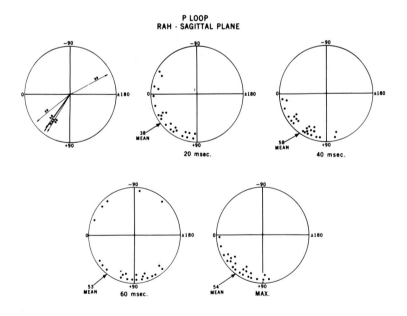

Fig. 12. Direction of the 20, 40, 60 msec. vectors and of the maximal deflection vector of the P loop in the left sagittal plane in patients with right atrial hypertrophy.

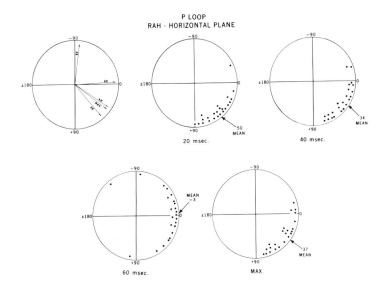

Fig. 13. Direction of the 20, 40, 60 msec. vectors and of the maximal deflection vector of the P loop in the horizontal plane in patients with right atrial hypertrophy.

T.M. - 6 F - TETRALOGY OF FALLOT

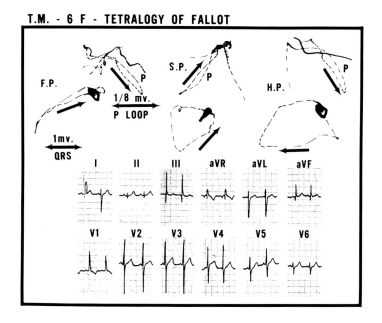

Fig. 14. Vectorcardiogram and electrocardiogram in a patient showing typical signs of right atrial hypertrophy secondary to Tetralogy of Fallot. Note the major anterior P loop deflection vector in the horizontal plane.

Scheuer et al. [9], along with Haywood and Selvester [1] demonstrated the superiority of the horizontal plane display for analysis of the P loop. The major advantages of the transverse coordinates include lesser overlapping or cross-over of vectorial forces along with a left-right and anterior-posterior spatial measurement on a single recording. From the anatomical and physiological standpoint the right-left atrial relationship is primarily that of an anterior-posterior orientation. It is therefore understandable that initial anterior displacement of the P loop might arise as a consequence of right atrial enlargement. On the other hand, major abnormal posterior P loop vector forces indicate left atrial hypertrophy. The normal P loop maximal deflection vector is oriented to the left, inferior, and posterior [10] as a consequence of the usual left atrial predominance, and increased left heart stroke work. Thus left atrial hypertrophy tends to exaggerate in part the usual appearance of the P loop. In order for right atrial forces to dominate the P loop, the right atrium must enlarge and in addition, overcome the normal posterior and leftward loop orientation. This is the apparent explanation for the approximately 1 unit discrepancy of mean deviations from the normal average posterior/anterior vector ratio noted in the presence of right and left atrial hypertrophy. That is, left atrial forces will amost always dominate under normal conditions and when left atrial hypertrophy is operative.

It was not the purpose of this study to describe in detail the salient features of bi-atrial hypertrophy. There are, however, a few points worthy of mention. A secure diagnosis of combined atrial hypertrophy can be made when both large anterior and posterior P vector forces are present as described here. On occasion, right atrial hypertrophy is suggested by normal initial vectors in the presence of an extremely posterior directed P loop.

It is concluded that the following criteria are useful for the diagnosis of right or left atrial hypertrophy.

Right Atrial Hypertrophy

1) The horizontal and sagittal planes are most valuable,
2) Abnormal anterior direction of the 40 msec. and of the maximal deflection vectors,
3) Increased magnitude of the maximal anterior deflection vector in the horizontal plane above 0.09 mv.,
4) Posterior/anterior vector ratio less than one,
5) Clockwise rotation of the P loop in the horizontal plane and
6) Duration of the P loop less than 100 msec.

Left Atrial Hypertrophy

1) The horizontal and sagittal planes are most valuable,
2) Normal direction of the 20, 40, 60 and of the maximal deflection vector of the P loop,
3) Increased magnitude of the posterior deflection vector in the horizontal plane above 0.09 mv.,
4) Normal or small magnitude of the anterior vectors,
5) Posterior/anterior vector ratio greater than two,
6) Figure-of-eight rotation or counterclockwise rotation in the horizontal plane and
7) Duration of the P loop greater than 100 msec.

SUMMARY

High gain, high frequency Frank P loop vectorcardiograms were recorded in 52 normal subjects, 28 patients with left atrial hypertrophy and 24 patients with right atrial hypertrophy. Magnification of the gated still P loop along with timed atrial vectorcardiography allowed optimal measurement of P loop duration, direction and magnitude. The most useful criteria for the diagnosis of right atrial hypertrophy are: maximal anterior deflection vector in the horizontal plane greater than 0.09 mv., posterior/anterior vector ratio smaller than 1, and duration of P loop less than 100 msec. In the case of left atrial hypertrophy the major diagnostic criteria are: posterior deflection vector in the horizontal plane greater than 0.09 mv., posterior/anterior vector ratio more than 2 and duration of the P loop exceeding 100 msec.

It is concluded that the Frank vectorcardiogram is useful for the non-invasive diagnosis of atrial hypertrophy.

REFERENCES

[1] L. J. Haywood and R. H. Selvester, Analysis of right and left atrial vectorcardiograms. Timed records of 100 normal persons, Circulation 33 (1966) 577.
[2] A. Benchimol and A. Pedraza, The timed Frank vectorcardiogram in the diagnosis of cardiac arrhythmias, J. Electrocardiol. 2 (1969) 363.
[3] A. Benchimol, Vectorcardiography (Williams and Wilkins Company, Baltimore, 1973).
[4] R. H. Selvester and L. J. Haywood, High gain, high frequency atrial vectorcardiograms in normal subjects and in patients with atrial enlargement, Amer. J. Cardiol. 24 (1969) 8.
[5] E. Frank, An accurate, clinically practical system for spatial vectorcardiography, Circulation 12 (1956) 737.

[6]   P. H. Langner, R. H. Okada, S. R. Moore,
        and H. L. Fies, Comparison of four orthogonal
        systems of vectorcardiography, Circulation 17
        (1958) 46.
[7]   R. H. Selvester, L. J. Haywood, and D. E.
        Griggs, Atrial enlargement in the diagnosis of
        heart disease, Circulation (Abstract) 22 (1960)
        806.
[8]   D. A. Brody, J. W. Cox, A. B. McEachran,
        H. H. Giles, and V. J. Ruesta, Spatial param-
        eters and shape factors of the normal atrial
        vectorcardiogram and its scalar components,
        Circulation 39 (1969) 229.

[9]   J. Scheuer, M. Kahn, S. Bliefer, E. Donoso,
        A. Grishman, The atrial vectorcardiogram in
        health and disease, Amer. Heart J. 60 (1960)
        33.
[10]   T. Sano, H. K. Hellerstein, and E. Vayda,
        P vector loop in health and disease as studied
        by the technique of electrical dissection of the
        vectorcardiogram (differential vectorcardiog-
        raphy), Amer. Heart J. 53 (1957) 854.

Vectorcardiography 3 I. Hoffman and R.I. Hamby eds.
© 1976 North-Holland Publishing Company - Amsterdam

THE P-LOOP IN INTRA-ATRIAL CONDUCTION DISTURBANCES

Olga Zoneraich and Samuel Zoneraich

From the Department of Medicine, Division of Cardiology, Queens Hospital Center,
The Long Island Jewish Medical Center and the State University
of New York, Medical School at Stony Brook, New York

In the last decade much attention has been focused on the electrocardiographic and vectorcardiographic findings of intraventricular conduction defects, concentrating on bifascicular blocks.

Atrial conduction disturbances remain a neglected problem. We are unaware of any published paper in the English literature dealing with vectorcardiographic features of intra-atrial conduction disturbances.

It is the purpose of this study to describe the vectorcardiographic findings in intra-atrial conduction disturbances and to try to correlate these findings (or patterns) with abnormalities in conduction at the atrial level.

Material and Methods

The study group consisted of 70 patients. They have been divided into two groups:

Group I: Thirty normal subjects served as a control group. They ranged in age from 18 to 60 years. Twenty were male and 10 female.

Group II: Forty patients with intra-atrial conduction disturbances were divided into two sub groups.

Sub group A: Twenty patients free of any cardiac condition. Their diagnoses included gastro-intestinal disease (6), cerebrovascular accident (CVA) (8), cancer (3), pneumonia (3). They ranged in age from 35 to 91 years. Fifteen were male and 5 female.

Sub group B: Twenty patients with known cardiac disease: ASHD (6), hypertension (5), rheumatic heart disease (4) and primary myocardial disease (5). Their age varied between 35 and 81 years. Fourteen were male and 6 female. Four patients also had diabetes mellitus as a second diagnosis (2 in A and 2 in B sub groups).

The diagnosis of intra-atrial conduction disturbance was based on a P-wave duration of 120 msec or more. All patients were in sinus rhythm.

The size of the left atrium was evaluated by echocardiography and roentgenograms. Echocardiography is considered an excellent non-invasive technique for evaluation of left atrial dimensions and is far superior to routine cardiac series [1]. Twelve lead electrocardiograms were recorded immediately before the vectorcardiograms were obtained. We used the Frank lead system [2]. Frontal, horizontal and right sagittal vectorcardiograms were recorded with Hart Electronics PV-5 Vectorcardiograph. By using an automatic adjustable beam blanking device, one can record less than a complete heart cycle. This permitted us to record a very clear vector P-loop.

The cut-off frequency response used in this study was 50 and 100 Hz. The vectorcardiographic loops were interrupted at a rate of 500 times per second. In all tracings, the inscription was interrupted by the large end of the time dash.

The study of atrial conduction disturbance requires a high degree of magnification. In our study, magnification averaged 3 cm. for 1/10 mv. Assessment of the P-wave duration is sometimes difficult. Therefore, we included, in our study, only those patients having a P-wave duration at least, 120 msec. The shape of the ECG P-wave presented the following patterns--bifid, dome shaped, peaked and flat. The following parameters were studied:

A) The P-loop patterns related to the four compared ECG P-contours.
B) The maximal P-loop vector (orientation and magnitude).
C) The sense of direction of the P-loop.
D) The localization of notches and conduction delays in each of the four patterns.

Results

Table 1 summarizes the data obtained in the control group (30 subjects).

The maximum vector of the P-loop is usually oriented inferiorly, posteriorly and to the left.

The sense of direction of the P-loop is counterclockwise (CCW) in the frontal plane, clockwise (CW) in the sagittal plane and appears as a figure of eight or CCW loop in the horizontal plane.

Table 1

P-loop in the normal subject

Plane	Direction	Sense of rotation	Magnitude
Frontal	65° to 90°	CCW	< 0.2 mv.
Horizontal	-40° to 5°	Fig. of 8 or CCW	< 0.1 mv.
Sagittal	85° to 100°	CW	< 0.2 mv.

The magnitude of the maximum vector is less than 0.2 mv. in frontal and sagittal planes. The P-loop is relatively smooth with a short conduction delay (seen at least in two planes) located between the initial 20 to 25 msec vectors. Two small notches can usually be seen in the P-loop, one in the efferent and the other in the afferent limb (figure 1).

In the horizontal plane the ratio between the posterior and the anterior maximum vector is less than 1. The magnitude of either one is less than 0.1 mv.

Group II. The vectorcardiographic P-loops in patients with intra-atrial conduction disturbances (noncardiac and cardiac patients) differed from those of the control group. The size, the shape of P-loop, the number of conduction delays and their location were different from Group I. We divided them into four patterns: A, B, C, D.

Pattern A. The electrocardiogram showed a dome shaped form (12 cases). The loss of details in the P-wave is evident in the standard electrocardiogram (L_2 figure 2). Projecting the P-wave on the orthogonal leads (X, Y, Z) we improve our ability to detect the notches and conduction delays. Fine details can be better studied by vectorial display which depicted an enlarged and distorted P-loop, with initial, mid, and terminal conduction delays and many bites and notches (figure 2).

The postero-anterior ratio of the P-loop in the horizontal plane increased in spite of a normal sized left atrium (figure 3).

When atrial enlargement was present a very large figure of eight loop with many cross overs (figure 4) was recorded.

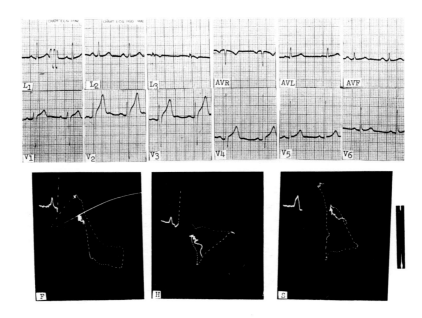

Fig. 1. A 35 year old normal subject. The electrocardiogram shows a P-wave duration of 0.10 sec. The P-loop is smooth. The maximum vector is oriented inferiorly posteriorly and to the left. An initial conduction delay is seen on the efferent limb between 20-25 msec vector. A second notch is seen on the afferent limb. In all tracings the vertical line indicates 1/10 of a mv.

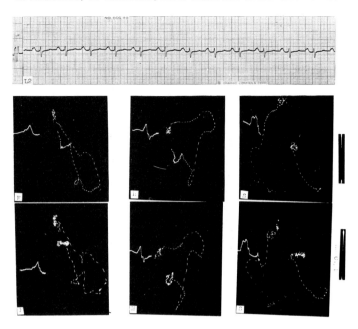

Fig. 2. A 79 year old male hospitalized with severe dehydration. Lead 2 of the electrocardiogram shows an enlarged P-wave with a duration of 0.14 sec with a dome shaped configuration. The vectorcardiogram (upper row) is recorded with a cut-off frequency of 50 hz. The lower tracings are recorded with a cut-off frequency of 100 Hz.

The vectorcardiogram shows a distorted P-loop with many bites, notches and conduction delays. The maximal vector has a normal orientation inferiorly posteriorly and mainly to the left. The P-wave is also projected on the X, Y and Z axes.

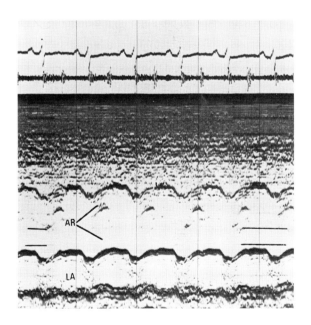

Fig. 3. The echocardiogram of the patient presented in figure 2 shows a normal sized left atrium with a postero-anterior diameter of 2.5 cm. LA = posterior wall of the left atrium. AR = aortic root.

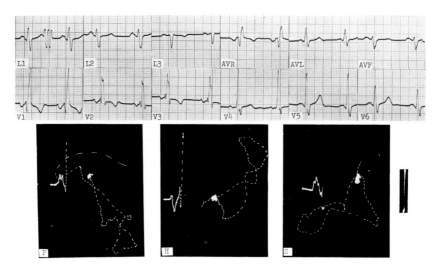

Fig. 4. A 53 year old male hospitalized with hypertension and congestive heart failure. The electrocardiogram shows a large P-wave with a duration of 0.16 sec. The P-loop is very large, with many bites, notches and conduction delays. In this case, intra-atrial conduction disturbances coexist with severe intraventricular blocks (right bundle branch block and left anterior hemiblock). The size of the left atrium was enlarged.

Pattern B. The electrocardiogram shows a bifid P-wave (17 patients). The two notches of the P-wave can be visualized in the standard 12 lead electrocardiogram and in the orthogonal leads but the fine, localized conduction delays can be analyzed only within the vectorcardiographic display (figures 5 and 6). These vectorcardiograms in the frontal and sagittal plane show a double peaked loop. As a rule, both parts of the loop are of nearly equal size (figure 5). The sense of direction in the frontal plane can be CW (figure 5). A figure of eight is frequently present in the horizontal and sagittal plane in this sub group (figure 5).

Pattern C. The electrocardiogram presents a peaked P-wave (5 cases). While the standard electrocardiogram shows only a small notch on the ascending limb of the P-wave, the P-loop presents richness and variety of notching (figure 7). These loops were recorded in patients who had myocardial infarction, pulmonary edema or CVA but who had normal sized left atria.

Pattern D. The electrocardiogram shows a flat P-wave (amplitude 1 mm or less) in 6 cases. The P-wave in standard electrocardiograms do not reveal fine details. The dense conduction delay throughout the entire loop is seen only in the P vectorcardiogram (figure 8). This pattern was recorded mainly in the very old (age 80 to 90 years).

Marked distortions make it impossible to accurately divide the vectorcardiographic loops of patients with intra-atrial conduction disturbances into initial and terminal vectors.

The maximum vector in the frontal and sagittal planes exceeded normal magnitudes, especially in patterns A and B.

The ratio between the posterior and anterior maximum vector in the horizontal plane was more than 1. In many recordings, the P-loop was distorted making it impossible to obtain any measurements of the maximum vector.

Discussion

Intra-atrial block or intra-atrial conduction disturbance is a well recognized electrocardiographic entity. It occurs in 13.5% as a fixed condition [6], 1.2% is intermittent in routine electrocardiograms. Intra-atrial block is present in non-cardiac patients as well as in subjects with known cardiac diseases.

High gain, high frequency vectorcardiograms detect conduction abnormalities at the atrial level [3, 4, 5] better than any other method.

Intra-atrial conduction disturbance means a delayed spread of the stimulus in any part of the atria [7]. This delay will produce a change in form and

duration of the P-wave. Brody et al. [8], in a very
sophisticated computerized study, determined the
P-wave duration in normal subjects to be 99.4 ± 12.5
msec. When the P-wave duration equals or exceeds
0.12 sec intra-atrial block is present. The most
difficult question is the location of the level of the
block. The pathways of the atrial depolarization remains a controversial issue.

The previously accepted theory of Lewis and co-
workers [9], that the atrial activation occurs tangen-
tially along the atrial wall, is now disputed. In the
last decade modern techniques used in anatomic, electrophysiologic and biochemical studies tried to prove
that a specific atrial conduction system does exist [10].

In 1907 Keith and Flock [11] suggested that direct muscular connections may exist between the
sinus and AV node.

Wenckebach [12] and Thorel [13] brought evidence supporting the presence of muscular bundles
connecting the SA node with the AV node. Bachman
[14] in 1916 described the inter-atrial bundle and
proved [15] that notching, bifurcation or splitting of
the P-wave of the electrocardiogram are due to
pathological changes of the interauricular bundle (direct injury or interference with its blood supply).
The controversy arises concerning the nature of the
specific atrial conduction system and of the anatomical structure of these muscular bridges which contain Purkinje fibers (with rapid conduction) and normal myocardial fibers (with slow conduction). The
constant form of the P-wave in normal individuals
suggests that the existence of a specific pathway allows the sinus impulse to depolarize the atria in a
specific manner. Hence, widening of the P-wave
suggests a delayed spread of excitation.

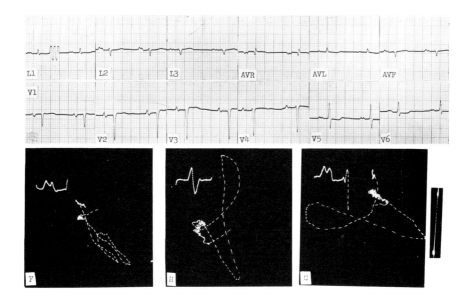

Fig. 5. A 58 year old male hospitalized with left ventricular failure due to primary myocardial disease. The
electrocardiogram shows a bifid P-wave with a duration of 0.14 sec. The vectorcardiogram shows a large double
peaked P-loop in the frontal plane and figure of eight in the sagittal and horizontal plane. The size of the left
atrium was at the upper limit of normal.

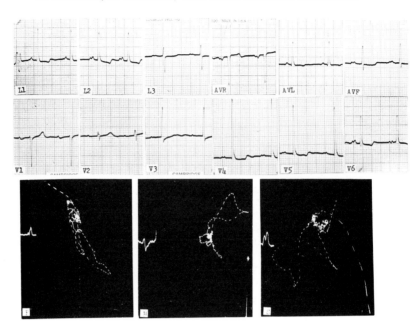

Fig. 6. A 79 year old female hospitalized with a CVA. The electrocardiogram shows a bifid P-wave with a duration of 0.14 sec. The vectorcardiogram shows a double peaked frontal P-loop with clockwise direction of both peaks. In the horizontal plane a very small appendage is oriented to the right and anteriorly. The entire P-loop is located postero-inferiorly and bites and notches are present. The size of the left atrium was normal.

The three internodal pathways and the interauricular bundle could each or all be partially affected, completely blocked or transiently involved.

When the widening of the P-wave is transient, an intermittent intra-atrial block is present.

The occurrence of ventricular fascicular blocks are more or less accepted today, but the existence of specific blocks due to abnormal conduction through the atrial tracts is disputed. Multiple cross over connections between these atrial-specific pathways make it more difficult to pinpoint the level of physiological or pathological conduction disturbance. We present four patterns of vectorcardiograms that correspond to four prevailing common electrocardiographic contours of the P-wave. The bifid contour, which is the most frequent in our study, may correspond to a lesion in the Bachman bundle at the level of the inter-atrial septum.

Different clinical entities may produce the same electrocardiographic and vectorcardiographic patterns. We recorded abnormal P-loops in patients with diabetes mellitus (figure 9). When atrial enlargement is present the size of the P-loop is larger (figure 4).

One cannot assess with certitude the separate contribution made by each of the two factors, conduction delay and hypertrophy, to the enlargement of P-loop. The same problem exists at the level of the left ventricle when left ventricular hypertrophy coexists with left bundle branch block.

When the anterior internodal tract was injured [16, 17], the duration of the P-wave increased significantly. It is tempting to speculate that, in patients with intra-atrial conduction disturbance and a dome-shaped or peaked P-wave, the anterior internodal tract could be involved in delaying the conduction. Blocking of a main conducting bundle may induce activation of latent cross-over pathways which in turn will depolarize the atrial in a distorted manner. The result of this activation will be a P-loop showing many bites, notches and conduction delays.

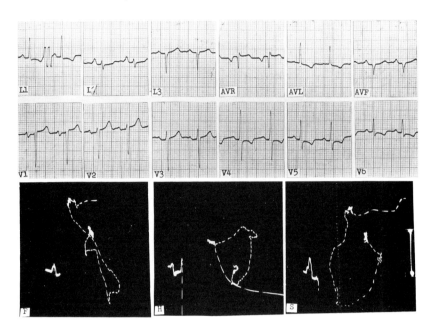

Fig. 7. A 45 year old male hospitalized with severe chest pain and pulmonary edema. The electrocardiogram shows a tall peaked P-wave in lead 2 with a duration of 0.12 sec. The vectorcardiogram shows a distorted P-loop with initial mid and terminal conduction delay, bites and notches. The posterior part of the P-loop is twice as large as the anterior part. The echocardiogram shows a normal sized left atrium.

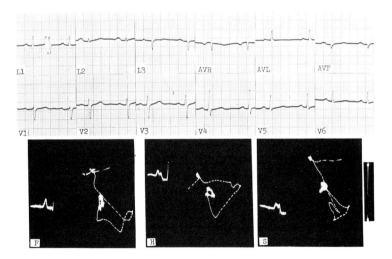

Fig. 8. An 89 year old male hospitalized with prostatic hypertrophy. The electrocardiogram shows a flat P-wave with a duration of 0.14 sec. The vectorcardiogram shows a P-loop of small magnitude. The maximal vector is less than 0.10 mv. Diffuse dense conduction delay is present. Bites and notches are also evident.

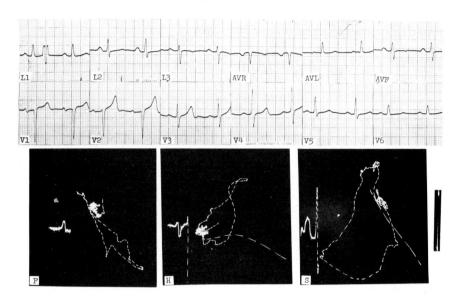

Fig. 9. A 55 year old male hospitalized with pneumonia and diabetes mellitus. The electrocardiogram shows a P-wave with a duration of 0.14 sec. The P-loop is loaded with notches and conduction delays. The major part of the P-loop is posteriorly located in spite of a normal sized left atrium.

Baruch et al. [18] described the P-loop in patients with mitral stenosis and related the distortions (high frequency components) to areas of fibrosis, inflammation and hypertrophy.

Legato et al. [19] reported the ultrastructural changes in the right atria of ten patients with intra-atrial block. The ultrastructural changes were more extensive when the P-wave duration was more than 140 msec. than in those with a duration of 120 msec.

They suggest that the lesser degree of block is probably due to sluggish conduction through the anterior internodal tract. In the elderly a sclerodegenerative process of the conduction tissue (Lenegre disease at the level of the atria ?) may produce severe intra-atrial block [20].

In patients with intermittent intra-atrial block a functional lesion in one or more of the specific pathways may transiently change the configuration of the P-loop.

Further investigation of atrial depolarization in progress as well as mapping the human atria will enable us to better define the correlation of abnormal electrocardiographic and vectorcardiographic patterns with specific abnormal conduction disturbances.

Summary

Frank P-loop vectorcardiograms were recorded in 30 normal subjects and in 40 patients with intra-atrial conduction disturbances (cardiac and non-cardiac patients). High magnification of the P-loop (0.1 mv = 3 cm.) permitted accurate measurement of the P-loop duration, magnitude and direction. High frequency recordings allowed optimal evaluation of the notches, bites and conduction delays in the P-loop.

Four vectorcardiographic patterns have been selected as counterparts of the four types of enlarged P-waves seen in electrocardiograms of patients with atrial conduction disturbances. When intra-atrial conduction disturbances coexisted with left atrial enlargement, the P-loop was larger and smoother. The role of partial or complete block in the specific internodal or inter-atrial pathways is discussed. High magnification, high frequency vectorcardiography of the P-loop seems to be the best available method for determining a specific pattern of intra-atrial conduction disturbance.

Acknowledgement

The authors are indebted to Dr. Renee Fleisher for reviewing the manuscript and to Miss Ada Fantroy, Mr. Floyd Jackson and Mrs. Karen Franklin for their technical assistance.

References

[1] H. Feigenbaum, Echocardiography (Lea and Febiger, Philadelphia, 1972), p. 147.

[2] E. Frank, An accurate, clinically practical system for spacial vectorcardiography, Circulation 3 (1956) 737.

[3] R. H. Selvester and L. Haywood, High gain, high frequency atrial vectorcardiograms in normal subjects and in patients with atrial enlargement, American J. Cardiol. 24 (1969) 8.

[4] A. Benchimol, Vectorcardiography (Williams and Wilkins Co., Baltimore, 1973), p. 35.

[5] C-Te Chow and R. Helm, Clinical vectorcardiography (Grune and Stratton, New York, 1967), p. 50.

[6] J. Legato and M. Ferrer, Intermittent intra-atrial block: Its diagnosis, incidence and implications, Chest 65 (1974), 243.

[7] J. Cohen and D. Scherf, Complete interatrial and intra-atrial block (atrial dissociation), Am. Heart J. 70 (1965) 23.

[8] A. Brody, R. C. Arzbaecher, D. Woolsey, and T. Sato, The normal atrial electrocardiogram: Morphologic and quantitative variability in bipolar extremity leads, Am. Heart J. 74 (1967) 4.

[9] T. Lewis, A. Oppenheimer, B. S. Oppenheimer, The site of origin of the mammalian heart beat; the pacemaker in the dog, Heart 2 (1910) 147.

[10] N. James and L. Sherf, Specialized tissues and preferential conduction in the atria of the heart, Amer. J. Cardiol. 28 (1971) 414.

[11] A. Keith and M. W. Flack, The form and nature of the muscular connections between the primary divisions of the vertebrate heart, J. Anat. Physiol. 41 (1907) 172.

[12] K. F. Wenckebach, Beitrage zur Kenntnis der menschlichen Herztatigkeit, Arch. Anat. Physiol. 1-2 (1907) 1.

[13] C. Thorel, Uber den Aufbau des Sinusknotens und seine verbindung mit der Cava superior und den wenkebachschen bundeln, Munchen Med. Wschr. 57 (1910) 183.

[14] G. Bachmann, The significance of splitting of the P-wave in the electrocardiogram, Ann. Int. Med. 14 (1941) 1703.

[15] G. Bachmann, The inter-auricular time interval, Am. J. Physiol., 41 (1916), 309.

[16] J. W. Holsinger, Jr., A. G. Wallace, and W. C. Sealy, The identification and surgical significance of the atrial internodal conduction tracts, Annals of Surgery 167 (1968), 447.

[17] A. L. Waldo, H. L. Bush, Jr., H. Gelband, G. Zorn, Jr., K. J. Vitikainen, and B. F. Hoffman, Effects on the canine P-wave of discrete lesion in the specialized atrial tracts, Circulation 29 (1971) 452.

[18] G. E. Burch and T. D. Giles, Atrial vectorcardiogram in mitral valve disease, Cardiology 58 (1973), 80.

[19] J. Legato, B. Bull, and M. Ferrer, Atrial ultrastructure in patients with fixed intra-atrial block, Chest 65 (1974) 252.

[20] S. Zoneraich and O. Zoneraich, Atrial tachycardia with high degree of intra-atrial block, J. Electrocardiology 4 (1971) 369.

SECTION 3.
PACEMAKERS AND CONDUCTION DISORDERS

Vectorcardiography 3 I. Hoffman and R.I. Hamby eds.

DYNAMIC VECTORCARDIOGRAPHY IN THE EVALUATION OF LEFT HEMIBLOCKS

Agustin Castellanos, Louis Lemberg, Ruey J. Sung, and Robert J. Myerburg

From the Division of Cardiology, Department of Medicine,
University of Miami School of Medicine, and the Section
of Electrophysiology, Jackson Memorial Hospital,
Miami, Florida, U.S.A.

Clinical Evaluation of the Hemiblock Patterns

Recent experimental studies [1, 2] have suggested that the trifascicular concept of intraventricular conduction popularized by Rosenbaum et al. [3] might be an oversimplification of a complex problem. Nevertheless there is clinical and experimental evidence suggesting that certain electrocardiographic and vectorcardiographic patterns result from abnormal left ventricular depolarization in turn produced by conduction defects affecting the divisions (or fascicles) of the left bundle branch [4].

How large a lesion has to be or at what level of the intraventricular conducting system must it be located in order to produce a hemiblock pattern has been a matter of debate and speculation [4].

However, it has to be held in mind that it is possible for some "focal" or "parietal" conduction disturbances (those located beyond the "Purkinje myocardial junction" or peripheral "gates") to produce similar (although perhaps not identical) QRS patterns [4]. According to Grant [5] there are several ways (short of post-mortem conducting system studies) by means of which it can be reasonably proven that a given QRS "deformity" is due to a specific conduction disturbance. The first is experimental. Similar QRS changes should be produced by placing appropriate lesions in the corresponding segment of the conducting system. Yet too much emphasis on this approach led many workers astray due to the differences between dog and man. Moreover, post-mortem conducting system studies, important as they are, do not give a perfect correlation with dynamic electrophysiological phenomena except, of course, when a structure is completely interrupted by fibrous tissue [3, 4].

Grant believed that a clinical method of uttermost importance was that tracings considered to be diagnostic of the defect under consideration should be "properly controlled" [5]. This meant that serial recordings should be available, before, after and (ideally) at the moment of appearance of the conduction disturbance. These postulates have been met in the case of the hemiblocks by the methods stressed by Grant as well as by the analysis of (intracardiac) post-surgical conduction disturbances and of tracings

showing spontaneous or electrically-induced aberration of supraventricular impulses [3, 4].

Unfortunately, the vectorcardiogram, which is a most useful tool for the study of intraventricular conduction defects, has not been extensively used for this purpose [6-11]. Contrary to common belief much work remains to be done in the field of intraventricular conduction. This presentation will deal with the contribution of dynamic vectorcardiography, an extension of the previously mentioned (Grant's) approach to the understanding of hemiblock patterns.

Post-Surgical Left Anterior Hemiblock (LAH)

Figure 1 shows the abnormal left axis deviation which can occur in some patients during total surgical repair of Tetralogy of Fallot [11]. This LAH-right bundle branch block (RBBB) pattern has been attributed to a lesion in the penetrating portion of the His bundle leading to bifascicular block or to a lesion in the anterosuperior division associated with right ventricular "parietal" or "focal" conduction delay produced by the ventriculotomy.

In any case the sudden shift of the frontal plane maximal QRS vector (FMV) abnormally to the left and superiorly most probably is due to a lesion in the specialized intraventricular conducting system which leads to a delay of activation of the anterosuperior regions of the left ventricle.

LAH and Right Bundle Branch Block (RBBB)

The presence of RBBB does not interfere with the diagnosis of LAH since the former conduction disturbance classically produces (mainly) terminal conduction disturbances which do not significantly change the direction of the FMV [12].

The initial QRS vectors are said not to be affected in clinical RBBB, in contrast to experimental RBBB [13]. However, it is best considered that the initial vectorial changes produced by RBBB are not detected by body surface recordings rather than to

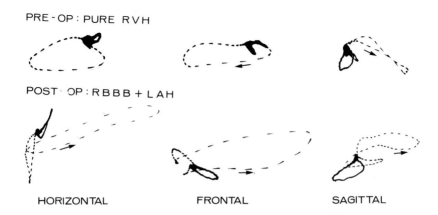

PRE-OP: PURE RVH

POST-OP: RBBB + LAH

HORIZONTAL   FRONTAL   SAGITTAL

Fig. 1. Post-surgical left anterior hemiblock (and RBBB) occurring after complete repair of Tetralogy of Fallot. The frontal plane QRS loop (Frank system) shows the typical features attributed to left anterior hemiblock.

consider them non-existent since some changes must occur in view of the fact that the contribution to septal depolarization of the impulse descending through the right bundle branch is no longer present [12]. Perhaps the "purest" form of iatrogenic RBBB (without hemiblock) is that produced by mechanical (catheter) stimulation since spontaneous, surgical or functional RBBB might occur associated with some degree of hemiblock which could be responsible for the initial vectorial abnormalities [4].

Other Causes of Abnormal Superior and Leftward Deviation of the FMV

Frontal plane QRS loops showing abnormal superior and leftward deviation of its FMV are seen in pulmonary emphysema, WPW syndrome (usually type B), pacing from the right ventricular apex or deep in the middle cardiac vein, hyperkalemia, left coronary arteriography (especially in patients without coronary artery disease) and inferior wall myocardial infarction (figure 2) [12].

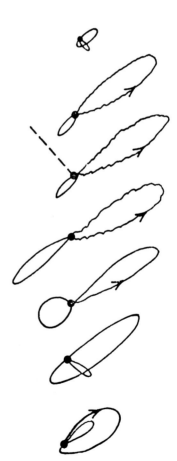

Fig. 2. Diagrammatic representation of various processes which can produce abnormal superior and leftwards deviation of the frontal plane maximal QRS vector. From top to bottom: pulmonary emphysema, WPW syndrome (pure Kent bundle conduction); right ventricular apical pacing, hyperkalemia, left coronary arteriography, left anterior hemiblock and inferior wall myocardial infarction.

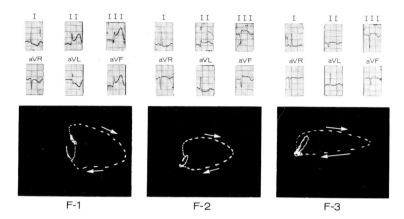

Fig. 3. Frontal plane QRS and ST-T changes occurring in a patient with extensive inferior wall myocardial infarction. Whereas the electrical axis (as determined from the standard electrocardiographic leads) shows a significant leftward shift from the left to the right panel, the frontal plane maximal QRS vector is deviated only slightly.

It is not known whether the abnormal location of the FMV seen in pulmonary emphysema, thoracic chest wall deformities and hyperkalemia results from LAH or a coexisting extracardiac or intracardiac process [12].

Of special significance is that abnormal superior and leftward deviation of the FMV can be induced by an acute, dye-induced, focal block occurring in the ordinary muscle of the anterosuperior left ventricular wall (which is the region perfused by the injected area) [14]. This possibility raises the interesting question as to whether other causes of acute or chronic "focal" block, such as produced by electrical injury or diffuse fibrosis, can also result in similar shifts of the FMV.

Differences between the Degree of Superior and Leftward Shift of the Electrical Axis and the FMV

It should be stressed that, with the Frank system, abnormal superior and leftward deviation of the FMV can be considered present with shifts superior (to the left of) 0° [12]. This contrasts with abnormal left axis deviation in the electrocardiogram which usually requires an axis shift of at least -30°.

This is due to the fact that the scalar Y lead of the Frank system differs from aVF because of the influence of the back (M) electrode. Which of these gives a better representation of the inferosuperior

or supero-inferior electrical forces is a subject that needs clarification.

Inferior Myocardial Infarction (IMI) with Abnormal Superior and Leftward Deviation of the FMV

Extensive IMIs can deviate the FMV in an abnormal superior and leftward direction [12, 15-17]. When this occurs the QRS loop shows CW rotation and the initial QRS vectors are also displaced abnormally superiorly. The amount of work required to be done in this area is clearly indicated by the scant information regarding the electrogenesis of the ventricular activation process in extensive IMI. (See figure 3.)

Presumably the septum should be involved in cases where the pre-infarction initial vectors were pointing inferiorly. Otherwise it is difficult to understand how these early forces (clearly not of posterior free wall origin) can be affected.

LAH and Left Ventricular Focal Block

QRS duration is not greatly prolonged in LAH. Terminal delays, if present, are not significant (less than 25 msec). When LAH is associated with a terminal delay greater than 30 msec, the resulting pattern probably reflects the association of LAH with left ventricular "focal" block (figure 4) [12, 18, 19].

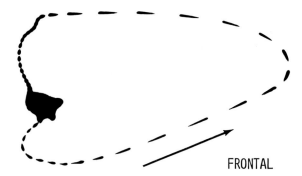

FRONTAL

Fig. 4. Frontal plane QRS loop showing left anterior hemiblock with terminal left ventricular "focal" block.

LAH and Left Ventricular "Focal" Block Obscuring a Previously Present RBBB

If the degree of focal block is very significant, for example, in the range of 50 msec, a previously present RBBB (with a right sided delay of 40 msec) can be hidden by the LAH combined with the left ventricular "focal" block (figure 5) [20]. This possibility is more prone to occur in patients with cardiomyopathy or extensive fibrosis due to coronary artery disease than in patients with chronic conducting system disease.

LAH with Inferior and Leftward Deviation of the Initial QRS Vectors

The initial QRS vector in LAH points inferiorly and to the right. A leftward, inferior and anterior orientation of the initial vectors can be due to a coexisting incomplete left bundle branch block or to LAH associated with a conduction delay in the postero-inferior division (figure 6, top) [21]. In both cases the impulse emerging from the right bundle branch would be responsible for the right-to-left direction of the early QRS forces. A similar orientation of the initial vectors has also been attributed to coexisting septal fibrosis or anteroseptal infarction.

In some cases the pattern of LAH coexisting with incomplete LBBB or conduction delay through the postero-inferior division is associated with a significant leftward oriented (exclusively terminal) conduction delay (figure 6, bottom) [21]. The latter probably represents an added left ventricular "focal" block [21].

Left Bundle Branch Block (LBBB) with Left Axis Deviation

The loops shown in figure 6 should not be confused with those attributed to "complete" LBBB with abnormal left axis deviation in which a medial delay (of at least 20 msec) is present [19].

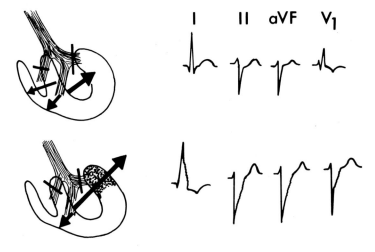

I   II   aVF   V₁

Fig. 5. Diagrammatic representation of how a left anterior hemiblock associated with a significant terminal left ventricular "focal" block (due to fibrosis) can mask a previously present right bundle branch block.

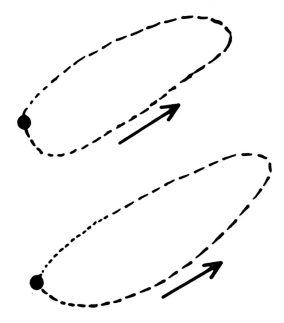

Fig. 6. Left anterior hemiblock with incomplete LBBB (top) and left anterior hemiblock with incomplete LBBB associated with left ventricular focal block (bottom) (frontal plane QRS loops). The horizontal plane is required in these cases to determine whether an anteroseptal infarction is or is not present.

Classical "complete" LBBB does not show abnormal left axis deviation presumably because the site from which the impulse emerges from the unblocked right bundle branch is not so low (caudal) as that from which it emerges when the so called right ventricular apex is paced or when LAH is present (figure 7).

Frontal plane QRS loops showing "complete" LBBB morphology with abnormal superior and leftward deviation of the FMV can result from [4]: (a) LAH with incomplete (high degree LBBB); (b) LAH with high degree left posterior hemiblock; (c) "complete" LBBB with a "focal" block in the free wall of the left ventricle and (d) "complete" LBBB with right superior hemiblock (figure 8) and "complete" LBBB with chronic lung disease or thoracic chest wall abnormalities.

LAH and Inferior Wall Myocardial Infarction (IWMI)

In these cases the frontal plane QRS loops shows abnormal superior deviation of the initial QRS vectors (due to the infarction) associated with a superior and leftward orientation of the FMV with C-CW rotation (due to LAH) [7, 9].

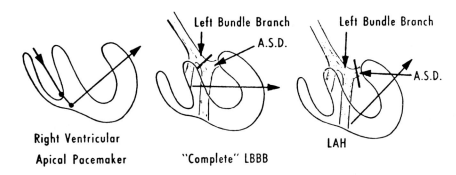

Fig. 7. Diagrammatic representation as to why classical "complete" left bundle branch block does not produce abnormal left axis deviation (middle schematic). The latter is attributed to the site of impulse exit from the right bundle branch, which is represented as occurring at a higher (more cephalic) level than during right ventricular apical pacing (left) or left anterior hemiblock (right) ASD = anterior superior division of the left bundle branch.

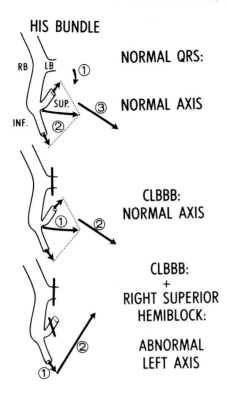

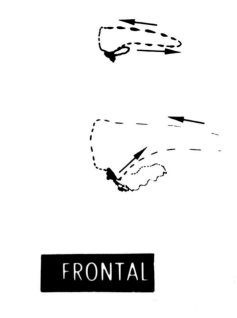

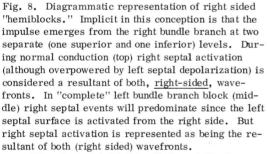

Fig. 9. Left anterior hemiblock associated with inferior wall myocardial infarction. The bottom loop is a magnification of the top one.

Fig. 8. Diagrammatic representation of right sided "hemiblocks." Implicit in this conception is that the impulse emerges from the right bundle branch at two separate (one superior and one inferior) levels. During normal conduction (top) right septal activation (although overpowered by left septal depolarization) is considered a resultant of both, right-sided, wave-fronts. In "complete" left bundle branch block (middle) right septal events will predominate since the left septal surface is activated from the right side. But right septal activation is represented as being the resultant of both (right sided) wavefronts.

When "complete" left bundle branch block co-exists with block in the superior division of the right bundle branch, right septal activation is a function of the more inferior division. In consequence the initial (septal), and subsequently the remaining depolarization occurs in an inferosuperior sequence.

This is shown statically in figure 9 and dynamically in figure 10. Pure IWMI is depicted in figure 10, left. Whereas the initial vectors point abnormally superiorly and to the left, the FMV is deviated to the left and inferiorly. The frontal plane QRS loop shows CW rotation. A coexisting LAH appeared suddenly one hour later. Therefore the FMV became deviated abnormally to the left and superiorly and the rotation changed from CW to C-CW. Of additional interest in the case is that the appearance of LAH abolished the ST-T loop changes produced by the acute IWMI [9]. This is an exception to the usual findings in recent IWMI when both processes coexist.

Rosenbaum et al. first observed that QRS changes in IWMI could be masked when LAH appeared [3].

A definite cause and effect relationship could be established in the case reported in the last cited reference because the conduction disturbance was intermittent. The tracings showed a beat-to-beat alternation between pure IWMI and pure LAH. The hemiblock changed lead aVF from a QS complex with a negative T wave to an rS complex with a positive T wave.

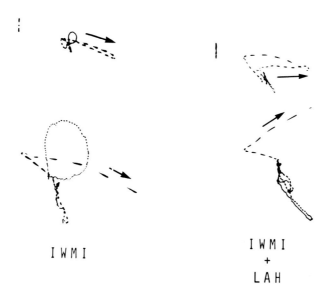

Fig. 10. Frontal plane loops in pure inferior wall myocardial infarction (left) and as left anterior hemiblock associated with inferior wall myocardial infarction (right).

These interesting findings were explained by the relationship between the anatomic location of the infarction and the first ventricular sites depolarized during LAH. According to Rosenbaum and colleagues [3], when the infarction appears after the conduction disturbance the inferiorly oriented vectors will be abolished if the necrosis extends into the ventricular muscle first activated in LAH, without modification of the subsequent ventricular activation process. Similar changes occur if the LAH appears after the infarction. On the other hand an IWMI not involving the portions of the ventricles which are first depolarized in LAH will be missed (or only suspected in the presence of suggestive ST-T abnormalities), regardless of whether it appears before or after the hemiblock. An analogous phenomenon is the abolition of the electrocardiographic changes characteristic of myocardial infarction by a complete left bundle branch block, another conduction disturbance which changes the direction of the initial vectors.

LAH and Antero-Septal
Myocardial Infarction

When an infarction of this location is associated with LAH the initial QRS vectors are oriented posteriorly, inferiorly and to the left [12]. The other features of LAH still persist.

LAH and Antero-Lateral
Myocardial Infarction

An infarction in this part of the heart can increase the duration of the early part of the QRS loop which is located in the right inferior quadrant [12] The abnormal superior and leftward deviation of the FMV as well as the C-CW rotation persists (figure 11).

LAH with Superior and Rightwards
Deviation of the FMV

Although LAH is usually identified with abnormal superior and leftward deviation of the FMV there are several processes in which LAH with superior and rightwards deviation of the FMV is seen [12]. This occurs in some patients when LAH coexists with: (a) extensive antero-lateral myocardial infarction (figure 12); (b) extensive infero-antero-lateral myocardial infarction (figures 13 and 14); (c) right ventricular hypertrophy, generally due to congenital heart disease; and (d) some types of RBBB (especially when coexisting with congenital or pulmonary heart disease). In all of these cases the frontal plane QRS loops show exclusive or predominant C-CW rotation. Because of the statements made in this section it appears that the most constant features of LAH are:

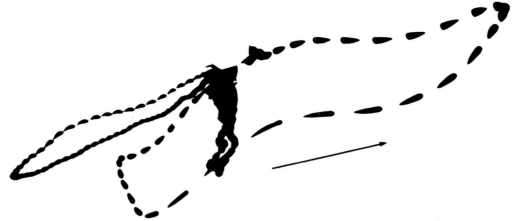

Fig. 11.   Left anterior hemiblock associated with anterolateral wall myocardial infarction.   (Frontal plane.)

(a) <u>superior</u> (generally leftward, but occasionally rightward) deviation of the FMV and (b) <u>C-CW rotation</u> of the QRS loop.

<u>LPH and IWMI</u>

This combination is characterized by abnormal superior deviation of the initial QRS vectors.   The FMV points inferiorly and to the right (figure 15). When the infarction is recent the ST-T loop is abnormally open (because of electrical injury) and shows an abnormal velocity of inscription (due to "electrical ischemia") [9] (figure 18).

Although the extremely abnormal superior deviation of the initial QRS vectors excludes right ventricular hypertrophy, some patients with cardiomyopathy (and even chronic conducting system disease without significant myocardial involvement) can present similar changes in the early part of the loop. This has been attributed to a coexisting initial "focal" block due to septal fibrosis or simply to the sui-generis type of intraventricular propagation characteristic of LPH.   Abnormal ST-T loop changes might differentiate between LPH due to inferior wall myocardial infarction and LPH produced by other processes.   However, as will be discussed below, the age of the infarction can not always be judged by <u>all</u> features of the ST-T loop.

It has been shown that in some patients in which LPH and IWMI coexist the duration of the (early) part of the loop (located superiorly) is not abnormal.   Thus the initial QRS changes characteristic of myocardial infarction are not present.

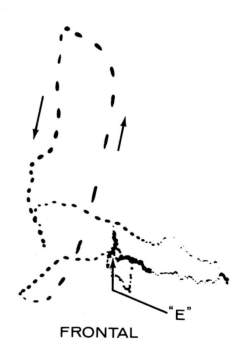

FRONTAL

Fig. 12.   Left anterior hemiblock (with RBBB) associated with extensive anterolateral wall myocardial infarction.   In this case the QRS loop is located in the right superior (not left superior) quadrant.   This was attributed to the infarction.   Note predominant counterclockwise rotation (due to left anterior hemiblock).

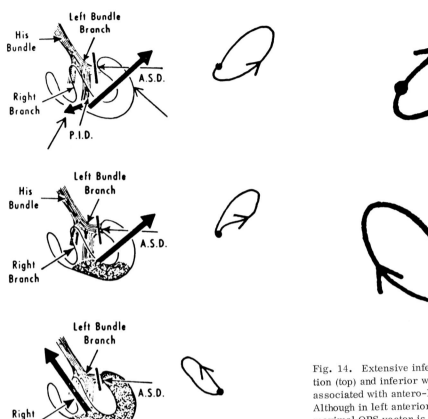

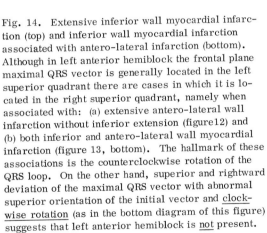

Fig. 14. Extensive inferior wall myocardial infarction (top) and inferior wall myocardial infarction
associated with antero-lateral infarction (bottom).
Although in left anterior hemiblock the frontal plane
maximal QRS vector is generally located in the left
superior quadrant there are cases in which it is located in the right superior quadrant, namely when
associated with: (a) extensive antero-lateral wall
infarction without inferior extension (figure 12) and
(b) both inferior and antero-lateral wall myocardial
infarction (figure 13, bottom). The hallmark of these
associations is the counterclockwise rotation of the
QRS loop. On the other hand, superior and rightward
deviation of the maximal QRS vector with abnormal
superior orientation of the initial vector and clockwise rotation (as in the bottom diagram of this figure)
suggests that left anterior hemiblock is not present.

Fig. 13. Diagrammatic representation of sequential
(frontal plane) QRS changes when a pure left anterior
hemiblock (top) is associated with inferior wall
myocardial infarctions (middle) and inferior and lateral wall myocardial infarctions (bottom).

This is illustrated dynamically in figure 17;
the first QRS complex in each panel depicts the basic
pattern displayed by supraventricular (either sinus
or A-V junctional) beats. Note the normal location
of the electrical axis. On the other hand, the second
ventricular complex in each panel (following premature atrial impulses) show different (increasing from
left to right) degrees of functional LPH.

The last QRS complex in this figure (with a
complete LPH pattern) is characterized by right axis

deviation. There are qR complexes and ischemic T
wave changes in II, III and aVF (the latter not
shown). The relationship between the size of the q
and that of the R in III is such that the presence of
IWMI is hard to recognize. But on the other hand
the ischemic T wave inversion in the inferior leads
suggests the appearance of acute ischemia that the
patient did not have.

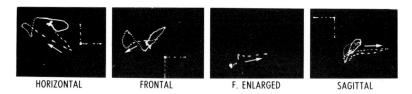

Fig. 15. Infero-posterior infarction with right bundle branch block and left posterior hemiblock.

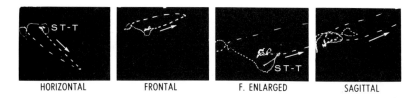

Fig. 16. (Same patient as in figure 15, one day later.) Whereas the horizontal and right sagittal QRS loops have not changed significantly the frontal plane is now suggestive of left anterior (not left posterior) hemiblock.

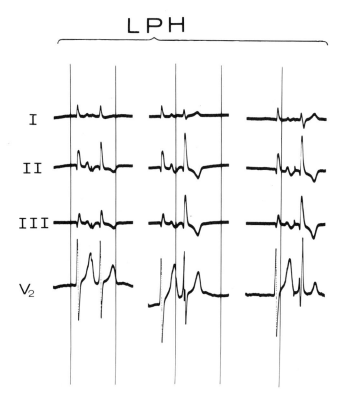

Fig. 17. Old inferior posterior wall myocardial infarction (first QRS complex in each panel) with increasing (from left to right) degrees of left posterior hemiblock (second QRS complex in each panel).

In contrast, figure 18 shows the frontal plane QRS loops in a patient with acute inferior wall myocardial infarction and LPH. Although the QRS loop does not show evidence of infarction (the initial 25 msec are not directed superiorly) this diagnosis is suspected by the abnormal ST-T loop. The latter is "open" and shows uniform speed of inscription.

LPH Coexisting with Anterior Myocardial Infarction

In these cases the frontal plane QRS loop shows the classical features of LPH whereas the antero-septal infarction is diagnosed from the horizontal plane. However, if the infarction extends somewhat into the free left ventricular wall and affects the areas first depolarized by the impulse emerging from the unblocked antero-superior division the initial vectors will not be directed superiorly [12]. According to the amount of muscle affected they will point inferiorly and either to the right or to the left as in figure 19. In the former cases they will be directed to the left after an initial rightward shift.

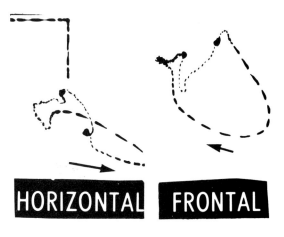

Fig. 18. Acute inferior wall myocardial infarction associated with left posterior hemiblock (right bundle branch block is also present). Whereas the QRS loop does not suggest inferior wall myocardial infarction (only left posterior hemiblock) the "open" ST-T loop favors the existence of recent injury in the inferior wall.

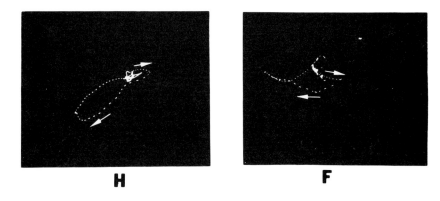

Fig. 19. Left posterior hemiblock (and right bundle branch block) in a patient with anterior myocardial infarction. Involvement of the area at which the impulse emerges from the unblocked antero-superior division of the left bundle branch abolished the initial superior electrical forces that generally occur in uncomplicated left posterior hemiblock.

However, if there is significant involvement of the anterolateral wall the initial vectors and the body of the QRS loop will be located in the right inferior quadrant (figure 20, bottom). The CW rotation characteristic of LPH remains. This feature is helpful to exclude pure extensive anterolateral wall myocardial infarction (figure 20, middle loop).

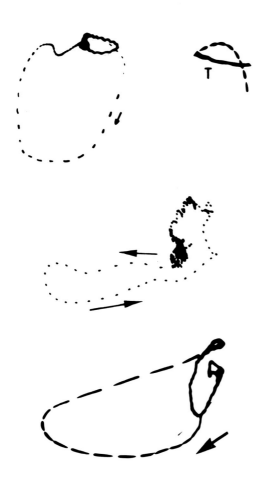

Fig. 20. Frontal plane QRS loops in pure left posterior hemiblock (top), pure extensive antero-lateral myocardial infarction (middle) and left posterior hemiblock associated with antero-lateral myocardial infarction (bottom).

Summary

Dynamic vectorcardiography, that is the analysis of sequential changes, occurring before or after the appearance of acute (organic or functional) hemiblock has proven a useful method in evaluation of the corresponding patterns. Left anterior hemiblock is characterized mainly by the superior orientation of the maximal frontal plane QRS vectors and counterclockwise rotation of the QRS loop. This knowledge is essential in understanding the electrogenesis of associated processes.

Important features of complicated left posterior hemiblock are the behavior of: (a) the initial QRS vectors and of the ST-T loop in inferior wall myocardial infarction; (b) the initial QRS vectors and QRS rotation in antero-lateral wall infarction and (c) the initial QRS vectors in antero-septal and left para-septal infarction.

Further studies are still required to corroborate the validity of these patterns.

References

[1]   R. J. Myerburg, K. Neilsson, and H. Gelband, Physiology of canine intraventricular conduction and endocardial excitation, Circulation Res. 30 (1972) 217.
[2]   R. Lazzara, N. Kahn, and B. K. Yeh, Conduction time in canine bundle branches evidence of interconnections amongs fibers, Fed. Proc. 30 (1971) 553.
[3]   M. B. Rosenbaum, M. V. Elizari, and J. O. Lazzari, The hemiblocks (Tampa Tracings, Oldsmar, Florida, 1970).
[4]   A. Castellanos and R. J. Myerburg, The hemiblocks in myocardial infarction (Appleton-Century-Crofts, New York, in press).
[5]   R. P. Grant, Peri-infarction block, Prog. Cardiovasc. Dis. 27 (1959) 237.
[6]   A. Benchimol, Vectorcardiography (Williams and Wilkins, Baltimore, 1973).
[7]   A. Benchimol and K. B. Desser, Coexisting left anterior hemiblock and inferior wall myocardial infarction. Vectorcardiography features, Am. J. Cardiol. 29 (1972) 7.
[8]   A. Castellanos, Jr., E. Chapunoff, C. A. Castillo, A. G. Arcebal, and L. Lemberg, The vectorcardiogram in left posterior hemiblock associated with inferior wall myocardial infarction, Chest 61 (1972) 221.
[9]   A. Castellanos, Jr., R. Chahine, E. Chapunoff, J. Gomez, and B. Portillo, Diagnosis of left anterior hemiblock in the presence of inferior wall myocardial infarction, Chest 60 (1971) 543.

[10] S. I. Cohen, S. H. Lau, E. Stein, M. W.
      Young, and A. N. Damato, Variations of aber-
      rant conduction in man. Evidence of isolated
      and combined block within the specialized con-
      ducting system, Circulation 38 (1968) 899.

[11] L. Lemberg, A. Castellanos, Jr., and A. G.
      Arcebal, The vectorcardiogram in acute left
      anterior hemiblock, Am. J. Cardiol. 28 (1971)
      483.

[12] L. Lemberg and A. Castellanos, Jr., Vector-
      cardiography. A Programmed Introduction,
      2d ed. (Appleton-Century-Crofts, New York,
      1975).

[13] D. Penaloza, R. Gamboa, and F. Sime, Ex-
      perimental right bundle branch block in the
      human heart. Electrocardiographic, vector-
      cardiographic and hemodynamic observation,
      Am. J. Cardiol. 8 (1961) 767.

[14] R. J. Smith, J. W. Harthorne, and C. A.
      Sanders, Vectorcardiographic changes during
      intra-coronary injections, Circulation 36 (1967)
      63.

[15] P. G. Hugenholtz, C. E. Forkner, and H. D.
      Levine, A clinical appraisal of the vectorcar-
      diogram in myocardial infarction. II. Frank
      lead system, Circulation 24 (1961) 825.

[16] A. Grishman and L. Scherles, Spatial vector-
      cardiography (Sanders, New York, 1952).

[17] R. Pryor and S. G. Blount, The clinical signif-
      icance of true left axis deviation. Left ventric-
      ular blocks, Am. Heart J. 72 (1965) 391.

[18] J. W. Mayer, A. Castellanos, Jr., and L.
      Lemberg, The spatial vectorcardiogram in
      peri-infarction block, Am. J. Cardiol. 11
      (1963) 613.

[19] E. Cabrera and A. Gaxiola, Teoria y practica
      de la electrocardiografia (La Prensa Mexicana,
      Mexico, D.F., 1966).

[20] M. B. Rosenbaum, J. Yesuion, J. O. Lazzari,
      and M. V. Elizari, Left anterior hemiblock
      obscuring the diagnosis of right bundle branch
      block, Circulation 48 (1973) 298.

[21] J. M. Calvino, L. Azan, and A. Castellanos,
      Jr., Estudio vectorcardiografico de los vectores
      iniciales de QRS anormalmente diugidos nacia
      la igurerda, Rev. Cubana Cardiol. 18 (1957)
      187.

Vectorcardiography 3 I. Hoffman and R.I. Hamby eds.
© 1976 North-Holland Publishing Company - Amsterdam

HIS BUNDLE ELECTRO-VECTORCARDIOGRAPHY IN

WOLFF-PARKINSON-WHITE SYNDROME AND ITS VARIANTS

Agustin Castellanos, Bolivar Portillo, Benjamin Befeler,
Ruey J. Sung, and Robert J. Myerburg

From the Division of Cardiology, Department of Medicine,
University of Miami School of Medicine, The Medical
Service, Veterans Administration Hospital, Section
of Clinical Electrophysiology, Jackson Memorial
Hospital, Miami, Florida, U.S.A. and the
Sanatorio Antituberculoso, Maracaibo, Venezuela

Introduction

Vectorcardiography is one of the various methods by means of which the electrical activity of the
heart can be studied. His bundle electro-vectorcardiography, that is, simultaneous recording of planar
loops, body surface electrocardiograms and intracardiac electrograms has enhanced our knowledge of the
pre-excitation syndromes in which the significance of
coexisting patterns of atrioventricular and intraventricular conduction are not clear [1-4].

Nomenclature

Kent bundle = Accessory A-V pathway (AP) extending
     from atria to ordinary ventricular muscle.
James bundle = AP extending from atria to "low"
     A-V node or "upper" His bundle.
Mahaim bundle = AP extending from His bundle or left
     bundle branch to the ordinary ventricular muscle.
Wolff-Parkinson-White (WPW) syndrome = Electro-
     cardiographic pattern characterized by a short
     P-R interval and an initial delay. This pattern
     usually is due to an AP of the Kent bundle type
     but can also result (rarely) from the combina-
     tion of James and Mahaim bundles.
Lown-Ganong-Levine (LGL) syndrome = Electrocar-
     diographic pattern characterized by short P-R
     and A-H intervals and, in absence of bundle
     branch block, by narrow QRS complexes. This
     pattern is probably due to an AP of the James
     bundle type.

All loops are horizontal plane projections obtained with the Frank system of electrode placement.

Wolff-Parkinson-White Type A
Presumably Due to an Accessory
A-V Pathway of the Kent Bundle
Type

In WPW syndrome various types of QRS mor-
phologies result from different modalities of A-V
conduction [1-6]. This is well seen in patients with
intermittent (especially rate-related) WPW syndrome.
Exclusive conduction through the normal (A-V node-
His bundle) pathway (without bundle branch block) is
characterized by normal P-R and H-V intervals, narrow QRS complexes and absence of initial delay (figure
1, left). Conduction through both normal and accessory

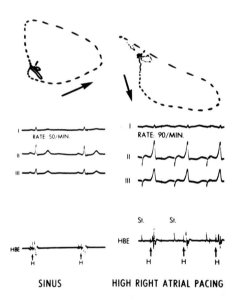

SINUS   HIGH RIGHT ATRIAL PACING

Fig. 1. Horizontal plane QRS loop (Frank system),
standard leads and His bundle recordings in a patient
with intermittent WPW syndrome type A. Whereas
the left sided panel depicts exclusive A-V node-His
bundle conduction, the right sided panel, obtained during atrial pacing at a rate of 90/min shows a minor
degree of "fusion" resulting from ventricular activation via both normal and abnormal A-V pathways.
Paper speed was 50/mm/sec. HBE = His bundle
electrographic lead. H = His bundle electrogram.
St = pacemaker artifact. (From Castellanos et al.,
Am. J. Cardiol. [1]).

pathways results in different grades of pre-excitation
(fusion QRS complexes with short P-R intervals).
Minor degrees of pre-excitation are characterized by
shortening of the H-V interval and slight increase in
QRS duration with appearance of a delta wave (figure 1,
right). In the horizontal QRS loop the (exclusively) initial delay is associated with an anterior shift of the
loop and preservation of the normal counterclockwise
(C-CW) rotation (figure 1, right).

    Increasing degrees of pre-excitation result in
wider QRS complexes. The initial delay becomes
more marked. The horizontal QRS loop shows a
greater anterior shift and a Figure-of-8 rotation (figure 2, left). Finally, when exclusive Kent bundle conduction occurs, fusion beats are no longer present
since ventricular activation occurs only through the
anomalous A-V connection. The His bundle (H) deflection appears <u>after</u> the onset of ventricular depolarization (figure 2, right). The bizarre horizontal QRS
loop--with diffuse delays (initial and terminal)--is
partly inscribed in the right anterior quadrant and
shows clockwise (CW) rotation.

    The terminal delay, oriented anteriorly and to
the right, is not due to right bundle branch block
(RBBB) but is an expression of the anomalous late
right ventricular depolarization which occurs when
an impulse propagates exclusively from a posterior
left ventricular site [1-4]. Similar features are seen
in beats arising spontaneously or iatrogenically (electrical pacing) in an equivalent posterosuperolateral
left ventricular area (figure 3).

    Figure 4 shows the different degrees of pre-excitation
that can occur in WPW type A (as seen in the horizontal plane projection). Black dots indicate the ventricular entrance of the accessory pathway. Open circles
represent the areas first depolarized by the impulse
descending through the posterior and anterior divisions of the left bundle branch and right bundle branch,
respectively.

    A minor degree of pre-excitation occurs in the
first (left sided) schematic since the ventricles are
activated from all four sites. In the second diagram
a greater degree of pre-excitation is seen. The wave-

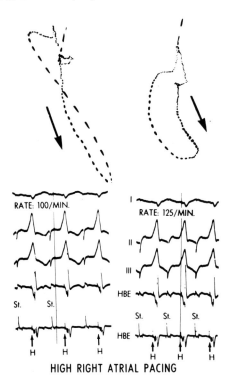

HIGH RIGHT ATRIAL PACING

Fig. 2. (Same patient as in figure 1). Increase in the
degree of pre-excitation produced by atrial pacing at
faster rates. In the right sided panel the H deflection
appears after the onset of QRS. (From Castellanos et
al., Amer. J. Cardiol. [1]).

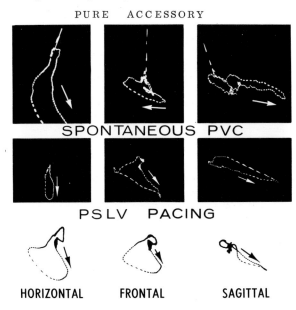

Fig. 3. Vectorcardiograms obtained during exclusive
accessory pathway conduction (WPW type A, during
rapid atrial pacing; top); spontaneous premature ventricular conduction (PVC) arising in the posterosuperolateral left ventricular (PSLV), and pacing from the
PSLV. In all three examples the rightward oriented
terminal delays are due to the late right ventricular activation due to the specific type of intraventricular conduction resulting from impulse initiation in a posterior
left ventricular site. The terminal delay therefore cannot be ascribed to right bundle branch block (RBBB).
(From Castellanos et al., Am. J. Cardiol. [1]).

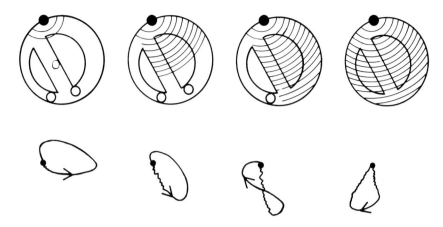

Fig. 4. Schematic representation of the changes of the horizontal QRS loop resulting from increasing (from left to right) degrees of pre-excitation in WPW type A.

front propagating from the pre-excited site has reached the area normally depolarized by an impulse traversing the posterior division. Hence, the ventricles are activated only from the pre-excited area, the anterior division and the right bundle branch. In the third schematic, activation is a function only of the pre-excited area and right bundle branch. The degree of pre-excitation therefore increases. Finally, the last (right sided) schematic shows exclusive Kent bundle conduction with ventricular activation a function only of impulses propagating from the pre-excited site.

The left sided panel in Figure 5 depicts exclusive conduction through the A-V node-His bundle pathway with normal intraventricular conduction and H-V intervals. On the other hand, the QRS complex in figure 5, right, is a fusion beat in which the forward H deflection is inscribed at the onset of ventricular depolarization. Note short P-R interval. The horizontal plane QRS loop shows an initial delay with a Figure-of-8 rotation.

Exclusive Kent bundle conduction occurs in figure 6, left. In the horizontal plane QRS loop (now with CW rotation) the initial delay is associated with a rightward oriented terminal delay. The P-R interval is short and the H deflection appears <u>after</u> the onset of ventricular depolarization. In figure 6, right, (same patient) the P-R is not short. The H-V interval is normal. The horizontal plane QRS shows the right-anterior terminal appendage classically attributed to RBBB. Therefore, this ventricular complex results from exclusive A-V node-His bundle conduction but with block in the right bundle branch.

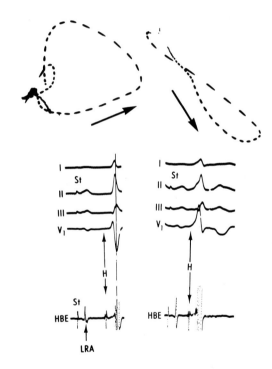

Fig. 5. Horizontal plane QRS loop, standard leads and His bundle recordings in a patient with intermittent WPW type A. The left sided panel shows exclusive A-V node-His bundle conduction. The left sided panel depicts a minor degree of pre-excitation resulting from ventricular activation via both, normal and accessory A-V pathways. (From Castellanos et al., Am. J. Cardiol. [1]).

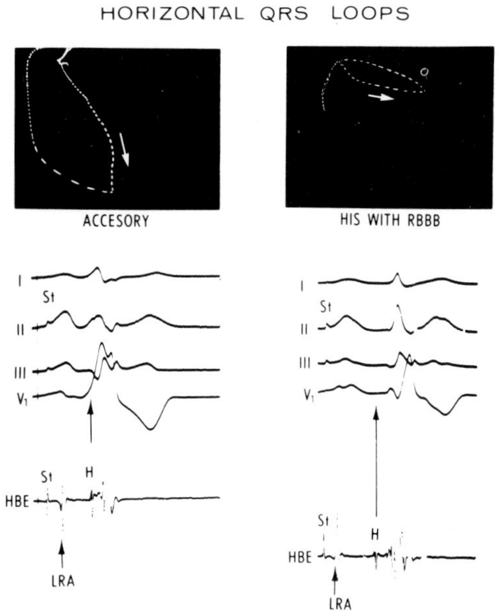

HORIZONTAL QRS LOOPS

ACCESORY

HIS WITH RBBB

Fig. 6. (Same patient as in figure 5.) Whereas the left sided panel shows exclusive Kent bundle conduction the right sided panel depicts exclusive A-V node-His bundle conduction with RBBB.

Differential Diagnosis of WPW Type A. In figures 2, 4 and 6, a rightward oriented terminal delay associated with an initial delay and short P-R interval is due to the sui generis type of (late) right ventricular activation pattern characteristic of WPW type A [1]. Similar loops are seen when a James bundle coexists with a Mahaim bundle and complete intra-Hisian, bilateral or trifascicular, block and when "WPW syndrome type A coexists with RBBB" [7]. Whereas in the former cases both A-H and H-V intervals are short, in the latter cases only the H-V interval is shorter-than-normal [2]. The differential diagnosis of the various processes which can produce initial and terminal delays is presented in Table 1 [2, 3].

WPW Type A Coexisting with RBBB. The left sided schematic in figure 7 shows the QRS loop which results from exclusive (normal) A-V node-His bundle conduction with RBBB. In the middle schematic, the posterior portions of the ventricles are activated from the pre-excited site [2, 3]. Here the wavefront emerging from the two divisions of the left bundle branch activates the left septal surface as well as the anterolateral left ventricular wall, and, after,

crossing the septum in a left-to-right direction, the anterior right ventricular free wall. Since the latter regions are activated as in the left sided schematic (when exclusive A-V node-His bundle conduction with RBBB occurred) it is apparent that the terminal delay in the middle loop is due to RBBB and not to the delayed right ventricular depolarization which occurs when the totality of the ventricles are activated from a pre-excited area (right sided schematic).

WPW Type A Morphology with Normal P-R Interval. The pattern of normal P-R interval, short H-V interval and initial delay in the vectorcardiogram could result from the presence of a Mahaim bundle, or from a Kent bundle associated with intra-atrial conduction defect. The dynamic response to pacing is diagnostic since the H-V interval does not change in the rare patients with Mahaim bundles [5, 6]. On the other hand, in those with Kent bundles the H deflection appears progressively after the onset of QRS when the atria are stimulated at increasing rates (table 1).

It should be stated that similar static electrocardiograms and vectorcardiograms are seen when initial left ventricular focal block (due to septal fibrosis or infarction) coexists with RBBB [3]. But in these cases the P-R and H-V intervals as well as the response to atrial pacing, are normal (figure 8 and table 1).

Lown-Ganong-Levine (LGL) Syndrome with RBBB. Finally, there is a short P-R-wide QRS syndrome in which the anteriorly placed horizontal loop shows an exclusively rightward oriented terminal delay [8]. The latter is probably due to the combination of a James bundle and RBBB if the A-H interval is short (figure 9). The coexistence of repetitive supraventricular tachycardias justifies the diagnosis of LGL syndrome with RBBB.

WPW Type B. The classification of WPW into types A and B should be made from beats showing exclusive AP conduction [2, 3]. This will avoid much of the confusion arising when the diagnosis of the type (A or B) of WPW is attempted from fusion beats.

Although different r/S ratios can be seen in V1 and V2 in patients with WPW type B, the latter can be subdivided into two major groups: those in which the Kent bundle ends anteriorly and those in which it ends posteriorly [2, 3].

Although in figures 10 and 11 the end of the Kent bundle is represented as "parietal" (occurring in the free right ventricular wall), it is important to stress that some Kent bundles open into the right septal surface.

Table 1

Differential diagnosis of syndromes producing initial leftward and
terminal rightward delays in the horizontal plane (QRS loop)

P-R	A-H	H-V	Atrial Pacing	Syndrome	Mechanism
S	N	S	↑ QRS	WPW type A (fusion)	Kent + NP
S	N	H after	= QRS H after V	WPW type A (pure)	Kent
S	N	S	↑ QRS	WPW type A (fusion) + RBBB	Kent = WPW type A with RBBB
S	S	S	= QRS	WPW type A (pure)	James + Mahaim + RBBB
N	N	S	= QRS	WPW type A	Mahaim + NP
N	N	N	= QRS	Initial focal block + RBBB	Septal fibrosis or antero-septal infarction + RBBB
N	N	S	QRS H after V	WPW type A + normal P-R	Kent + intra-atrial conduction defect
–	–	–	–	Spontaneous EVB	↑ automaticity, or reentry in PLV
–	–	–	–	Electrical EVB	Pacing of PLV

Abbreviations:
↑ : Increase in QRS duration
↟ : No change in QRS duration
S : Short
N : Normal
NP: Normal (A-V node-His bundle-bundle branch) pathway

RBBB : Right bundle branch block
BBBB : Bilateral bundle branch block
EVB : Ectopic ventricular beat
PLV : Posterior wall of left ventricle

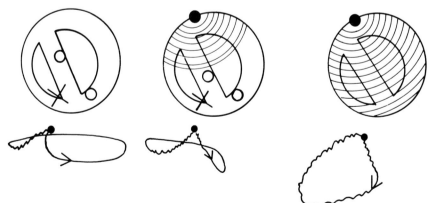

Fig. 7. Exclusive A-V node-His bundle conduction with RBBB (left), and exclusive Kent bundle conduction (WPW type A, right). The middle schematic shows block in the right bundle branch (WPW type A coexisting with RBBB).

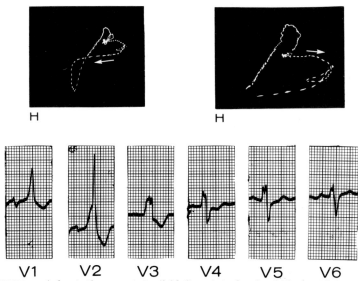

Fig. 8. "Pseudo" WPW type A due to the association of left ventricular focal block with RBBB. The P-R interval is normal. His bundle recordings and atrial stimulation are required for confirmation.

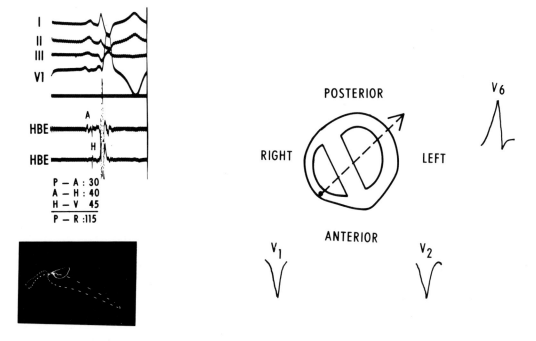

Fig. 9. "Pseudo" WPW type A occurring in a patient with LGL syndrome with RBBB. Note that the horizontal QRS loop only shows the terminal (rightward and anterior) delay characteristic of RBBB. The short P-R and A-H intervals (with normal H-V intervals) suggest the presence of an AP of the James bundle type.

Fig. 10. WPW type B with an anterior (parietal) right ventricular entrance producing predominantly negative complexes in V1 and V2. The initial delay points posteriorly and to the left.

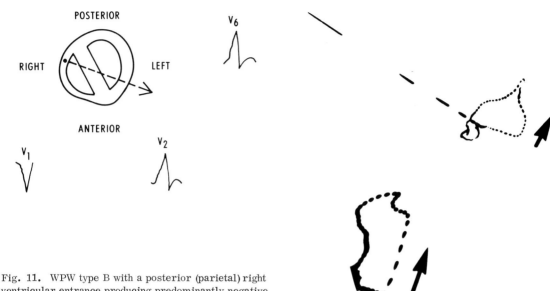

Fig. 11. WPW type B with a posterior (parietal) right ventricular entrance producing predominantly negative deflections in V1 and positive in V2. The initial delay points anteriorly and to the left. In classical WPW type A the initial delay points also anteriorly and to the left. But the anterior tilt is more significant than in this example. The diagnosis of the type (A or B) of WPW syndrome is best made from beats resulting from exclusive conduction through the Kent bundle.

In general, an anterior "parietal" entrance shows, during exclusive Kent bundle conduction, an r/S ratio smaller than 1 in both V1 and V2 (figure 10). A posterior "parietal" entrance yields ratios smaller than 1 in V1 and greater than 1 in V2 (figure 11).

During WPW type B with an anterior entrance the horizontal QRS loop shows diffuse delays when exclusive Kent bundle conduction occurs. A terminal delay oriented to the left and posteriorly (figure 12, bottom) is simply a consequence of the anomalous and delayed left ventricular activation which occurs when an impulse propagates from an ectopic right ventricular site [1-4]. Similar horizontal loops are recorded when the right ventricular apex is stimulated (figure 12, top) [1-4]. However, a terminal delay oriented to the right in presence of WPW type B suggests that the latter is associated with RBBB [1-4].

WPW Type B Coexisting with RBBB. Classically it is believed that the late right ventricular activation that characterizes RBBB will be neutralized by right ventricular pre-excitation (WPW type B) [10]. This produces a pseudo-normalization (narrowing) of the QRS complex. But the statement made above is correct only when the Kent bundle ends anteriorly in

Fig. 12. WPW type B with anterior parietal entrance (bottom). This horizontal loop resulted from exclusive Kent bundle conduction. The terminal (leftward and posterior) delay is not due to LBBB but to the specific type of activation pattern which occurs when an impulse propagates from an ectopic right ventricular site, regardless as to whether the impulse reached this area through an accessory pathway (bottom) or was induced electrically (top). In the latter, the large deflection located in the right posterior quadrant is the (unipolar) pacemaker stimulus artifact.

the right ventricle relatively close to the site from which the impulse traversing the right bundle branch would have otherwise emerged (figure 13, left).

WPW type B coexisting with RBBB has been attributed to the more "central" or "peripheral" site of block in the right branch [11]. This assumption need not always be used to explain the coexistence of WPW type B with RBBB [2, 3, 12, 13]. For example, if the Kent bundle ends posteriorly in the right ventricle, small degrees of pre-excitation will not prevent the anterior portions of the right ventricle from being activated by the wavefront which (after having emerged from the divisions of the left branch) crossed the septum in a left-to-right direction (figure 13, right) [3, 13].

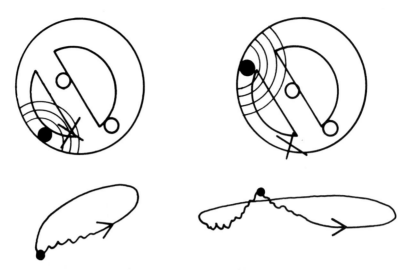

Fig. 13. WPW type B with RBBB. The latter conduction disturbance is hidden when the Kent bundle ends close to the site from which the impulse emerges from the right bundle branch (left sided schematic). This occurs because the impulse emerging from the Kent bundle pre-excites the areas which, in presence of RBBB, would otherwise have been activated by the impulse propagating (in a left-to-right fashion) from the divisions of the left bundle branch. In the right sided schematic a WPW type B with a posterior parietal entrance does not abolish the RBBB pattern because the conduction time from the pre-excited site to the anterior right ventricle is greater than the conduction time from the left septal surface to the latter. In other words, the terminal delay is (as in uncomplicated RBBB) a function of the impulse emerging from the divisions of the left bundle branch.

Moreover, if the Kent bundle ends in the right septal surface slow propagation might occur from the pre-excited area through the septal mass in a posterior and leftward direction only [13]. If conduction time from the pre-excited area to the free right ventricular wall is slower than conduction time from the left septal surface to the free right ventricular wall, WPW type B will not abolish the delayed activation of the right ventricle produced by RBBB.

The relationship between RBBB and WPW type B presumably with an anterior (septal) entrance is illustrated in figure 14 [2, 3]. The bottom horizontal loop shows the leftward initial and terminal delays characteristic of WPW type B (exclusive Kent bundle conduction). The P-R interval was short and the H deflection appeared after the onset of ventricular depolarization. Exclusive normal pathway conduction with RBBB (note terminal appendage oriented to the right) is seen at the top of figure 14. At this moment both P-R and H-V intervals were normal. On the other hand, the middle loop shows the coexistence of the initial delay diagnostic of WPW syndrome type B associated with the rightward oriented delay related to the RBBB. Thus, although right ventricular pre-excitation did occur, it was not of enough magnitude to prevent activation of some right anterior (septal or parietal) areas by the impulse emerging from the left septal surface.

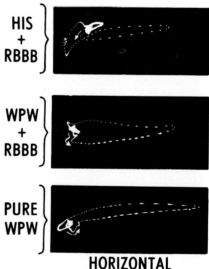

HORIZONTAL

Fig. 14. Intermittent WPW type B with an anterior entrance. The top loop was recorded during exclusive A-V node-His bundle conduction with RBBB. The bottom loop depicts the pattern occurring during exclusive Kent bundle conduction. The loop in the middle (obtained during conduction through both pathways) shows the initial delay characteristic of WPW type B and the terminal rightward delay due to some degree of RBBB.

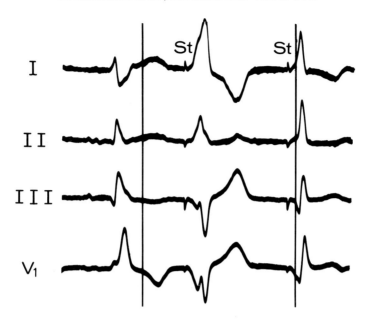

Fig. 15. Electrocardiogram obtained from a patient with RBBB while simulating (by pacing from the right ventricular septal myocardium) right ventricular pre-excitation. Whereas the first QRS complex shows RBBB, the second one depicts "pseudo" septal WPW type B (pure paced beat). Finally, in the third (fusion) ventricular complex, right ventricular pre-excitation (note q wave in V1 following pacemaker stimuli artifact) did not abolish the R wave in V1 which resulted from late activation of the anterior right ventricle by the impulse propagating (in a left-to-right direction) from the divisions of the left bundle branch. (From Castellanos Jr. and Castillo, Brit. Heart J. [13]).

This assumption was supported by the findings observed during simulated right septal pre-excitation [13]. In figure 15, the first (sinus) QRS complex shows a RBBB pattern. The second ventricular beat results from exclusive stimulation of the ordinary ventricular muscle of the right ventricular inflow tract (simulated right septal WPW type B with exclusive Kent bundle conduction). Thus the pacemaker stimulus is followed by a wide QRS complex with a predominantly negative deflection in V1. In contrast the last complex results from the fusion of a supraventricular with a ventricular beat (simulating WPW type B with A-V node His bundle conduction with RBBB). Although right septal pre-excitation occurs (note negative deflection in V1) the electrical forces move almost exclusively posteriorly and to the left therefore allowing the impulse propagating from the left septal surface to produce the late R in V1.

Summary

His bundle electro-vectorcardiography, the simultaneous recording of planar loops, body surface electrocardiograms and intracardiac (His bundle) electrograms proved to be most valuable in the study of Wolff-Parkinson-White syndrome and its variants. Dynamic recordings during atrial pacing at progressively higher rates allowed identification of QRS morphology resulting from exclusive A-V node-His bundle conduction, exclusive Kent bundle conduction and conduction through both pathways (A-V node-His bundle and Kent bundle).

Differences between the terminal rightward delay seen in WPW type A; WPW type A coexisting with RBBB and in Lown-Ganong-Levine with RBBB can be readily determined.

In WPW type B a terminal leftward delay occurs during exclusive Kent bundle conduction. In contrast a terminal rightward delay suggests the association of WPW type B with RBBB.

Diagnosis of the type (A or B) of WPW syndrome should be made from beats resulting from exclusive Kent bundle conduction only.

References

[1] A. Castellanos Jr., A. S. Agha, B. Portillo, and R. J. Myerburg, Usefulness of vectorcardiography combined with His bundle recordings and cardiac pacing in evaluation of the pre-excitation (Wolff-Parkinson-White) syndrome, Am. J. Cardiol. 30 (1972) 623.

[2] A. Castellanos Jr., L. Lemberg, and B. W. Claxton, Wolff-Parkinson-White syndrome generalities, Chest 65 (1974) 307.

[3] L. Lemberg and A. Castellanos Jr., Vectorcardiography. A programmed introduction. 2d ed. (Appleton-Century-Crofts, New York, 1975).

[4] A. Castellanos Jr., A. S. Agha, and B. Portillo, Vectorcardiographic significance of co-existing initial and terminal delays in pre-excitation syndrome, Circulation 44: No. 4: (II) 63, October 1971.

[5] C. A. Castillo and A. Castellanos Jr., His bundle recordings in patients with reciprocating tachycardia and WPW syndrome, Circulation 47 (1970) 271.

[6] A. Castellanos, E. Chapunoff, C. A. Castillo, O. Maytin, and L. Lemberg, His bundle electrograms in two cases of WPW (pre-excitation) syndrome, Circulation 41 (1970) 389.

[7] A. Castellanos Jr., J. W. Mayer, and L. Lemberg, The electrocardiogram and vectorcardiogram in WPW associated with bundle branch block, Am. J. Cardiol. 10 (1962) 657.

[8] B. Befeler, A. Castellanos, J. Aranda, R. Gutierrez, and R. Lazzara, Intermittent bundle branch block in patients with accessory atrio-His or atrio-AV nodal pathways, Brit. Heart J. (in press).

[9] E. Cabrera, J. Feldman, and F. C. Olinto, Estudio electro y vectorcardiografico de un caso de WPW con bloqueo de rama derecha, Arch. Inst. Card. Mex. 29 (1959) 404.

[10] R. Gamboa, D. Penaloza, F. Sime, and N. Banchero, The role of right and left ventricles in the ventricular pre-excitation (WPW) syndrome, Am. J. Cardiol. 10 (1962) 650.

[11] W. M. Gersony and D. D. Ekery, Concealed right bundle branch block in presence of type B ventricular pre-excitation, Am. Heart J. 77 (1969) 660.

[12] P. G. C. Robertson, D. Emslie-Smith, K. G. Lowe, and H. Watson, The association of type B ventricular pre-excitation and right bundle branch block, Brit. Heart J. 25 (1963) 755.

[13] A. Castellanos Jr. and C. A. Castillo, His bundle recordings in right bundle branch block co-existing with iatrogenic right ventricular pre-excitation, Brit. Heart J. 34 (1972) 153.

Figures 1, 2, 3, and 5 reproduced with permission from the American Journal of Cardiology.

Figure 15 reproduced with permission of the British Heart Journal.

Vectorcardiography 3 I. Hoffman and R.I. Hamby eds.

PATHOLOGICAL FINDINGS IN PATIENTS WITH LEFT ANTERIOR HEMIBLOCK

J. C. Demoulin and H. E. Kulbertus

From the Department of Morbid Anatomy and the Division of Cardiology,
Department of Internal Medicine, University of Liege
School of Medicine, Liege, Belgium

Introduction

The concept of left hemiblocks was introduced in the clinical field by Rosenbaum et al. in 1968 [1]. According to the description by these authors, the left branch subdivides into two discrete subbranches which function and can be blocked separately.

The electrocardiographic and vectorcardiographic manifestations of conduction blockade along the anterior and posterior subdivisions are well known; they are mainly characterized by the QRS frontal axis shifts which they produce [1, 2].

No agreement has been reached so far as regards the pathological lesions underlying the patterns of left hemiblocks. Some authors state, for example, that left anterior hemiblock is consistently related to damage of the anterior subdivision of the left branch [3, 4, 5]. Others insist that they have been unable to confirm the specific location of the lesions in this kind of conduction disturbance [6, 7, 8].

The purpose of this presentation is to summarize data which were gathered in our Institution since 1969 and relate to the histopathological basis of left anterior hemiblock.

Techniques and Material

All data reported in this paper have been obtained by histological examination of serial sections of the septum. Details regarding the technical aspects of the study have been previously described [9, 10]. Let us just mention that, in our laboratory, for the study of the left bundle branch, the septum is sectioned serially in a plane parallel to the atrioventricular ring. This angle of cutting provides transverse sections of the peripheral portion of the left branch and therefore makes it easier graphically to reconstruct their geometry.

In addition to the straightforward microscopical observation, stereological techniques have recently been introduced, especially with a view to approach, on a quantitative basis, the study of the fibrotic involvement of the conducting system in cases of left bundle branch block or hemiblock [11]. The point-counting method described by Weibel was selected [12].

This technique permits calculating the relative volumetric density of fibrosis which is observed at any given level of the left bundle branch structures. Details regarding its applications and describing the statistical treatment of the data have been previously published [11].

To date, 49 normal human hearts were examined and used to investigate the normal anatomy of the left branch. Ten hearts from patients with chronic left anterior hemiblock were also studied. The diagnosis of left anterior hemiblock was made from the electrocardiogram, using the following criteria, slightly modified from Rosenbaum et al. [1].

1. QRS duration shorter than 120 msec
2. leftward deviation of the main QRS axis higher than $-30°$
3. qR morphology in leads I and aVL and rS in leads II, III and aVF.

Patients with acute myocardial infarction, congenital heart disease or valvular heart disease were excluded.

Results

a. Normal anatomy of the left branch

The obtained results confirmed that the left branch gives off a thin, and elongated anterior ramification and a wider posterior one. These two subdivisions course towards the corresponding papillary muscle. An important contingent of midseptal fibers was also observed in all cases (figure 1). The latter fibers were grouped into a third, easily identified subbranch in about 65% of the cases (type I). They formed a complicated network covering the midseptal surface (type II) in about 25% of the cases and were directly given off by the posterior ramification in about 10% of the observations (type III). The various offshoots of the left bundle branch consistently showed multiple peripheral anastomoses.

The general picture which emerges from these anatomical data is that the left ventricular Purkinje network is composed of three main, widely interconnected parts, consisting of the anterior subdivision, the posterior subdivision and the midseptal fibers. The same overall configuration (with similar considerable individual variations) can be observed in the dog by iodine staining of the conducting tissue (figure 2).

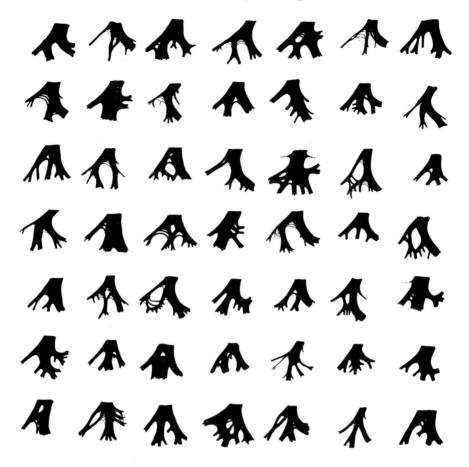

Fig. 1. Diagrammatic sketches describing the left bundle branch geometry in 49 normal human hearts.

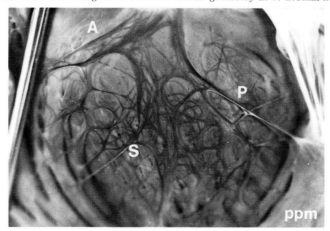

Fig. 2. Left bundle branch visualized in a dog's heart by iodine-staining of the conducting tissue. The anterior (A) and posterior (P) groups of fibers are seen to course towards the corresponding papillary muscle. They give off small rami which join over the mid-septal surface to form a third (septal, S) fascicle. The rich interconnecting network can clearly be observed. ppm: posterior papillary muscle.

A similar description of the left bundle branch geometry has also been proposed by others [7, 13, 14, 15] and is in agreement with the electrophysiological data obtained by Durrer et al. [16] and Myerburg et al. [17]. In view of this, the histopathological lesions seen in cases with left anterior hemiblock will be described in terms of anterior, posterior and midseptal lesions.

b. Qualitative findings in cases of LAHB

The histological features of ten cases with chronic left anterior hemiblock [9, 10] are summarized in table 1. They indicate that this electrocardiographic pattern is associated with left bundle branch pathology but that the lesions are much more widely distributed than expected. They generally involve most of the left sided conducting tissue and a clearcut predominance of the anterior lesions can be seen in only one-half of the cases.

c. Quantitative approach

With a few to confirm these data, stereological measurements were made to compare 8 hearts from patients with chronic left anterior hemiblock with 8 hearts from control subjects of the same age group, devoid of cardiac pathology or conduction disturbances. At gross anatomic examination, the two groups were similar as regards the lesions of the main coronary arteries and the fibrocalcific changes of the left side of the cardiac skeleton. The stereological data, reported at length elsewhere [11], are summarized in tables 2 and 3.

It seems apparent from these data that although some fibrosis develops in the left bundle branch with increasing age, the amount of fibrosis is consistently higher, at all levels, in patients with left anterior hemiblock (table 2).

Pooling together the data from the 8 patients with chronic left anterior hemiblock, it seems that there is a tendency for the anterior fibers to be more severely involved by the fibrotic replacement than the rest of the conducting tissue. The midseptal fibers, in their turn, seem more severely damaged than the posterior ones. However, the statistical analysis performed in each case separately indicates that a predominance of the anterior lesions can be statistically demonstrated in only one-half of the cases. In the remainder, fibrosis seems evenly distributed throughout the three groups of fibers (table 3).

Discussion

Our data confirm that the pattern of left anterior hemiblock is associated with significant histopathological alterations of the left conducting system and that it may therefore be considered as a reliable sign of left bundle branch disease.

In contrast to what might have been initially expected, the lesions are hardly ever limited to an anterior locus and generally involve most of the left sided conducting system. An anterior predominance of the fibrotic replacement can be observed in only one-half of the studied cases.

Table 1

Pathological findings in 10 cases of LAHB

N°	Description of lesions	Anterior fibers	Midseptal fibers	Posterior fibers
1	Fibrosis	+++	+	−
2	Fibrosis	+++	++	++
3	Amyloidosis	+++	++	+
4	Fibrosis; inflammation	+++	++	++
5	Fibrosis	+++	++	++
6	Fibrosis	++	++	++
7	Fibrosis; focal necrosis	++	++	++
8	Fibrosis; focal necrosis	++	++	++
9	Fibrosis; focal necrosis	++	++	++
10	Fibrosis	+	+	++

+++ total or subtotal interruption; ++ severe lesions; + moderate or mild lesions; - no significant lesion.

Table 2

Mean density of fibrosis (%)

Groups	Anterior fibers	Midseptal fibers	Posterior fibers	Mean values	Variance analysis
Patients without conduction disturbances (8 cases)	25.4	23.2	24.6	24.4	N.S.
Patients with chronic LAHB (8 cases)	63.5	51.1	43.0	51.6	$p < 0.001$
	$p < 0.001$	$p < 0.001$	$p < 0.001$	$p < 0.001$	

Table 3

Mean density of fibrosis in patients with chronic LAHB (%)

N^o	Anterior fibers	Midseptal fibers	Posterior fibers	Variance analysis
1	57.4	42.3	54.7	N.S.
2	64.9	61.5	45.1	$p < 0.01$
3	78.2	52.4	46.0	$p < 0.025$
4	38.1	50.1	50.6	N.S.
5	57.1	40.7	39.3	N.S.
6	68.2	58.5	34.4	$p < 0.001$
7	75.8	42.5	16.4	$p < 0.01$
8	69.0	75.9	65.3	N.S.
Whole group	63.5	51.1	43.0	$p < 0.001$

It is our belief that these data remain perfectly consistent with the concept of left hemiblocks. Indeed, in the presence of evenly distributed lesions, one can anticipate that the physiological disturbance will primarily involve the anterior ramification which is the thinnest of the three.

Furthermore, our findings are also in good agreement with the observations made by Myerburg et al. [17]. These authors, from studies performed on dogs, indicate that to produce an experimental left anterior hemiblock on an isolated preparation, one has to interrupt concomitantly not only the anterior subbranch, but also most of the median,

interconnecting fibers. They conclude that if the human heart behaves in a similar fashion, the so-called hemiblock patterns are likely to correspond to diffuse lesions of the left bundle branch. The histological observations amply support their hypothesis.

Finally, our data provide a better explanation for the fact that the association of a left anterior hemiblock with a right bundle branch block is a common forerunner of complete atrio-ventricular block. This clinical observation would have been difficult to account for should the lesions in left anterior hemiblock be strictly limited to an anterior locus. On the contrary, it is easily understood if one is aware of the diffuse, often severe lesions of the left branch which can be found in this kind of conduction disturbance.

References

[1] M. B. Rosenbaum, M. V. Elizari, and J. O. Lazzari, Los Hemibloqueos. Paidos. Buenos Aires.

[2] C. J. Rothberger and H. Winterberg, Experimentelle Beitrage zur Kenntnis der Reiztleitungstorungen in den Kammern des Saugetierherzens, Z. ges exp. Med. 5 (1917) 264.

[3] R. L. Hawley and R. Pryor, Quantitative and electrocardiographic correlation of the conduction system of the yeart (abstract), Am. J. Cardiol. 15 (1965) 132.

[4] M. V. Elizari, Estudio histopatologico del sistema de conduccion en cuatro casos de miocarditis cronica chagasica. VII Congreso arg. Cardiol. Buenos Aires (quoted by Rosenbaum, Elizari, and Lazzari, 1968, ref. 2), 1967.

[5] M. Sugiura, R. Okada, K. Hiraoka, and S. Ohkawa, Histological studies on the conduction system in 14 cases of right bundle branch block associated with left axis deviation, Japan. Heart J. 10 (1969) 121.

[6] M. L. Entman, E. H. Estes, and D. B. Hackel, The pathologic basis of the electrocardiographic pattern of parietal block, Am. Heart J. 74 (1967) 202.

[7] L. Rossi, Sistema di conduzione trifascicolari ed emiblocchi di branca sinistra. Considerazioni anatomiche ed estopatologiche, G. Ital. Cardiol. 1 (1971) 55.

[8] M. Blondeau and J. Lenegre, Bloc atypique de la branche droite, Masson Ed. Paris (1970).

[9] J. C. Demoulin and H. E. Kulbertus, Histopathological examination of concept of left hemiblock.

[10] H. E. Kulbertus, The concept of left hemiblocks revisited. A histopathological and experimental study. Advances in Cardiology 14 (1975) 126.

[11] J. C. Demoulin, L. J. Simar, and H. E. Kulbertus, Quantitative study of left bundle branch fibrosis in left anterior hemiblock. A stereological approach, Am. J. Cardiol., in print.

[12] E. R. Weibel, G. S. Kistler, and W. E. Scherle, Practical stereological methods for morphometric cytology, J. Cell. Biol. 30 (1966) 23.

[13] H. N. Uhley, Some controversy regarding the peripheral distribution of the conduction system, Am. J. Cardiol. 30 (1972) 919.

[14] H. K. Hecht, C. E. Kossman, R. W. Cholders, R. Langendorf, M. Lev, K. M. Rosen, R. D. Pruitt, R. C. Truex, H. N. Uhley, and T. B. Watt, Atrioventricular and intraventricular conduction, Am. J. Cardiol. 31 (1973) 232.

[15] G. A. Medrano, C. P. Brenes, A. De Micheli, D. Sodi-Pallares, El bloqueo simultaneo de las subdivisiones anterior y posterior de la rama izquierda del haz de His (bloqueo bifascicular). Y su associacion con bloqueo de la rama derecha (bloqueo trifascicular), Arch. Inst. Cardiol. Mex. 40 (1970) 752.

[16] D. Durrer, R. Th. van Dam, G. E. Freud, M. J. Janse, F. L. Meijler, and R. C. Arzbaecher, Total excitation of the isolated human heart, Circulation 41 (1970) 899.

[17] R. J. Myerburg, K. Nilsson, and H. Gelband, Physiology of canine intraventricular conduction and endocardial excitation, Circ. Res. 30 (1972) 217.

Vectorcardiography 3 I. Hoffman and R.I. Hamby eds.
© 1976 North-Holland Publishing Company - Amsterdam

ANTERIOR CONDUCTION DELAY: A POSSIBLE CAUSE

FOR PSEUDO DORSAL INFARCTION

Irwin Hoffman, Jawahar Mehta, Joseph Hilsenrath, and Robert I. Hamby

From the Department of Medicine, Cardiology Division - ECG-VCG Section,
Long Island Jewish-Hillside Medical Center, New Hyde Park, New York,
School of Medicine, Health Sciences Center, State University of
New York at Stony Brook, Stony Brook, New York and the
ECG-VCG Department, South Nassau Communities
Hospital, Oceanside, New York

Abnormal anterior QRS forces are frequently encountered in right ventricular hypertrophy or true dorsal myocardial infarction. A variety of criteria have been reported for identifying such cases [1-5]. Nevertheless, the diagnosis of true dorsal infarction has been unsatisfactory in our hands because of relatively poor correlation with appropriately localized coronary artery obstruction or ventriculographic dysfunction of the posterior wall [6]. Ha et al. [7] have confirmed this difficulty in separating normal subjects with prominent anterior forces from abnormals who present with the appropriate coronary angiographic and ventriculographic defects.

We present herein a hypothesis "Anterior conduction delay," which may explain prominent anterior QRS forces in patients apparently free of coronary disease or right ventricular hypertrophy. In addition, this theory also may explain the occasional observation of prominent anterior QRS forces in patients whose coronary disease is localized in the left anterior descending artery and whose ventricular dysfunction is localized in the anterior wall of the left ventricle.

In the six cases presented herein, sequential electrocardiographic and clinical evidence is described which points to anterior conduction delay as a possible explanation for prominent anterior QRS forces.

Case Reports

Case 1. A 44-year-old man was referred to the Long Island Jewish-Hillside Medical Center because of unstable angina with persistent chest pain and abnormal electrocardiogram. His 12 lead ECG (figure 1) displayed prominent R waves in V2-3 with T inversion in leads I, AVL and V4-6. The ECG interpretation was dorsal myocardial infarction with lateral wall ischemia. A vectorcardiogram (figure 2) showed the QRS loop displaced prominently to the left and anterior, with the anterior forces having a duration of 50 msec. The T loop was directed to the right and anterior. The VCG was also interpreted as dorsal wall infarction and lateral ischemia.

The patient underwent coronary arteriography and was found to have almost complete obstruction of the left anterior descending artery, but normal right and left circumflex vessels. The left ventricular angiogram showed anterior wall asynergy, but normal movement of all other segments. At the time of coronary bypass surgery, the anterior wall of the left ventricle was discolored. A saphenous vein bypass was placed between the aorta and the left anterior descending artery. Post-operatively, the patient sustained a myocardial infarction. The 12 lead ECG was repeated two days post-operatively (figure 3). The tall precordial R waves had completely disappeared. ST elevations were present in V2-6 and T inversions in leads V4-6. These findings are classic for acute anterior wall myocardial infarction.

Case 2. A 71-year-old woman was admitted to South Nassau Communities Hospital on 1/20/70 because of congestive heart failure. Her horizontal and frontal plane vectorcardiograms are depicted in figure 4 (left). The frontal loop is superior to the E point with largely counterclockwise rotation, except for the early forces which are abnormally left, superior and clockwise. This combination is typical of inferior wall infarction complicated by left anterior hemiblock [8]. The patient returned two years later on 3/23/72 because of congestive heart failure. Her VCG was repeated and is shown in figure 4 (right). The superior and counterclockwise frontal plane loop had disappeared. Instead an abnormally left, superior, clockwise frontal loop appeared, typical for inferior myocardial infarction uncomplicated by left anterior hemiblock. The horizontal loop was quite normal with counterclockwise rotation and completely normal duration of initial anterior forces. The very prominent anterior forces noted in figure 4 (left) had disappeared along with the left anterior hemiblock.

Case 3. A 45-year-old man was first seen because of incapacitating angina in 1961. Coronary angiography was performed at the Cleveland Clinic and showed only localized disease in the left anterior descending artery. At that time, the patient received a single internal mammary implant using a myocardial tunnel. He was greatly improved after surgery.

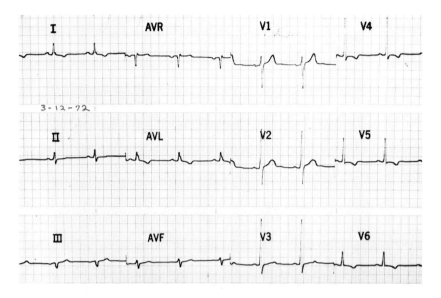

Fig. 1. Case 1. Twelve lead ECG showing prominent anterior
forces and T inversion in I, AVL and V4-6.

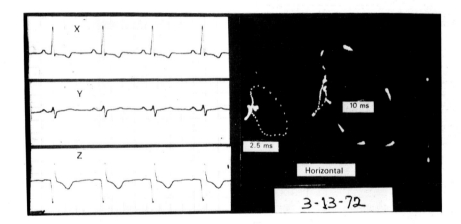

Fig. 2. Case 1. VCG horizontal plane showing QRS loop mainly
to left and anterior.

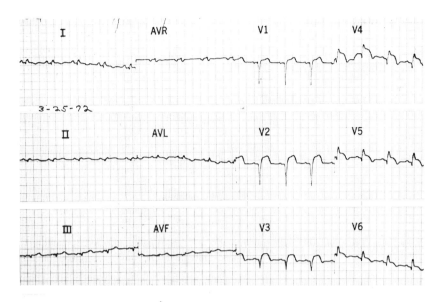

Fig. 3. Case 1. ECG after bypass surgery. Note the loss of prominent anterior forces and development of anterior infarction pattern.

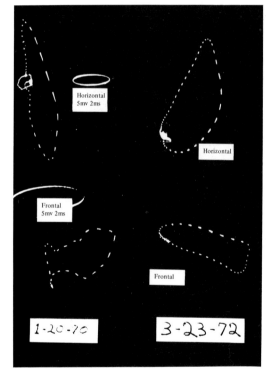

Fig. 4. Case 2. VCG - 1/20/70 - Early QRS forces are left, superior and clockwise in frontal plane and late forces are counterclockwise. 3/23/72 - Late counterclockwise forces have disappeared. Note loss of prominent anterior forces in horizontal loop.

Repeat angiogram done in 1974 showed a patent graft and a recession of left anterior descending artery obstruction to 40%. The right coronary and circumflex arteries were again free of disease.

Twelve lead ECG and VCG (figures 5 and 6) done in 1974 were unchanged from preoperative records. The prominent anterior R waves in V1-3 and in horizontal and saggital loops are evident. These findings originally led to an erroneous diagnosis of dorsal wall infarction.

Case 4. A 46-year-old man was first seen for progressive angina of six months duration. ECG (figure 7) revealed prominent R waves in V1-3 and T wave inversion in V1-4, which was interpreted as "dorsal wall infarction with lateral ischemia."

Vectorcardiogram (figure 8) was interpreted as consistent with the ECG diagnosis. Left ventricular angiogram revealed anterior hypokinesia. On coronary angiography, 90% obstruction of the left anterior descending artery was seen. The right and circumflex coronary arteries were normal. The patient underwent successful bypass to the left anterior descending artery. Postoperative ECG revealed persistent prominent R waves in anterior chest leads with T inversion in V1-6.

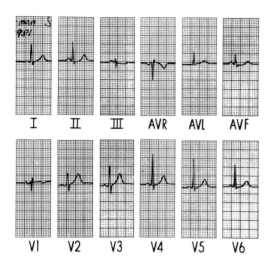

Fig. 5. Case 3. ECG showing prominent anterior forces--interpreted as dorsal wall infarction.

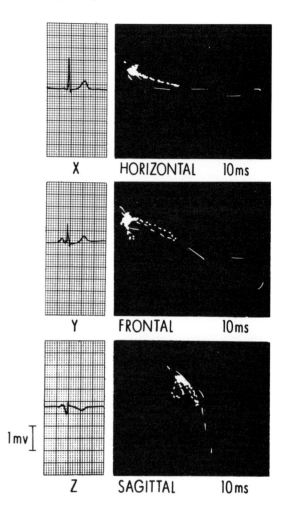

Fig. 6. Case 3. VCG--Note the prominent anterior forces.

Case 5. A 49-year-old woman was first seen with unstable angina. She had a history of two previous myocardial infarctions. ECG and VCG (figures 9 and 10) were interpreted as "dorsal wall infarction with lateral ischemia." Cardiac catheterization revealed only anterior wall hypokinesia with significant obstruction in the left anterior descending and circumflex arteries. Bypass grafts were placed on the left anterior descending and circumflex marginal vessels. Postoperative ECG and VCG were unchanged from preoperative recordings.

Case 6. A 47-year-old man was referred for cardiac catheterization and bypass because of unstable angina. Preoperative ECG (figure 11a) revealed prominent R waves in the anterior chest leads. VCG (figure 12) was also interpreted as dorsal wall infarction. Angiographic studies revealed 90% obstruction of the left anterior descending artery only. The patient received a single bypass graft to the left anterior descending artery. Postoperatively, the patient sustained an anterior wall infarction (figure 11b) with loss of prominent anterior forces. This patient had an ECG-VCG evolution similar to Case 1.

Discussion

In five of these six cases undergoing angiography, prominent anterior QRS forces coexisted with obstructive disease in the left anterior descending artery and ventricular dysfunction of the anterior wall of the left ventricle. The right coronary or circumflex arteries were involved in only two of the five cases. These observations confirm previous findings of inappropriate coronary and ventriculographic abnormalities in patients whose VCGs were consistent with dorsal wall infarction [6, 7]. This contrasts with our experience in patients with ECG and VCG evidence of anterior or inferior infarction in whom fairly good correlation were obtained with demonstrable obstructive disease in appropriate arteries and localized dysfunction of the left ventricle [9].

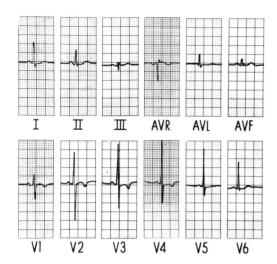

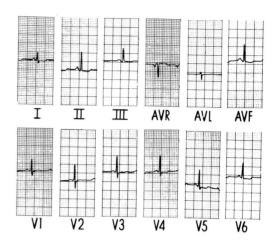

Fig. 7. Case 4. ECG--showing prominent R waves in V_{1-3} and T inversion V_{1-4}.

Fig. 9. Case 5. ECG showing prominent anterior forces with T low or diphasic in I, AVL and V_{3-6}.

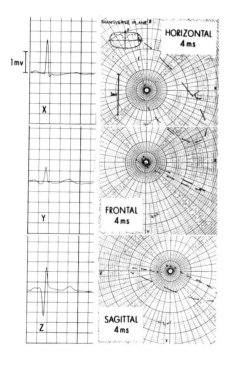

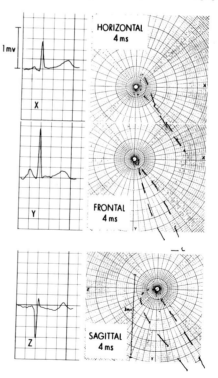

Fig. 8. Case 4. VCG--showing QRS loop directed anteriorly and to the left. VCG--diagnosis "dorsal wall infarction."

Fig. 10. Case 5. VCG interpreted as "dorsal wall infarction with lateral ischemia."

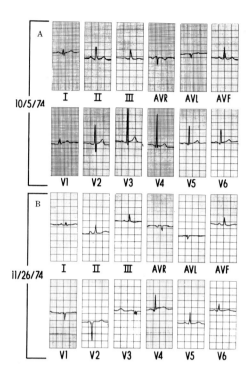

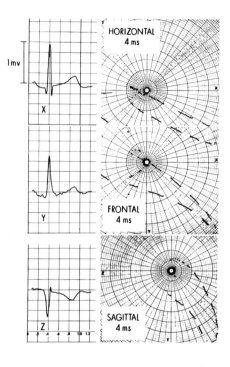

Fig. 11a and 11b. Case 6. ECG--10/5/74--Promi-
nent anterior forces are evident, 11/26/74. After
bypass surgery, prominent anterior forces disappeared and a new anterior wall infarction evolved.

Fig. 12. Case 6. VCG--before surgery, revealed
anterior QRS shift.

This paradox may be explained by conduction
delay in the anterior wall due to ischemia of the conduction system. It is well known that ECG axis shift
to the right, left, superior or inferior may result
secondary to disorders in the fascicular conducting
system.

An anatomic basis for the anterior conduction
delay theory may be found in the work of Demoulen
and Kulbertus [10] who have demonstrated that the
left bundle branch system may well be trifascicular
rather than bifascicular, with a distinct set of fibers
directed anteriorly and supplying the anterior wall of
the left ventricle. It is our belief that ischemic disease of this anterior division may result in a perma-
nent or intermittent anterior shift of the QRS complex
of the electrocardiogram or vectorcardiogram, simulating the ECG-VCG pattern of dorsal myocardial infarction or right ventricular hypertrophy.

In the cases presented, neither the localization
of the coronary artery disease, nor the obvious ventricular disease, correspond with the electrocardiographic diagnosis of "true dorsal infarction."
Rather, it seems evident that the electrocardiographic picture observed preoperatively was related
to the patients' anterior wall disease. A conduction
delay located in the anterior wall of the left ventricle
could well result in an anterior shift of QRS. Addi-
tionally, after infarction of this area, as in cases 1
and 6, following unsuccessful bypass grafting, death
of the involved muscle could result in complete absence of precordial R waves as noted in the postoperative electrocardiograms. Had the prominent
anterior forces been the result of right ventricular
hypertrophy, or of dorsal myocardial infarction,
some persistence of anterior forces would have been
expected even after the patient sustained his anterior
infarction.

If, indeed, prominent anterior QRS forces can result from anterior left ventricular wall defect, it is reasonable to anticipate that in some cases this conduction delay will be intermittent. Case 2 illustrated that during left anterior hemiblock--an established variety of left ventricular conduction delay--her anterior forces were unusually prominent. When the left anterior hemiblock disappeared, the prominent anterior forces also disappeared. Thus, in this 71-year-old woman with established coronary artery disease and old inferior infarction, prominent anterior forces were mistakenly interpreted as diagnostic of dorsal infarction when they probably were the result of transient conduction delay involving the anterior wall. Transient ischemia may also be responsible for shifting the QRS and T axes. This has been documented by Fernandez et al. [11] and Smith et al. [12] during selective coronary angiography, which causes a transient ischemia of the conduction system.

It should be emphasized that anterior conduction delay may shift the QRS complex forward regardless of the etiology of the conduction disorder. It has been demonstrated that the abnormal left superior axis shift (left anterior hemiblock) seen in patients with ostium primum defects probably results from shortening of the left posterior division. Similarly, the picture of anterior conduction delay could logically result from a disproportion in the lengths of several fascicular divisions of the left bundle branch system with the "anterior" fascicle being the longest. This explanation may possibly apply to the small percentage of normal patients who present with ECGs and VCGs indistinguishable from true dorsal infarctions, as reported by Hilsenrath et al. [6] and Ha et al. [7].

It may likewise be anticipated that any of the multiple etiologies for ventricular conduction delays (ischemia, tachycardia, trauma, degeneration, etc.) may be expected occasionally to result in anterior fascicular delay either alone or combined with other types of ventricular conduction delay.

Recognition that anterior conduction delay may be responsible for anterior QRS shifts may prevent incorrect diagnoses and allow better correlation of the ECG-VCG findings with clinical and laboratory findings.

The figures in this paper are reproduced with permission of the Journal of Electrocardiology.

References

[1]   E. S. Lipman, and E. Massie, Clinical scalar electrocardiography, 5th ed. (Year Book Medical Publishers, Chicago, 1965).

[2]   P. Toutouzas, P. Hubner, G. Sainani, and J. Shillingford, Value of vectorcardiogram in diagnosis of posterior and inferior myocardial infarction, Brit. Heart J. 31 (1969) 629.

[3]   I. Hoffman, R. C. Taymor, M. H. Morris, and I. Kittell, Quantitative criteria for the diagnosis of dorsal infarction using the frank vectorcardiogram, Am. Heart J. 70 (1965) 295-304.

[4]   G. VanHerpen, A. V. G. Bruschke, and A. W. Hanssen, The correlation between the coronary arteriogram and other diagnostic parameters, Proc. XIth International Vectorcardiography Symposium (North Holland Publishing Company, 1970), p. 352.

[5]   T. C. Chou and R. A. Helm, Clinical vectorcardiography (Grune & Stratton, New York, 1967).

[6]   J. Hilsenrath, R. E. Hamby, and I. Hoffman, Pitfalls in the prediction of coronary artery disease from the electrocardiogram or vectorcardiogram, J. Electrocardiology 6(4) (1973) 291-302.

[7]   D. Ha, D. I. Kraft, and P. D. Stein, The anteriorly oriented horizontal vector loop. The problem of distinction between direct posterior myocardial infarction and normal variation, Am. Heart J. 88 (1974) 408-16.

[8]   A. Benchimol and K. B. Desser, Coexisting left anterior hemiblock and inferior wall myocardial infarction--vectorcardiographic features, Am. J. Cardiol. 29 (1972) 7-14.

[9]   R. E. Hamby, I. Hoffman, J. Hilsenrath et al., Clinical hemodynamic and angiographic aspects of interior and anterior myocardial infarction in patients with angina pectoris, Am. J. Cardiol. 34 (1974) 513-19.

[10] J. C. Demoulen and H. E. Kulbertus, Histopathological examination of conception of left hemiblock, Brit. Heart J. 34 (1972) 807-14.

[11] F. Fernandez, L. Scebat, and J. Lenegre, Electrocardiographic study of the left intraventricular hemiblock in man during selective coronary angiography, Am. J. Cardiol. 26 (1970) 1-5.

[12] R. F. Smith, J. W. Hawthorne, and L. A. Sanders, Vectorcardiographic changes during intracoronary injections, Circulation 36 (1967) 63-76.

Vectorcardiography 3 I. Hoffman and R.I. Hamby eds.
© 1976 North-Holland Publishing Company - Amsterdam

WOLFF-PARKINSON-WHITE SYNDROME IN INFANTS AND CHILDREN
Vectorcardiographic Patterns with and without Associated Cardiac Defects

B. Lynn Miller and B. E. Victorica

From the University of Florida College of Medicine, Department of
Pediatrics (Cardiology), Gainesville, Florida 32610

This paper can best begin with the following definitions:

1. Wolff-Parkinson-White (WPW) Syndrome--Electrovectorcardiographic (ECG-VCG) findings of a slow initial ventricular activation with widening of the QRS and a PR interval that is shorter than normal or shorter than the PR interval in the same patient when there is normal atrioventricular (A-V) conduction, thus a form of ventricular pre-excitation via an accessory or anomalous A-V pathway.

2. Bundle of Kent--An accessory A-V pathway, muscular fibers with continuity between atrium and ventricle that are eccentric to the normal A-V conduction system.

3. Lown-Ganong-Levine Syndrome--A form of ventricular pre-excitation combining a short PR interval with a normal-width QRS resulting from atrial fibers, usually called James fibers, which by-pass the proximal A-V nodal delay and then connect with the specialized ventricular conduction system.

4. Delta vector--The initial slowly inscribed portion of the QRS loop on the VCG similar to the delta wave on the ECG, usually of low-amplitude and beginning near the end of the P loop.

5. Type A WPW--Defined in the VCG as the WPW syndrome in which the mean delta vector is directed anteriorly regardless of the orientation of the remainder of the QRS loop.

6. Type B WPW--Defined in the VCG as the WPW syndrome in which the mean delta vector is directed at 0° or posteriorly regardless of the orientation of the remainder of the QRS loop.

The WPW syndrome [1] is a congenital anomaly of the atrio-ventricular (A-V) conduction with pre-excitation of the ventricles via an accessory pathway. An abnormal sequence of ventricular activation begins eccentrically. All cases manifest slowly inscribed initial QRS forces which, although usually oriented leftward, may be either anterior or posterior. The middle and terminal QRS forces are variably altered. After recognition of the WPW syndrome in the ECG-VCG these basic tools for the diagnosis of structural heart disease are generally abandoned in any specific case apart from the correlation of the conduction abnormality with specific heart defects, most notably with Ebstein's anomaly of the tricuspic valve [2], and more recently with prolapsing mitral valve leaflets [3].

In a previous report [4] we found certain consistencies in the VCG in patients with WPW with and without associated heart defects. The patients were considered to have Type A WPW when the mean delta vector was oriented anteriorly regardless of the remainder of the QRS loop and Type B when the delta vector was oriented posteriorly. Using this approach we found those patients without associated heart disease to have a concordant mean QRS vector, whether WPW Type A or Type B (figure 1, top left and top right). In contrast were those patients with associated heart disease who had a discordant mean QRS vector, whether WPW Type A or Type B (figure 1, bottom left and bottom right). The one exception was patients with Ebstein's anomaly of the tricuspid valve who showed a WPW Type B concordant pattern. This present report extends our previous Grishman cube VCG study to a total of 30 patients and presents the findings with the Frank orthogonal lead system in 18 patients. Approximately 40% of the cases in each group had associated heart defects.

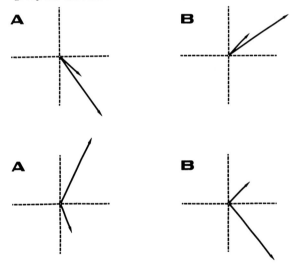

Fig. 1. Diagrammatic representation of the orientation of the delta vector (shorter arrow) and the mean QRS vector (longer arrow) in the horizontal plane in WPW syndrome: top left) Type A without associated heart defects; bottom left) type A with associated heart defects; top right) type B without associated heart defects or with Ebstein's anomaly; and bottom right) type B with other severe cardiac defects. The length of the arrows does not indicate magnitude.

It does appear that there is further clinically useful information available in the VCG in patients with WPW syndrome. Certain hypertrophy patterns are apparent and others are obscured and this is predictable on taking into consideration the anterior or posterior orientation of the delta vector.

Material and Methods

The study group includes all patients evaluated at the University of Florida Teaching hospital who had a diagnosis of WPW made when they were less than 15 years old and in whom VCGs were available. Most patients were seen at this institution on several occasions. There were 35 patients in all, of whom 13 (37%) had associated cardiac defects and 22 (63%) did not.

Eighteen patients were previously reported in a study of the Grishman Cube System VCG in WPW [4]. In the present report, detailed VCG data are analyzed using either Grishman, Frank or both systems on 17 additional patients, and the Frank system data (not previously shown) are given for five patients who were in the previous Grishman system study. Clinical data are shown in Tables 1a and 1b for these 23 patients and the five who were previously reported are identified. All together we studied 30 patients with WPW syndrome by Grishman VCG technic, 18 in the previous report and 12 additional cases. Eighteen patients had Frank VCGs for analysis.

The Frank orthogonal lead system VCGs [5] were obtained with Marquette 3-channel data carts as a part of the computerized system which is employed routinely at this institution [6]. The X-Y-Z scalar leads and the 3 planar vector loops were produced with an incremental plotter by the computer. The initial 0.04 seconds of the QRS loop and the P and T loops were amplified three times for better visibility. The velocity and direction of inscription of the loops was indicated by numbers, each unit representing 10 milliseconds. The Grishman cube system VCGs [7] were obtained with a Sanborn Visoscope model 569-A and a Hewlett Packard 196-A oscilloscope camera. The electron beam was interrupted every 2.5 seconds and the direction of inscription was indicated by shaped dots with the blunt edge leading. In both the Frank and the Grishman tracings, the vector loops were recorded in frontal (F), horizontal (H) and right sagittal (S) planes.

Analysis of the VCGs included measurement of the direction of the mean delta vector defined in the VCG as the initial portion of the QRS loop which is slowly inscribed in contrast to the subsequent portion of the loop. The mean delta vector and the mean QRS vector directions were measured in the H and F planes

to the nearest 5 degrees. The usual ECG reference frame 0^0 to $+180^0$ measured in a clockwise manner below and 0^0 to -180^0 in a counterclockwise manner above the transverse axis was employed for the F plane and the same reference frame was superimposed on the H plane. The H plane was viewed from above with the patient's left on the viewer's right. Also, the direction of inscription of the QRS loop was noted in the H and F plane as clockwise (CW), counterclockwise (CCW) or figure-of-eight.

For further analysis the cases were separated into two groups by the orientation of the delta vector. When the mean delta vector was oriented anteriorly, the ventricular pre-excitation was considered Type A WPW and when the delta vector was oriented at 0^0 or posteriorly, it was considered Type B WPW as in our earlier report [4]. The cases were then analyzed as to concordance, either anterior or posterior, of the mean delta and mean QRS vectors. The angles between the mean delta vector and the mean QRS vector in the H plane was determined in each case and were then separated into those with less than 45^0 delta to QRS angle and those with 45^0 or greater. The VCG data with these parameters were correlated with the presence of associated heart defects if any. Further consideration was given to the expected ventricular dominance pattern whether due to hypertrophy or hypoplasia as determined by the non-electrocardiographic (non-ECG) data.

Electrocardiograms (ECGs) consisted of the standard 12-leads with the additional right and left precordial lead, V3R and V7 in most cases. ECGs were obtained with direct writing recorders at 25 mm./second and in some cases 50 mm./second paper speed. Analysis of the ECGs included measurement of PR interval and of QRS duration in standard lead II. The QRS morphology was tabulated for leads V1, V2 and V6. Rhythm abnormalities although not a primary concern in this report were also noted.

Results

The ECG-VCG parameters measured are shown for each case in Table 2 and in a similar form in the previous report [4].

The assessment of the accuracy of two possible criteria for the diagnosis of associated heart defects is presented in Tables 3a and 3b.

Analysis of the Grishman VCG in the WPW Syndrome

There were 30 cases in this group and 18 (60%) had no evidence of heart defects.

TABLE 1a

Clinical Data in Patients with WPW Syndrome without Associated Heart Defects

Case No.	Age/Sex	Signs/Symptoms	Associated Defects Excluded by	Treatment
1	birth/M	tachycardia	clinical examination	digoxin
2	1 M/F	tachycardia, failure	clinical examination	digoxin
3	1 M/F	tachycardia, failure	clinical examination	digoxin
4	5 W/F	spells	clinical examination	digoxin
5	6 W/M	tachycardia, seizure	clinical examination	digoxin
6	2 M/F	tachycardia, failure	clinical examination	cardioversion, digoxin
7	4 M/F	murmur	clinical examination	none
8	1 Y/M	tachycardia, fever	clinical examination	digoxin
9	8 Y/M	syncope, dizziness	clinical examination	none
10	11 Y/M	murmur	clinical examination	none
11	12 Y/F	murmur	clinical examination	none
12	13 Y/F	seizure	clinical examination	none
13	14 Y/M	tachycardia, dizziness	catheterization	digoxin, quinidine propranolol, operation

In Table 1a and 1b, cases are sequenced by age of patient at diagnosis. Cases #2, 3, 14, 19, and 21 were included in previous report as Cases 1, 2, 13, 14, and 16.

TABLE 1b

Clinical Data in Patients with WPW Syndrome with Associated Heart Defects

Case No.	Age/Sex	Signs/Symptoms	Associated Heart Defects Diagnosis	Confirmed by	Treatment
14	13 D/M	cyanosis	total anomalous pulmonary venous return	catheterization	digoxin
15	2 M/M	failure tachycardia	ventricular septal defect aortic insufficiency	catheterization/ operation	operative repair digoxin
16	2 M/F	failure	non-obstructive cardiomyopathy	catheterization	digoxin
17	3 M/M	murmur, spells	ventricular septal defect pulmonic stenosis	catheterization	digoxin
18	3 M/M	cyanosis, failure	transposition of the great arteries ventricular septal defect	catheterization	digoxin
19	5 M/F	tachycardia	Ebstein's anomaly	catheterization	digoxin quinidine
20	1 Y/F	failure	non-obstruction cardiomyopathy	clinical examination	digoxin
21	4 Y/F	murmur tachycardia	Ebstein's anomaly ventricular septal defect (small)	catheterization	none
22	14 Y/F	dyspnea post-op tachycardia	atrial septal defect	catheterization/ operation	operative repair digoxin, propranolol quinidine

TABLE 2

Electrovectorcardiographic Analysis of the WPW Syndrome

| | Frank Orthogonal Lead System | | | | | | Grishman Cube Lead System | | | | | | QRS Morphology | | |
| | Horizontal Plane | | | Frontal Plane | | | Horizontal Plane | | | Frontal Plane | | | | | |
Age	Mean Delta	Mean QRS	Loop Inscription	Mean Delta	Mean QRS	Loop Inscription	Mean Delta	Mean QRS	Loop Inscription	Mean Delta	Mean QRS	Loop Inscription	V1	V2	V6
Without Associated Cardiac Defects															
1 2Y	+ 60	+ 95	CW	+ 70	+160	CW	+ 90	+115	CW	+ 15	−165	CCW	Rs	Rs	Rs
2 1M	− 25	− 60	CCW	+ 30	+ 20	CW	− 70	− 60	8	+ 35	+ 25	CCW	rS	rS	R
3 8Y	+ 80	+120	CW	+100	+ 75	CW	+ 50	+130	CW	+ 60	+120	CW	Rs	Rs	Rs
4 5W	+ 45	− 30	CCW	+ 25	+ 35	CW	--	--	--	--	--	--	rS	rS	Rs
5 6W	+ 55	− 30.	CW	− 15	− 5	CCW	− 50	− 40	8	+ 20	+ 10	CCW	rS	rS	Rs
6 2M	+100	+115	CW	−150	−115	8	--	--	--	--	--	--	Rs	Rs	R
7 4M	--	--	--	--	--	--	+ 35	+ 50	8	− 20	+ 5	CW	RsR	R	R
8 1Y	− 40	− 45	CW	− 25	− 30	CCW	--	--	--	--	--	--	QS	Rs	Rs
9 8Y	+ 35	+ 40	CW	+ 20	− 5	CW	+ 5	+ 20	CW	+ 5	− 10	8	Qrs	Rs	Rs
10 11Y	+ 65	+ 55	8	− 25	+ 60	CW	+ 30	+ 45	CW	− 50	− 45	8	Rs	Rs	RS
11 13Y	+ 65	+ 55	CCW	+ 70	+ 55	CCW	+ 55	+ 65	CW	+ 50	+ 65	CW	Rs	RS	R
12 13Y	+ 30	+ 15	CCW	− 10	− 60	CCW	--	--	--	--	--	--	qR	Rs	R
13 14Y	+ 75	+ 35	CCW	− 30	+ 20	8	+ 45	+ 55	CCW	− 85	− 15	CW	RS	Rs	R
With Associated Cardiac Defects															
14 2W	+ 15	+ 70	CW	− 30	− 65	CCW	− 20	+ 25	CW	− 60	− 70	CCW	qRS	Rs	Rs
15 2M	+ 50	+ 10	CCW	− 45	− 40	8	+ 60	+ 10	CCW	− 40	− 25	8	RS	Rs	Rs
16 3M	--	--	--	--	--	--	− 50	− 40	8	− 5	− 15	CCW	rS	rS	Rs
17 3M	--	--	--	--	--	--	+ 5	− 50	8	+ 20	+ 15	8	rS	RS	Rs
18 2Y	--	--	--	--	--	--	+ 15	+ 85	CW	− 15	− 85	CCW	R	R	Rs
19 7Y	− 25	− 40	CCW	− 10	+ 20	CW	− 90	− 30	CW	− 70	− 5	CW	rS	R	Rs
20 1Y	+ 90	− 55	8	−115	+ 25	CW	--	--	--	--	--	--	rS	rS	R
21 15Y	− 5	− 15	CW	− 25	− 10	CW 8Y	− 90	− 35	CW	− 60	− 25	CW	rS	rS	R
22 14Y	+ 80	+115	8	+115	+110	8	+ 50	+120	CW	+ 30	+165	CW	Rs	Rs	Rs

Age = Age at date of tracing which was tabulated.

Mean delta vector and mean QRS vector direction measured 0 to +180° anteriorly and 0 to −180° posteriorly in the horizontal plane, and 0 to +180° inferiorly and 0 to −180° superiorly in the frontal plane.

CW and CCW = predominantly clockwise or counterclockwise inscription, respectively.

8 = complex or figure of eight inscription.

Cases #2, 3, 14, 19 and 21 were included in previous report (see text) as Cases #1, 2, 13, 14 and 16 respectively.

TABLE 3 (a and b)

Accuracy of Two Criteria for Diagnosis of Associated
Heart Defects in the WPW Syndrome

	Type A Delta Anterior		Type B Delta Posterior		Total
3a. Grishman Cube System	17 cases		13 cases		30 cases
Without Associated Heart Defects	12 cases		6 cases		18 cases
1) Delta–QRS ant./post. direction					
concordant	12	100%	6	100%	
discordant	0		0		
2) Delta–QRS angle in H plane					
less than 45°	8	67%	5	83%	
45° or more	4		1		
With Associated Heart Defects	5 cases		7 cases		12 cases
1) Delta–QRS ant./post. direction					
concordant	3		4		
discordant	2	40%	3	43%	
2) Delta–QRS angle in H plane					
less than 45°	0		2		
45° or more	5	100%	5	71%	
3b. Frank Orthogonal System	14 cases		4 cases		18 cases
Without Associated Heart Defects	10 cases		2 cases		12 cases
1) Delta–QRS ant./post. direction					
concordant	8	80%	2	100%	
discordant	2		0		
2) Delta–QRS angle in H plane					
less than 45°	8	80%	2	100%	
45° or more	2		0		
With Associated Heart Defects	4 cases		2 cases		6 cases
1) Delta–QRS ant./post. direction					
concordant	3		2		
discordant	1	25%	0	0%	
2) Delta–QRS angle in H plane					
less than 45°	2		2		
45° or more	2	50%	0	0%	

WPW Type A (Grishman)--Without Associated
Heart Defects--12 cases.

In all 12 cases (100%) with an anterior mean
delta vector (by definition), the mean QRS vector was
also anterior, i.e., concordant (see Table 3a). A
mean delta vector to mean QRS vector angle of less
than 45° in the H plane was a less consistent finding
with several exceptions.

The mean delta vector orientation was between
+5° and +90° in the H plane in the 12 cases under consideration and the mean QRS vector was between +20°
and +130° with two cases being greater than +90°.
The inscription of the QRS was CW in six, CCW in
four and figure of eight in two.

Case 3 (figure 2, left) shows a pattern that likely represents ventricular activation only through the
accessory pathway. Case 9 (figure 3, left) shows a
frequent pattern of Type A WPW with a leftward anterior H plane QRS loop and CW inscription in this instance. In other cases with a similar basically narrow
loop CCW or figure-of-eight inscription was seen. In
these cases, the F plane commonly showed a mild left
axis deviation of the mean QRS forces. Case 1

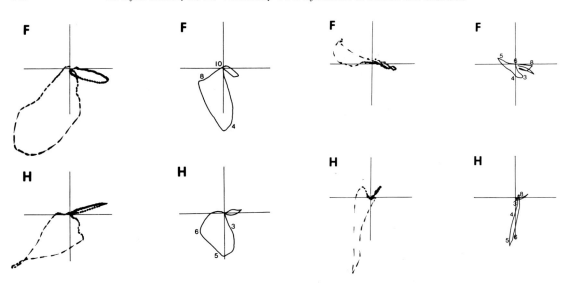

Fig. 2. WPW type A without associated cardiac defects left) Case 3 Grishman VCG right) Case 3 Frank VCG. In this and all subsequent vectorcardiograms, H = horizontal plane and F = frontal plane. The Grishman cube system tracings are formed of shaped dots with the blunt edge leading; each dot represents 2.5 msec. The Frank system tracings are formed of continuous lines with each number increment indicating 10 msec.

Fig. 4. WPW Type A without associated defects in Case 1 at two years old left) Grishman VCG, right) Frank VCG.

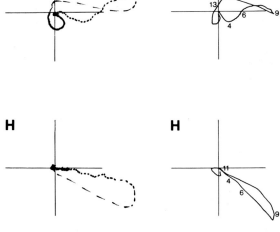

Fig. 3. WPW Type A without associated defects in Case 9 left) Grishman VCG, right) Case 9 Frank VCG.

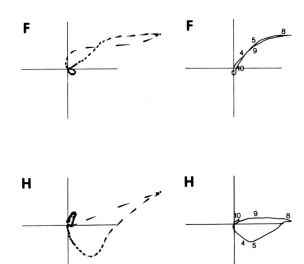

Fig. 5. WPW Type A with associated defects in a two month old with ventricular septal defect, Case 15 left) Grishman VCG, right) Frank VCG. Note maximal QRS forces oriented posteriorly, and superior mean QRS vector.

(figure 4, left) is less usual in the narrow anterior and slightly rightward H plane QRS loop and the slightly superior low amplitude F plane QRS loop. Also, the end of the delta vector is less distinct in this two-year-old patient as has been noted in younger infants.

WPW Type A (Grishman)--With Associated Heart Defects--five cases.

Two of the five patients (one from the previous report and Case 17 of this series) showed a discordant mean delta-mean posterior QRS vector angle.

Case 15 of this series showed a slightly anterior mean QRS vector with a posterior maximal QRS vector (figure 5, left). Cases 18 and 22 showed the mean QRS concordant at +85° and +120° respectively. The expected ventricular hypertrophy pattern in these cases according to non-ECG data (necropsy, cardiac catheterization, etc.) were abnormal left ventricular dominance or hypertrophy (LVH) for the previously reported case of double-inlet left ventricle (by necropsy) and bi-ventricular hypertrophy (BVH), left-greater-than-right for Cases 15 and 17. Pure right ventricular hypertrophy (RVH) was present in Cases 18 and 22 of the present series. In each case, the middle and terminal QRS forces were oriented in a direction compatible with the expected hypertrophy pattern.

The mean delta-to-QRS angle was greater than 45° in all five cases (100%) but it was also wide in four (33%) of the 12 patients without heart disease. Thus in Type A WPW a narrow delta-QRS angle was seen only in patients without associated heart disease. A wide delta-QRS angle was seen in all those with associated heart defects and in some patients without associated heart defects.

Type B WPW (Grishman)--Without Associated Heart Defects--six cases.

All six cases had the mean QRS vector oriented posteriorly, i.e., concordant with the mean delta vector (see table 3). The H plane delta-QRS angle was less than 45° in five of the six cases.

The H plane delta vector was between -5° and -90°. The mean QRS vector was between -30° and -60°. The QRS loop inscription was CW in four and CCW in two. In the F plane the mean QRS showed a mild left axis deviation ranging from +10° to -20° in five patients, with the remaining patient having a normal mean QRS axis of +60°.

Case 2 (figure 6, left) shows a small initial anterior portion of the delta vector but the slowing involves the entire efferent limb of the loop and both the mean delta and mean QRS are posteriorly oriented.

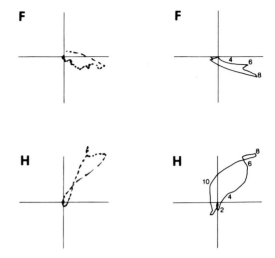

Fig. 6. WPW Type B without associated defects in Case 2 at one month of age left) Grishman VCG, right) Frank VCG. Initial slowing extends throughout efferent limb of QRS.

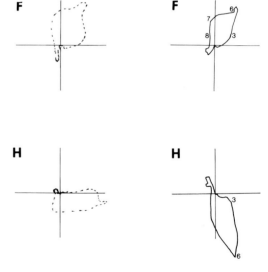

Fig. 7. WPW Type B with associated defects in Case 14, by Grishman left, but WPW type A by Frank, right. This two-week-old infant had total anomalous pulmonary venous return.

Type B WPW (Grishman)--With Associated Heart Defects--seven cases.

The mean QRS was anterior, i.e., discordant to the delta vector in three of the seven patients. One of these was Case 14 (figure 7, left) who had a mean delta at -20° and a mean QRS at $+25^\circ$. This was a two-week-old infant with an expected hypertrophy pattern of pure RVH and the other two cases had defects which would cause pure RVH or BVH, right-greater-than-left.

Of the four cases in whom the mean QRS was posterior, i.e., concordant, three patients had Ebstein's anomaly of the tricuspid valve. Figure 8, left, and Figure 9, left are from Cases 19 and 21 and show the features characteristic of WPW in Ebstein's anomaly of the tricuspid valve. (a) The delta vector is leftward, posterior and superior; (b) the mean QRS forces are concordance in the H plane. Frequently there is also mild left axis deviation of the major QRS forces in the F plane. The remaining patient in whom the mean QRS was posterior, and therefore concordance, Case 16, would be expected in the absence of WPW to show LVH as judged from the clinical data. The mean delta-QRS angle was 45° or greater in five (71%) of the cases.

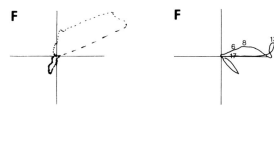

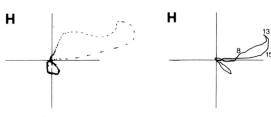

Fig. 9. WPW Type B with associated heart defects, Ebstein's anomaly of the tricuspid valve, Case 21, left) Grishman VCG at 8 years old and right) Frank at 15 years old.

The mean delta vector ranged from -20° to -90° and the mean QRS from $+70^\circ$ to -40°. The QRS loop inscription was CW in five, CCW in one, and figure-of-eight in one. In the F plane, the mean QRS was between $+25^\circ$ and -25° in five patients with one patient having the mean QRS at $+55^\circ$ and the other at -70°, the latter being associated with open CCW inscription (figure 7, left).

Analysis of the Frank VCG in the WPW Syndrome

There were a total of 18 cases for consideration in this group. Fourteen of these (78%) had no associated heart defects.

Type A WPW (Frank)--Without Associated Heart Defects--10 cases.

In eight cases, the mean QRS vector was oriented anteriorly, i.e., concordant with the mean delta vector. The delta-QRS angle in the H plane was narrow at less than 45° in the same eight patients (see figures 2-4, right). Case 12 (figure 10a), in addition to the concordant anterior delta and mean QRS vectors in the H plane, shows a superior QRS loop with open CCW inscription in the F plane, a left anterior hemiblock pattern. The tracings in figure 10b are from a 14-year old, Case 13, who had severe recurrent

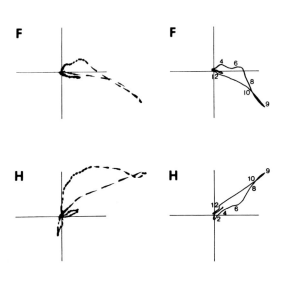

Fig. 8. WPW Type B with associated heart defects, Ebstein's anomaly of the tricuspid valve, Cast 19, seven years old. Left) Grishman VCG, Right) Frank VCG.

paroxysmal tachycardia and was operated upon subsequently (at another institution) to interrupt the accessory A-V pathway with partial effectiveness and a residual lessened degree of pre-excitation.

Two patients, Cases 4 and 5, had a discordant mean QRS vector and a wide delta-QRS angles in the H plane, 75° and 85° respectively. These are findings that using the criteria from the Grishman experience would suggest an associated cardiac defect, i.e., false-positive cases. The WPW pattern present at five weeks old in Case 4 (figure 11a) had evolved at four months old (figure 11b) to a short PR interval with a normal QRS, i.e., a Lown-Ganong-Levine syndrome. Case 5 (figure 12) showed the mean delta oriented anteriorly and the mean QRS posteriorly at -30°. The Grishman VCG in Case 5 showed concordant delta and QRS mean vectors due in part to a more prolonged delta which started anteriorly but continued posteriorly not unlike Case 2 (figure 6). Case 8 (figure 12b) is similar but the delta vector is slightly posterior, Type B WPW, and the delta and mean QRS vectors are concordant. It may be that a different line of separation rather than 0° will prove more reliable for this system.

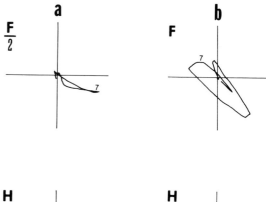
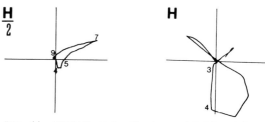

Fig. 11. WPW Type A without associated heart defects, a) Frank VCG at five weeks old; note discordant mean delta and mean QRS in H plane.
b) Frank VCG at four months old, resolution of WPW. Case 4.

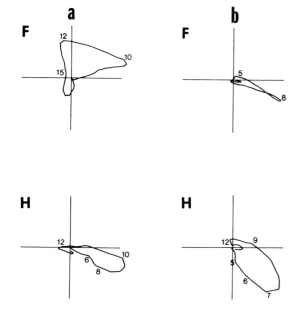

Fig. 10. WPW Type A without associated heart defects a) Case 12, Frank VCG 13 years old. Note open counterclockwise superior QRS loop in F plane
b) Case 13, Frank VCG 13 years old with severe tachycardia problem.

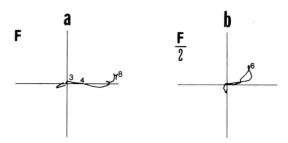
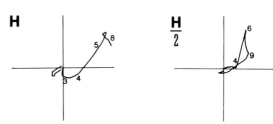

Fig. 12. WPW without associated heart defects,
a) Type A with discordant mean delta and mean QRS (an incomplete loop) in Case 5, six weeks old
b) Type B with concordant delta and mean QRS in Case 8, one year old.

The mean delta vector was between $+30^{\circ}$ and $+100^{\circ}$ in this group and the mean QRS was between $+120^{\circ}$ and -30°. Case 6 with the delta vector at $+100^{\circ}$ showed an Rs in ECG lead V-6 but a slurred q wave with a qRS in V7. Case 6 was an infant who presented with paroxysmal tachycardia and on reversion to sinus rhythm showed the WPW pattern.

Type A WPW (Frank)--With Associated Heart Defects--4 cases.

One of these patients had a posterior mean QRS vector, i.e., discordant to the delta vector. Case 20 (figure 13 a and b) showed some variation in the WPW pattern but consistently an anterior delta vector and large posterior QRS forces. The direction of the QRS forces was consistent with the expected hypertrophy pattern according to non-ECG data, namely LVH. Three cases with associated heart defects had concordant anterior mean delta and mean QRS vectors. Case 14 (figure 7, right) was a two-week-old infant who in view of the clinical data should have pure right ventricular hypertrophy. Case 15 (figure 5, right) was a two-month-old infant with expected bi-ventricular hypertrophy, and Case 22 (not shown) was a 14-year-old girl with expected right ventricular volume overload. In these three cases the appropriate hypertrophy pattern in the absence of the WPW syndrome would result in important anterior QRS forces and in all three the mean QRS was anterior.

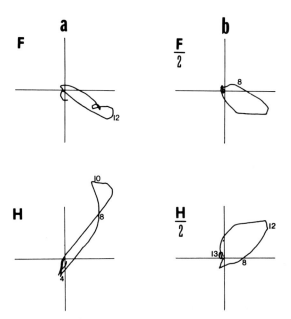

Fig. 13. WPW Type A with associated heart defects a and b serial tracings in Case 20, one year old with non-obstructive cardiomyopathy, note discordant mean delta and mean QRS vectors in H plane.

Type B WPW (Frank)--Without Associated Heart Defects--2 cases.

Both patients showed a posterior concordant mean QRS vector and a narrow delta-QRS angle in the H plane. Case 2 is shown in figure 6, right, and Case 8 is shown in figure 12b. Both cases showed a mild left axis deviation in the F plane with a mean QRS at $+20^{\circ}$ in Case 2 and at -30° in Case 8.

Type B WPW (Frank)--With Associated Heart Defects--2 cases.

These two cases also showed concordant posterior mean QRS vector and a narrow delta-QRS angle. The delta vector was superior at -10° and -25° and the mean QRS vector was slightly superior in one case and slightly inferior in the other. Both patients had Ebstein's anomaly of the tricuspid valve and the tracings were not unlike those from some patients with WPW Type B without associated heart disease. However, there is a consistency of type of WPW in these cases with the delta vector not only leftward and posterior but slightly superior.

Discussion

The classification of the WPW syndrome into Types A and B utilizing the major QRS deflection in the right precordial leads of the ECG was proposed in 1945 by Rosenbaum et al. [8]. However, as pointed out by Lowe et al. [9], the direction of the delta vector instead of the major QRS force has been employed widely, Type A meaning an anterior orientation of the delta and Type B designating a posterior orientation of the delta vector. The instantaneous 0.03 second QRS vector has been used [3] in a similar manner. When WPW is present without associated heart defects, the delta and major QRS forces in the VCG are generally concordant, either anterior or posterior, and the two approaches to classification would yield the same type. However, in the presence of associated cardiac defects, the delta and QRS forces may show anterior-posterior discordancy. In these cases, not only would the classification be different depending on whether the delta or major QRS were employed, but, of more importance, a positive aid to the diagnosis of the underlying heart disease may be overlooked.

WPW when uncomplicated by associated heart defects shows mean QRS forces that are in almost all instances oriented in a similar direction to the delta vector. When the delta vector was anterior the mean QRS was anterior in all cases in the Grishman series and in 80% in the Frank series. When the delta vector was posterior the mean QRS was posterior in all cases in both the Grishman and Frank series. The delta-QRS angle was narrow at less than 45° in the majority of cases but there were several exceptions.

In the presence of associated heart defects, WPW with an anterior delta vector showed a mean QRS vector that was discordanct in two (40%) of the Grishman series and one of the four (25%) of the Frank series. Consideration of the expected ventricular dominance or hypertrophy pattern as based on non-ECG data shows that in the absence of WPW these cases would be expected to have a pure left ventricular hypertrophy or a bi-ventricular hypertrophy, left greater than right pattern. Thus, it appears that the abnormal left ventricular dominance is influencing the mid and terminal QRS forces and is manifest in the QRS loop. The three cases not detected as abnormal had either pure right ventricular hypertrophy or bi-ventricular hypertrophy. The delta QRS angle was wide at 45° or greater in all five patients of WPW and associated heart disease in the Grishman series and in two of the four patients in the Frank series.

In the presence of WPW with a posterior delta vector, three of the seven cases (43%) showed the mean QRS to be anteriorly oriented in the Grishman series. All three had non-ECG data compatible with right ventricular dominance. Of the other four cases, three had Ebstein's anomaly of the tricuspid valve, an anomaly which has shown a great consistency of Type B with posterior concordant mean QRS forces [3, 9] due either to the unusual constancy of the location of the accessory A-V pathway or due to left ventricular hypertrophy and/or right ventricular hypoplasia. The other patient had a diagnosis of non-obstructive cardiomyopathy and would be expected to have a pure left ventricular hypertrophy pattern with leftward and posterior mean QRS forces in the absence of WPW as indeed were present during the WPW. There were only two cases of Type B WPW with associated heart defects in the Frank series, too few to reach any conclusions, but both showed the mean QRS vectors directed posteriorly, i.e., concordant and both patients had Ebstein's anomaly of the tricuspid valve. The delta-QRS angle was wide in the majority (72%) in the Grishman series but was not wide in the only two patients in the Frank series in this subgroup.

Consideration of the patients with WPW and with associated heart defects overall suggests that LVH may be appreciated in the presence of WPW Type A, and RVH obscured. In contrast, RVH may be apparent in WPW Type B whereas LVH is not.

Summary

There are certain consistent findings of diagnostic utility and theoretical interest which may be summarized as follows:

1. In WPW without associated heart defects the mean delta and mean QRS vectors are either concordant anterior or concordant posterior with rare exception. Further the angle between the delta and QRS is less than 45° in most cases.

2. When there are associated cardiac defects in WPW the mean delta and mean QRS vectors may be discordant, approximately 40% of cases in this study, suggesting the presence of the defect. Moreover, the delta-to-QRS angle is 45° or greater in the majority of cases.

3. In the presence of cardiac defects and WPW the mean QRS vector is generally oriented in a direction appropriate to the expected ventricular hypertrophy, or abnormal ventricular dominance. LVH may be present when the mean QRS is posterior in the face of an anterior delta vector. RVH is likely when the mean QRS is anterior in spite of a posterior delta vector.

4. Since ventricular hypertrophy can influence the direction of the major QRS forces the common practice of classifying on the basis of the delta vector, Type A anterior and Type B posterior seems preferable to the original suggestion that it be on the basis of the major QRS force.

5. The finding of a Type B concordant pattern with a superior delta orientation when Ebstein's anomaly of the tricuspid valve is accompanied by WPW remains reliable.

References

[1] L. Wolff, J. Parkinson and P.D. White, Bundle branch block with short P-R interval in healthy young people prone to paroxysmal tachycardia. Am Heart J. 5 (1930) 685.

[2] G. L. Schiebler, P. Adams, Jr., and R. C. Anderson, The Wolff-Parkinson-White syndrome in infants and children. A review and a report of 28 cases. Pediatrics 24 (1959) 585.

[3] J. J. Gallagher, M. Gilbert, R. H. Svenson, W. C. Sealy, J. Kasell, and A. G. Wallace, Wolff-Parkinson-White Syndrome; the problem, evaluation and surgical correction. Circulation 51 (1975) 767.

[4] B. L. Miller and B. E. Victorica, The vectorcardiogram of the Wolff-Parkinson-White Syndrome in infancy and childhood. In: I. Hoffman (ed.), Vectorcardiography 2 (North-Holland, Amsterdam, 1971), p. 597.

[5] E. Frank, An accurate clinically practical system for spacial vectorcardiography. Circulation 13 (1956) 737.

[6] M. Ariet, L. Crevasse, and T. Kennedy, Systems analysis of computerized EKG processing center. Submitted to the Journal of Electrocardiology. In press.

[7] A. Grishman, R. Borun, and H. L. Jaffee, Spatial vectorcardiography: Technique for the simultaneous recording of the frontal, sagittal and horizontal projections. Am. Heart J. 41 (1951) 483.

[8] F. F. Rosenbaum, H. H. Hecht, F. N. Wilson, F. D. Johnston, The potential variations of the thorax and the esophagus in anomalous atrio-ventricular excitation (Wolff-Parkinson-White Syndrome). Am. Heart J. 29 (1945) 281.

[9] K. G. Lowe, D. Emslie-Smith, C. Ward, and H. Watson, Classification of ventricular pre-excitation Vectorcardiographic study. Brit. H. Jour. 37 (1975) 9.

[10] D. Bialostozky, G. A. Medrano, L. Munoz, R. Contreras, Véctorcardiographic study and anatomic observations in 21 cases of Ebstein's malformation of the tricuspid valve. Am. J. Cardiol. 30 (1972) 354.

Vectorcardiography 3 I. Hoffman and R.I. Hamby eds.
© 1976 North-Holland Publishing Company - Amsterdam

NEW VECTORCARDIOGRAPHIC FINDINGS IN PATIENTS WITH
MYOCARDIAL INFARCTION AND ARTIFICIAL PACEMAKERS

Samuel Zoneraich and Olga Zoneraich

From the Department of Medicine, Division of Cardiology, Queens Hospital Center,
Long Island Jewish Medical Center and the State University of New York
Medical School at Stony Brook, New York

The diagnosis of myocardial infarction in the presence of left bundle branch block (LBBB) remains a matter of controversy.

Observations obtained from animal experiments have proven that in LBBB the mean vector representing the initial phase of myocardial depolarization is directed anteriorly to the left and inferiorly. The right to left septal activation which follows will be oriented to the left, inferiorly and posteriorly. Finally, during the last phase of activation the wave front is directed to the left, posteriorly and either superiorly or inferiorly.

In previous reports [1, 2], we presented evidence that an artificial pacemaker, inserted in the apex of the right ventricle, induces a QRS vectorcardiographic (VCG) pattern similar but not identical to clinical LBBB.

The main difference between clinical LBBB and the VCG pattern produced by endocardial stimulation of the right ventricular apex lies in the orientation of the initial and maximal vector. The initial vector in the induced pacemaker complex is always oriented superiorly and to the left. As a rule, the maximum QRS vector is inscribed in the left superior and posterior octant, very close to the sagittal plane. Thus, it appears that natural LBBB vectorcardiographic patterns could not be duplicated by artificial ventricular electrical stimulation. Changes in the position of the catheter tip will bring about variations in the electrical axis of QRS loops [3].

Right ventricular epicardial stimulation of the apical area induces vectorcardiographic patterns similar to those obtained with endocardial pacemakers.

The morphology of the QRS loop induced by left ventricular stimulation resembles the vectorcardiographic pattern recorded in patients with sinus rhythm and complete right bundle branch block (RBBB).

Common vectorcardiographic patterns in patients with transvenous pacemakers and myocardial infarction

A transvenous pacemaker causes an initial delay of the vectorcardiographic QRS loop lasting 20 to 30 milliseconds which is not seen in natural LBBB. The initial delay following the stimulus artifact is felt to represent the time required for the ventricular depolarization to activate a certain amount of muscle before entering the specific conducting system [4]. In unipolar stimulation, it is sometimes difficult to recognize the beginning of ventricular activation. On the other hand, a plausible explanation for the terminal delay during ventricular electrical pacing is yet to be found.

In evaluating the configuration of the pacemaker induced vectorcardiographic loop, one must be aware of possible distortions caused by the pacemaker artifact. Large unipolar spikes, especially, could distort the QRS loop as well as the ST segment. Bipolar spikes caused by average electrical intensity current do not as a rule distort the baseline.

Myocardial Infarction and Clinical LBBB

The spatial vectorcardiogram is considered helpful in the diagnosis of myocardial infarction, complicated by LBBB. De Pasquale and Burch [5] felt that by comparing the time courses of depolarization in patients with normal myocardium and LBBB with the time course of depolarization in those with LBBB and myocardial diseases, the spatial VCG might identify underlying lesions. Necropsy and clinical findings in support of this concept have been reported by Deglaude and Laurens [6], Wenger and Hupka [7], and recently by Walsh [8]. Experimental data were provided by Bisteni and coworkers [9] in studies on dogs.

There seems to be some basic agreement concerning the abnormal direction of the vectorial forces of QRS loops which point away from the infarcted zone. When the lower two-thirds of the septum were severely involved, the wave of depolarization was directed first to the right and the horizontal VCG had a clockwise direction. On the other hand, the initial vectors were oriented to the left and posteriorly when only the lower third of the septum was involved [8].

Myocardial Infarction and LBBB Pattern Induced by Artificial Pacemaker

The question is whether reliable information regarding the existence of necrotic areas within the myocardium could be obtained in humans by recording the VCG during transvenous right ventricular pacing. In our laboratory during the last nine years we studied the VCG patterns of the pacemaker beat produced in myocardial infarction [10, 11, 1].

All 50 patients representing our study group were admitted to the coronary care unit. Complete electrocardiograms and VCGs (Frank system) were obtained in all patients before and after insertion of the pacemaker, using the equipment (Cambridge and Hart Electronics) and the techniques previously reported [2, 11]. The initial data obtained by us were subsequently supported by others in clinical [12] and experimental studies [13].

A. Antero-septal and antero-lateral myocardial infarction distorted the pacemaker induced VCG loop causing similar changes to those observed in natural LBBB and antero-septal or antero-lateral wall myocardial infarction. The 20 msec initial vector was displaced to the right in antero-septal wall myocardial infarction (figure 1). In extensive anterior wall myocardial infarction, the centripetal limb was pushed to the right (figure 1). The presence of previous conduction disturbances like RBBB did not affect this pattern.

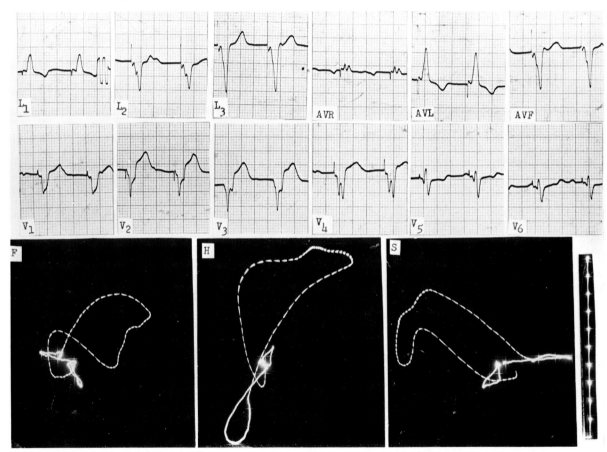

Case 1. Fig. 1. Pacemaker ECG, top, shows Q waves in L_1, a_{VL}, V_5 and V_6 suggesting septal and anterior wall myocardial infarction. Pacemaker VCG, bottom: There is displacement of the initial 20 msec vector to the right. The centrifugal and centripetal limb are displaced to the right. ST-T vector shows acute changes.

All VCG recordings were recorded with Hart Electronics PV_5 vectorcardiograph. VCG loops were interrupted at the rate of 500 times per second by the large end of the time dash.

B. As a rule, the initial vector was displaced to the left and anteriorly in posterior or in postero-diaphragmatic wall infarction. The orientation of the centripetal limb was less affected in this group than in anterior wall myocardial infarction.

C. Massive diaphragmatic myocardial infarction displaced the initial vectors superiorly, to the left or to the right.

D. The electrical diagnosis of acute myocardial infarction cannot be made in patients admitted with complete atrio-ventricular block and idioventricular rhythm. The extent and location of the myocardial infarction is detected by pacing the apex of the right ventricle. The resulting VCG will show LBBB pattern, distorted by the underlying myocardial infarction as described above (figure 1).

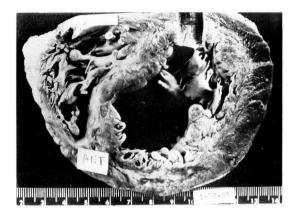

Case 1. Fig. 2. Necropsy specimen of case 1 shows extensive acute and subacute septal and anterior wall myocardial infarction.

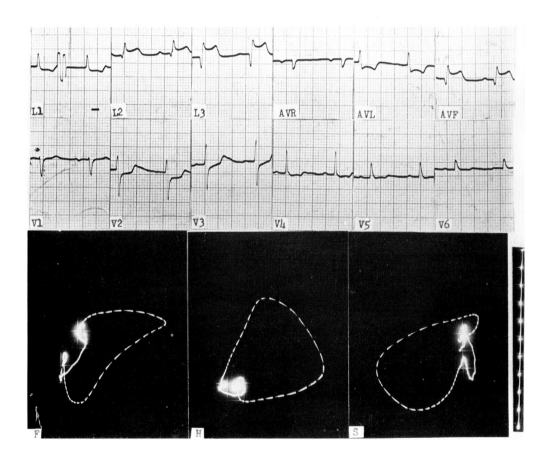

Case 2. Fig. 3. ECG and VCG before insertion of the pacemaker, showing acute changes of diaphragmatic myo-cardial infarction.

Figure 1 shows the pacemaker ECG and VCG of a 68-year-old patient admitted to the CCU because of acute myocardial infarction and complete heart block with idioventricular rhythm. Criteria for antero-septal and possible inferior wall myocardial infarction are present in the pacemaker ECG (QS in L_2, L_3, and aVF and Q wave in L_1, aVL, V_5 and V_6). VCG shows displacement of the initial vectors to the right and slightly anteriorly. Necropsy (figure 2) confirmed the presence of a massive transmural infarction of the septum and antero-inferior wall.

E. A large ST vector could be observed in LBBB and acute myocardial infarction. The pacemaker artifact does not eliminate it (figures 3 and 4).

Castellanos et al. [14] reported abnormal ST segment elevation in the ECG following the stimulus-QR pattern in two of four patients with recent anterior wall myocardial infarction and artificial ventricular pacing.

German et al. [15] felt that while the ECG diagnosis of an old myocardial infarction associated with clinical LBBB is disputable, the diagnostic value of large ST elevation during the acute episode of myocardial infarction is quite helpful. Thus, a large ST gradient when present, is of diagnostic significance in pacemaker ECG and VCG.

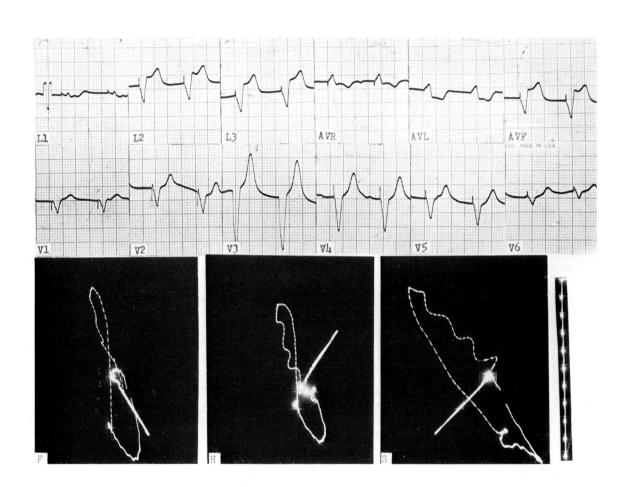

Case 2. Fig. 4. After insertion of right ventricular pacemaker. ST-T elevation is present in L_2, L_3 and aVF of ECG (top). ST-T vector is present also in pacemaker VCG. The undulatory pattern in centrifugal limb might be produced by unipolar stimulus artifact.

F. Malplacement of the catheter electrodes for right ventricular endocardial stimulation is easily recognized by pacemaker ECG and VCG (figures 5 and 6), and no chest x-ray is mandatory for confirmation. As observed in this patient, the frontal loop is oriented inferiorly indicating a superior right ventricular location of the pacemaker electrode. In such malplacement of the catheter the VCG loop fails to disclose the typical signs of myocardial infarction because the catheter tip does not reach the infarcted area of the septum. Accordingly (figures 5 and 6), one must bear in mind that an incomplete infarcted septum and a normal right septal surface will not produce a typical VCG pattern of LBBB and myocardial infarction.

However, an unusual orientation of the initial vectors in patients with pacemaker induced LBBB and myocardial infarction may be present in spite of normal positioning of the catheter electrode. This pattern could be observed in the tracings (figures 7 and 8) of a patient with extensive antero-lateral wall myocardial infarction, RBBB and left posterior hemiblock, in whom a transvenous pacemaker was inserted in the right ventricular apex. The correct position of the tip of the pacemaker was confirmed radiologically.

The pacemaker ECG shows tall R waves in V_1 and V_2 raising the question of electrode malplacement. VCG, however, shows in the frontal plane a left

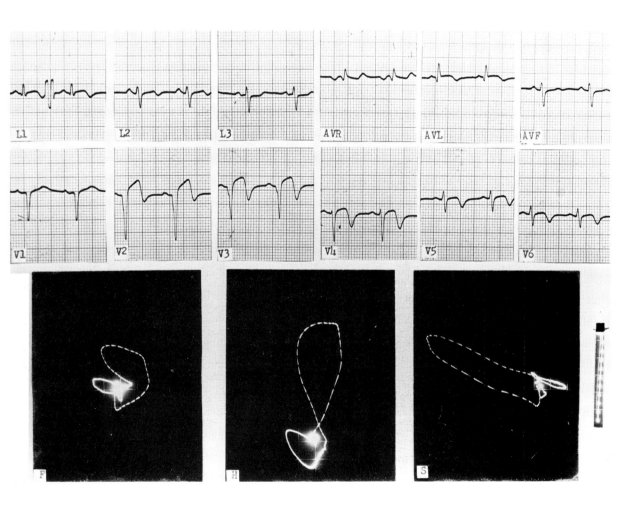

Case 3. Fig. 5. ECG and VCG before pacemaker implantation shows antero-septal wall myocardial infarction and left anterior hemiblock.

superior orientation of the QRS loop usually seen in right apical transvenous pacemakers. The abnormal orientation of the initial vectors in the horizontal plane--to the right and anteriorly--account for the narrow and tall R found in V_1 and V_2 on ECG. A plausible explanation of these findings is the presence of a small island of viable tissue in the right septum causing the small right and anterior appendage.

G. In some cases with severe necrosis and possible old fibrosis, VCG loops were very distorted with notches, bites and multiple conduction delays similar to those reported from this laboratory [16, 17] in naturally occurring ventricular extra-systoles in patients with myocardial infarction.

Kulbertus and Levan Rutten [12] accorded a special diagnostic significance to (1) displacement of the initial portion of QRS and (2) displacement of the afferant limb outside the left superior and posterior octant or of a significant departure from a smooth contour ("Bites out" or "pigtail curls"). Whereas the former changes were attributed to septal lesions, the latter were caused by the presence of infarcted segments within the left ventricle.

H. Assessment of the orientation of the stimulus artifact failed to bring supplementary information regarding the existence or localization of necrotic areas within the myocardium.

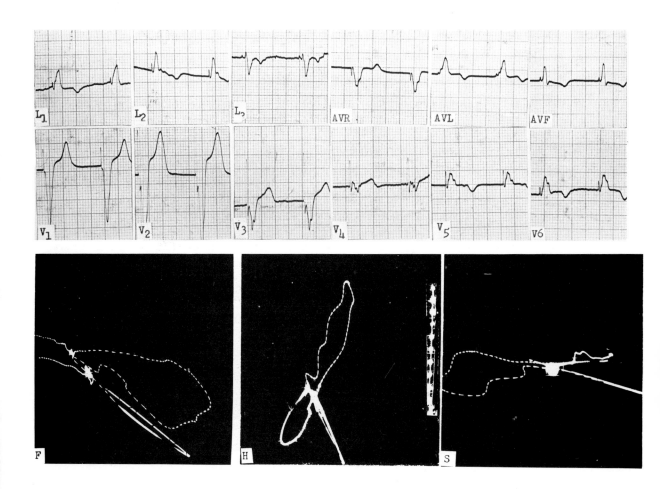

Case 3. Fig. 6. Shows an inferior oriented maximal vector of QRS loop in the frontal plane caused by malplacement of the electrode.

Conclusions

It is our opinion that the vectorcardiogram proved to be a very useful technique for detection of underlying myocardial necrosis in patients with artificial pacemakers (fixed or demand). In the presence of a known infarction, specific vectorcardiographic patterns are providing clues as to the site of myocardial lesions. Follow-up vectorcardiograms in these patients would help to detect new myocardial damage when important shifts of previous patterns occur. Vectorcardiography is the single non-invasive technique detecting the presence, location and extent of myocardial necrosis in patients with myocardial infarction, complete atrioventricular block and idioventricular rhythm.

Acknowledgment

The authors wish to express their gratitude to Miss Ada Fantroy, Mrs. Karen Franklin and Mr. Floyd Jackson for their assistance.

References

[1] O. Zoneraich and S. Zoneraich, Vectorcardiography of ventricular ectopic beats in patients with coronary artery disease. In: S. Zoneraich (ed.), In-non-invasive methods in cardiology (Charles C. Thomas, Publisher, Springfield, 1974), pp. 284-95.

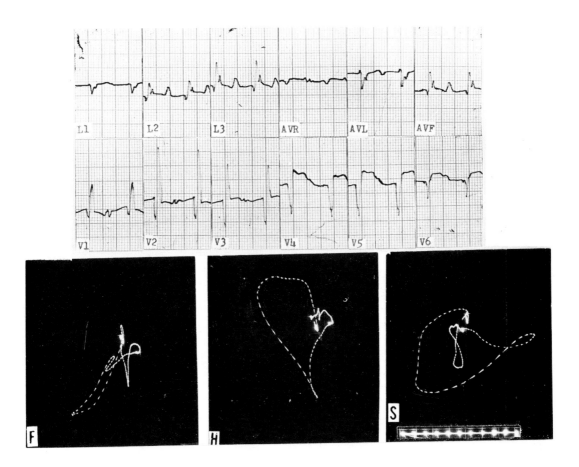

Case 4. Fig. 7. ECG and VCG before pacemaker insertion shows extensive antero-lateral infarction, RBB and LPH (left posterior hemiblock).

[2] O. Zoneraich, S. Zoneraich, and A. Douglas,
     The vectorcardiographic findings in patients
     with artificial pacemakers, Diseases of the
     Chest 53 (1968) 436.

[3] A. Castellanos, Jr., O. Maytin, L. Lemberg,
     and C. Castillo, Unusual QRS complexes pro-
     duced by pacemaker stimuli, Am. Heart J. 77
     (1969) 732.

[4] J. W. Lister, D. H. Klotz, S. L. Jomain,
     J. H. Stuckey, and B. F. Hoffman, Effect of
     pacemaker site on cardiac output and ventricu-
     lar activation in dogs with complete heart block,
     Am. J. Cardiol. 14 (1964) 494.

[5] N. De Pasquale and G. E. Burch, The spatial
     vectorcardiogram in left bundle branch block
     and myocardial infarction, with autopsy studies,
     Am. J. of Med. 29 (1960) 633.

[6] L. Deglaude and P. Laurens, Diagnostic vec-
     torgraphique de l'infarctus du myocarde associe
     d'un bloc de branche, Arch mal. coeur 47
     (1954) 579.

[7] R. Wenger and K. Hupka, Vectorcardiograph-
     ishe untersuchungen bei patienten mit schenkel-
     block und Herzmuskelinfarct, Cardiologia 29
     (1956) 196.

[8] T. J. Walsh, The Frank vectorcardiogram in
     left bundle branch block with myocardial infarc-
     tion. In: I. Hoffman (ed.), Proc. Long Island
     Jewish Hosp. Symposium, Vectorcardiography
     2 (North-Holland, Amsterdam, 1971), p. 232.

[9] A. Bisteni, G. A. Medrano, A. De Michelli, and
     D. Sodi-Pollares, Experimental myocardial in-
     farction in the presence of bundle branch block.
     In: I. Hoffman (ed.), Proc. Long Island Jewish

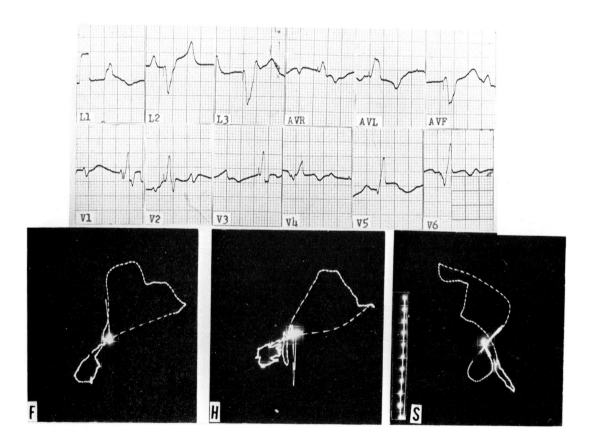

Case 4. Fig. 8. ECG and VCG after apical right ventricular pacing. Tall R wave in V_1-V_3 of ECG is represented in VCG by an initial appendage oriented anteriorly and to the right.

Hosp. Symposium, Vectorcardiography 1965 (North-Holland, Amsterdam, 1966), p. 226.

[10] O. Zoneraich and S. Zoneraich, Pacemaker vectorcardiography in patients with myocardial infarction and intraventricular conduction defects, J. Electrocardiology 4 (1971) 1.

[11] O. Zoneraich and S. Zoneraich, Pacemaker vectorcardiography in patients with myocardial infarction and intraventricular conduction defects. In: I. Hoffman (ed.), Proc. Long Island Jewish Hosp. Symposium, Vectorcardiography 2 (North-Holland, Amsterdam, 1971), p. 317.

[12] E. H. Kulbertus and F. Leval-Rutten, Vectorcardiographic study of QRS in patients with transvenous pacemakers and myocardial infarction, J. Electrocardiology 7 (1974) 27-33.

[13] E. L. Rothfeld, I. R. Zucker, and U. Ahuja, Electrical diagnosis of myocardial infarction in the paced dog heart, J. Electrocardiology 6 (1973) 27.

[14] A. Castellanos, Jr., R. Zoble, M. P. Procacci, J. R. Myerburg, and V. B. Bercovits, ST-QR pattern: New sign for diagnosis of anterior myocardial infarction during right ventricular pacing, Brit. Heart J. 35 (1973) 1161.

[15] L. German, O. P. Bahl, and E. Massie, Intermittent left bundle branch block. A study of the effects of left bundle branch block on the electrocardiographic patterns of myocardial infarction and ischemia, Am. Heart J. 85 (1973) 332.

[16] O. Zoneraich and S. Zoneraich, Ventricular bigeminy. In: P. Ryland (ed.), Proceedings of the twelfth international colloquium vectorcardiographicum (Presse Academique Europeennes, Bruselles, 1971), pp. 641-46.

[17] O. Zoneraich and S. Zoneraich, Bigeminal rhythm, vectrocardiographic pattern in coronary artery disease, J. Electrocardiology 5 (1972) 265.

SECTION 4.
COMPUTER APPLICATIONS

Vectorcardiography 3 I. Hoffman and R.I. Hamby eds.
© 1976 North-Holland Publishing Company - Amsterdam

COMPUTER DIAGNOSIS OF THE ELECTROCARDIOGRAM
AND VECTORCARDIOGRAM

Hubert V. Pipberger

From the Veterans Administration Research Center for Cardiovascular Data
Processing, Veterans Administration Hospital; and the Departments of
Clinical Engineering and Medicine, The George Washington
University Medical Center, Washington, D.C.

An attempt will be made to review the present status of computer diagnosis of orthogonal electrocardiograms (ECGs) and vectorcardiograms (VCGs). As implied by the title of this conference, "Clinical Vectorcardiography 1975," computer analysis of standard 12-lead ECGs will not be included in this discussion. Since a review of the subject in depth and great detail goes beyond the scope of this presentation, I will try to concentrate on some of the highlights. By necessity, I will have to dwell more on the system developed in the Veterans Administration than on others since I am personally more familiar with this computer program, having been intimately involved in its development since the late fifties.

The most complete and up-to-date reference source for ECG computer analysis is at present probably the proceedings of the Conference on ECG and VCG Data Processing, held by the International Federation for Information Processing [1].

With one exception [2], all operational computer systems for orthogonal ECGs or VCGs are based on the Frank-lead system [3-7]. This development is in line with the general trend toward adoption of the Frank-lead system which now appears to represent the most attractive compromise between accuracy and practicality.

A significant conceptual departure from available lead systems has been reported by Kornreich [8-10] who will expand on his approach later in this conference. Recognizing that neither the standard 12-lead ECG nor orthogonal-lead systems contain all the electrocardiographic information which can possibly be obtained from the body surface, an increasing number of investigators in recent years have recorded so-called body surface maps from more than one hundred closely spaced electrode sites on the human thorax. Since such a recording method is very time-consuming and not practical for clinical

application, Kornreich applied a data reduction method which led to a decrease in the number of leads from more than one hundred to nine. No information is given up in this data reduction process, and it can be assumed that the 9-lead system contains not only the information contained in standard and orthogonal leads but in addition all the residual information obtainable from the total body surface maps. Dr. Kornreich will elaborate in more detail on some of his methods and on his very promising results. Since both his data reduction methods and the diagnostic classification procedures are based on computer methodology, his contribusion to this conference fits well in this session on "Computer Applications."

Systems Design

A typical recording and processing station for ECG computer analysis is shown in figure 1. Three orthogonal leads are recorded simultaneously from the patient. They may be stored temporarily on tape reels or tape cassettes on the mobile recording cart. The alternative is transmission from the cart via direct wire connection or telephone line to a data receiving facility at the computer site. Problems related to telephone transmission of electrocardiographic data have been reviewed recently by Berson [11].

If data are transmitted in FM form, as is most often the case, they need to be demodulated at the receiving station. Subsequently, the analog recordings need to be converted into digital form [12] to become processable by the computer.

The first sections of computer analysis programs are common to all systems although they may differ greatly in detail. First, beginnings and ends of the various wave forms need to be identified through so-called wave recognition programs. Since the first such program was reported [13], the general approach to this problem has become fairly uniform. The rate of change of single leads or of spatial magnitude curves is most widely used for this purpose. Once P, QRS, and T waves have been properly identified, a measurement program is applied to determine time intervals and amplitudes of these complexes. A variety of electrocardiographic measurements form the basis of

Supported in part by Research Grant No. HL 15047 from the National Heart and Lung Institute, National Institutes of Health, U.S. Public Health Service, Bethesda, Maryland.

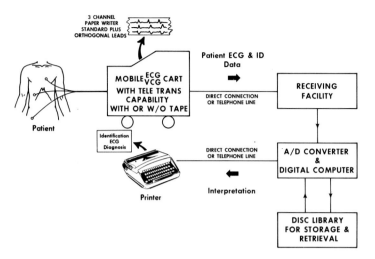

Fig. 1. Outline of a typical ECG data processing system. For further detail, see text.

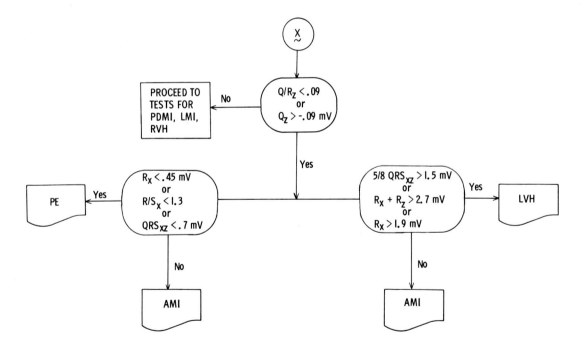

Fig. 2. Example for decision-tree logic used in all first-generation programs. If the Q/R ratio or Q amplitude in lead Z exceeds the limits of normal, anterior myocardian infarction (AMI), pulmonary emphysema (PE), and left ventricular hypertrophy (LVH) need to be considered. The additional measurements are to differentiate between these three diagnostic entities. (From Pipberger et al. [15] by permission of the American College of Cardiology.)

the diagnostic programs which are to be discussed in more detail later.

Results of the computer analysis are returned to the recording station via telephone line or via direct wire connection. A line-printer or teletype-writer is commonly used to reproduce the computer results.

For storage and retrieval of old records, disk drives have been found most advantageous, particularly when short-access times to old records are required for serial record comparison programs.

Diagnostic Classification Programs

Differences between the various available programs are largest in their approach to diagnostic classification. Since speaking of computer hardware in terms of first-, second-, and third-generation computers in ascending order of complexity has become customary, the classification of ECG computer programs into those of first and second generation [14, 15] has also been proposed. In the former, simulation of diagnostic methods, currently used by cardiologists, are simulated. An example is shown in figure 2. If the Q/R amplitude ratio in lead Z is less than 0.09 or the Q_z amplitude is greater than -0.09 mV, the diagnosis of anterior myocardial infarct (AMI) is considered. Since such findings also can be encountered in left ventricular hypertrophy (LVH) and pulmonary emphysema (PE), additional measurements are required to rule out these entities. The logic is best described as a decision tree.

In second-generation programs attempts have been made to take advantage of the computer's capability to use large numbers of ECG measurements simultaneously in order to improve the precision of diagnostic classification. Here the computer can truly be considered as an extension of human capabilities. Multivariate statistical techniques represent the method of choice for this approach.

First-generation programs [2, 4-7] have the advantage that most or all of the criteria used are familiar to electrocardiographers. Furthermore, the diagnostic logic is relatively easy to follow. Obviously, of course, the program performance can only be as good as the criteria used both in terms of sensitivity and specificity. The latter characteristic was found most critical in most of the early programs where excessive numbers of normals were classified as abnormal. Considering the overall diagnostic accuracy of only slightly more than 50 percent in Simonson's test of ten expert vectorcardiographers [16], one cannot realistically expect a much higher rate when criteria of the experts are programmed for computer analysis.

As mentioned earlier, in second-generation programs multivariate analysis based on large numbers of ECG measurements is used with the aim of improving diagnostic accuracy. In the program developed in the Veterans Administration [17], a total of 110 variables are used for P, QRS, ST, and T analysis respectively. Use of such large numbers of variables requires an extensive data base since the number of cases used in the program development has to be at least 20 times larger than that of the variables [18]. In order to avoid bias, the diagnoses of the cases used have to be based exclusively on non-ECG information; such as, catheterization data, ventriculograms, direct observation during surgery, post-morten information, or other documented solid data. Such a data base, comprising many thousands of cases, has been established through a Veterans Administration cooperative study with eight hospitals participating.

For each individual case, the multiple variables are combined to form a so-called patient vector which is then compared with the statistics derived from all the cases in the data base. Using a likelihood ratio test in a Bayesian classification scheme [17], the probability to belong to a given diagnostic category is computed for each case. A typical computer printout obtained from a patient with essential hypertension is shown in Table 1. The probability of having LVH was found to be very high (87 percent). P-wave analysis indicated a probability for left atrial overload of 58 percent as compared to 31 percent for being normal. The remainder of the diagnostic statements are self-explanatory.

Table 1

Typical computer printout from the record of a patient with long-standing Hypertensive Cardiovascular Disease (HCVD)
The probabilities are expressed as percentages.

ID	07094107	DATE	1/31/73
RACE	BLACK	AGE	50

HEART RATE   63/MIN
SINUS RHYTHM, MULTIPLE PVCs
FIRST DEGREE AV-BLOCK

QRS DIAGNOSTIC PROBABILITIES
LEFT VENTRICULAR HYPERTROPHY   87

COMPATIBLE WITH BIVENTRICULAR HYPERTROPHY

P WAVE PROBABILITIES
LEFT ATRIAL OVERLOAD   58
NORMAL   31
RIGHT ATRIAL OVERLOAD   11

DIGITALIS EFFECT

In Bayesian classification schemes, prior probabilities are used to compute posterior probabilities. These prior probabilities are based on the information provided in the ECG request form. The categories (Table 2) which are listed were kept as broad as possible to indicate only tentative clinical diagnoses which are under consideration. Checking one or more of these categories leads automatically to the selection of a set of prior probabilities for computation of the posterior probabilities. This approach may appear at first sight unfamiliar to the clinician until he realizes that this method is exactly that which he is using daily. A simple example may suffice to explain this approach to the diagnostic problem. When faced with an infant with chest pain, coronary artery disease (CAD) is only a very remote possibility to cause the pain. The prior probability for CAD, therefore, can be set very low. In a middle-aged or elderly man with chest pain, this situation is entirely different, and the prior probability for CAD needs to be set considerably higher. This is done automatically by the computer on the basis of the check marks on the ECG request form which are dialed in with the patient's identification number and transmitted to the computer with the ECG proper.

Table 2

Comparison of computer classification results with results of conventional 12-lead ECG analysis in a series of 1,192 patients [15]

| | ECG Diagnosis | | |
	Correct	Partially Correct	Incorrect
Computer Analysis (3-lead ECG)	86%	5%	9%
Physicians' Interpretation (12-lead ECG)	68%	4%	28%

Since second-generation programs represent a departure from more familiar ECG analysis routines, their clinical application can pose certain problems in terms of physician acceptance especially in the beginning. Dr. Richman will elaborate further on some of the practical aspects of routine application later in this session.

Computer Program Performance

There are basically three types of computer program evaluations. In the first and most simplistic approach, the program designer uses the same diagnostic criteria which were incorporated in the program and compares his own readings with that of the computer. Ideally, the agreement should be 100 percent, and any discrepancies have to be ascribed to technical failures in the wave recognition or measurement programs. Most of the early program evaluations were of this type. It has to be clearly understood, however, that diagnostic performance is not tested at all in type I evaluations since no objective yardstick is used for comparison, and the criteria used may or may not be efficient. It appears unfortunate that such studies have even continued to the recent past. To quote an example, Crevasse and Ariet [19] reported as recently as 1973 an accuracy rate for the diagnosis of LVH of 98 percent by computer and 96 percent by human observers. Since the same LVH criteria were used by both, no conclusions on diagnostic accuracy can be drawn from this study. When these same LVH criteria were tested by their originators [20] in 150 autopsy cases with LVH, the accuracy rate was only 60 percent. From this report, one may conclude that the accuracy rate of the computer was probably 98 percent of 60 percent or more precisely 59 percent.

In type II evaluations, computer results are compared with the readings of physicians who may use their own criteria. In one reported example [21] disagreements between computer and human observers reached almost 50 percent. Here again it is not possible to state who was right and who was wrong.

In type III evaluations, the diagnostic computer performance is tested against independent, objective evidence for the presence of cardiac abnormalities. To our knowledge, only the Veterans Administration program has been subjected to such tests, although several type III studies are presently in progress elsewhere. In the most recent Veterans Administration study [15], 1,192 cases were selected for testing because their clinical diagnoses could be firmly established on the basis of independent or non-ECG information. Only 21 percent of the patients were free of cardiovascular abnormalities. Classification results are shown in Table 2. The computer readings were not only compared against independent diagnostic evidence but also against interpretations of the standard 12-lead ECG obtained from two experienced electrocardiographers. The computer results in terms of correct interpretations exceeded those of the two readers by 18 percent. The effect of prior probabilities was investigated in the same study. They led to an improvement in diagnostic accuracy by approximately 20 percent.

A breakdown of results is shown in Table 3. Greatest improvements were found in cases with Hypertensive Cardiovascular Disease (HCVD) and Chronic Obstructive Lung Disease (COLD) where the recognition rate could be more than doubled.

Table 3

Breakdown of classification results in 1,092 cases without ventricular
conduction defects (QRS duration < 0.122 sec.)

| Diagnostic Entity | No. of Cases | ECG Interpretation | | | | | |
| | | Correct | | Partially Correct | | Incorrect | |
		3-lead %	12-lead %	3-lead %	12-lead %	3-lead %	12-lead %
Normal	173	98	93	1	0	1	7
Myocardial Infarct	418	85	79	3	0	12	21
Hypertensive Cardiovascular Disease	146	84	26	9	1	7	73
Valvular Heart Disease	171	96	68	1	1	3	31
Chronic Obstructive Lung Disease	75	81	29	3	0	16	71
Disease not related to cardiovascular system	73	91	92	1	0	8	8
Combination of more than one of above categories	36	22	14	75	61	4	25
TOTAL	1,092	87	68	5	2	8	30

From these results, advanced statistical classification techniques appear to improve ECG diagnosis by a substantial margin. As mentioned earlier, certain difficulties may be encountered with such methods because they are still unfamiliar to most clinicians. Furthermore, it is not always obvious which criteria have led to a given diagnosis since many are used in combination. Their interactions are not always easy to interpret. The computer printouts on the other hand have been kept as simple as possible in order to enable the non-cardiologist to make full use of them.

Computer Selection of Single or Multiple Criteria

A fortuitous by-product of the criteria selection for multivariate analysis was the identification of optimal criteria which can be easily used by hand. More than 300 different ECG measurements [22] were computed for each record in the data base in order to identify the most efficient ones and to eliminate those which were redundant. To our surprise and I hope not to the dismay of vectorcardiographers, measurements from scalar orthogonal leads were most often superior to those derived from vector loops. An example is shown in Table 4 for records from patients with COLD. The first four measurements led to a recognition rate of 77 percent with 8 percent false positives; i.e., normals which were erroneously classified as abnormal. Addition of the four best vector measurements increased the sensitivity from 77 percent to 82 percent with a concomitant increase in

false positives from 8 percent to 19 percent. The gain in sensitivity was thus completely offset by the loss in specificity. A similar experience was made in most diagnostic entities, and from a practical standpoint, analysis of scalar orthogonal leads is preferred first before proceeding to analysis of vector loops. A listing of very simple but useful criteria is given in Table 5. It has to be realized that they were selected from hundreds of measurements and tested on thousands of records. Erikssen et al. [23] tested the infarct criteria on a large sample of documented cases and compared the results with those obtained from conventional 12-lead ECG criteria. An improvement in diagnostic accuracy of approximately 20 percent could be achieved by using the orthogonal lead criteria. Such findings are not an indication of greater information content in orthogonal leads as compared to the conventional 12-lead ECG. They demonstrate, however, that systematic studies on criteria performance in large record samples can improve the accuracy of the ECG. Had large-scale studies of this type been performed on conventional 12-lead records, it is safe to assume that improvements similar to those achieved for orthogonal leads could also have been obtained.

Automated Comparison of Serial Electrocardiograms

Comparisons of old and recent ECG records represent an essential part of clinical electrocardiography. Important diagnostic clues can often only

Table 4

Selected scalar and vector measurements to discriminate between records from
patients with Chronic Obstructive Lung Disease (COLD) and normal patients

Measurements	Normal Limits (96% range)	Recognition Rate (cumulative)	False Positives (cumulative)
R_x	<0.51 mV	57%	2%
R/S_x ratio	<1.43	63%	3%
R_x peak time	<0.032 sec	66%	6%
R/S_y ratio	<0.80	77%	8%
Maximum QRS_{xy} angle	>71°	80%	12%
Maximum QRS_{yz} amplitude	<0.60 mV	81%	13%
Maximum QRS_{xz} amplitude	<0.74 mV	82%	14%
Maximum QRS_{xz} angle	<245°	82%	19%

be obtained by serial analysis. An efficient storage and retrieval system represents a prerequisite for comparisons. Of the various available storage media, such as analog tape, digital tape, magnetic disks, or drums, the disk appears most efficient due mainly to its short access time. A combination of disk and tape storage may reduce the cost of the storage system.

For record comparisons proper, three different approaches have been described [24-26]. Due to the substantial variations in ECG measurements of serial tracings, Pryor et al. [24] limited their comparisons essentially to final diagnostic statements. Dunn [25] compared both measurements and diagnoses with the latter being expressed in terms of probabilities. Measurements are listed only when they exceed day-to-day or year-to-year variability, previously determined both in normals and abnormals [27, 28]. As an option, serial probability changes can be displayed on the cathode-ray tube of a computer terminal [29]. This display was found particularly useful in the follow-up of patients with HCVD where the effect of antihypertensive therapy is reflected in the serial ECG changes.

Macfarlane et al. [26] described a comparison system which is primarily oriented toward ECG changes found in CAD. Up to two previous ECGs are stored on disk, and the most-recent record is compared with the old ones. Abnormalities of Q, ST, and T are stored for this comparison.

Further work in the analysis of serial ECG changes becomes increasingly important in long-term follow-up studies of patients in epidemiological

studies. Besides a few scattered observations in the literature, no systematic trend analysis studies have been reported which might lead to an estimate of the prognostic information content of the ECG. Computer analysis appears as the method of choice in such studies for two reasons. First, the number of serial records to be analyzed is extremely large, and this should preferably be done by automated means. Second, detailed analysis of trends may prove very difficult by visual inspection only. Advanced statistical techniques may be necessary to detect hidden trends in the follow-up which again necessitates computer means.

Numerical Analysis versus
VCG Display

During the last three decades, a major trend in electrocardiography was toward new methods of data display, and the VCG proved to be one of the most popular display forms. Although we have all learned much from vectorcardiographic studies, there may be less emphasis on loop displays in the coming years. More and more results will be presented in numerical form, and the display will become more a tool for gross overview of data and teaching. Kornreich's approach to the diagnostic problem is typical for this trend. His 9-lead system which contains more information than the conventional 12-lead or orthogonal lead systems is abstracted into a series of numbers which, properly weighted, are combined to a single, multidimensional patient vector which has little or no relationship to the familiar reference frames of other lead systems. Although this is not the time and place

Table 5

ECG measurements which can be easily obtained by hand and which proved very efficient in routine ECG readings. The criteria were selected from more than 300 variables tested by computer. Note that the majority of the measurements were obtained from scalar leads. Unless indicated otherwise, all criteria indicate amplitudes. No sensitivity data for LVH are given because they vary largely depending on the severity of the underlying disease.

	Normal Limits	Sensitivity	False Positive
Anterior Infarct			
Q/R_Z ratio	< 0.10	71%	3%
R_Z duration	> 0.08 sec	79%	5%
Posterodiaphragmatic Infarct			
Q/R_y ratio	> .25	70%	2%
Q_y duration	> .03 sec	72%	2%
Q_y	< -.25 mV	75%	4%
Lateral Infarct			
Q/R_X ratio	> .17	98%	2%
Left Ventricular Hypertrophy			
R_X	>1.9 mV		2%
R_Z	>1.7 mV		5%
$R_X + R_Z$ *	>3.1 mV		6%
QRS_{XZ}	>2.2 mV		7%

*A limit of 1.7 mV corresponds to the Sokolow criterion:
S V1 + R V5 or V6 > 3.5 mV.

Right Ventricular Hypertrophy			
R_X	< .50 mV	31%**	2%
R/S_X ratio	<1.3	60%	4%
Q/R_Z ratio	>1.2	71%	6%
R_Z	< .3 mV	77%	7%

**Sensitivity in Mitral Stenosis.

Chronic Obstructive Lung Disease			
R_X	< .50 mV	57%	2%
R/S_X ratio	<1.3	63%	4%
Maximum QRS_{XY}	< .8	74%	9%
Maximum P_{XY} angle	>92°	80%	11%

to begin the swan song of vectorcardiography and other related displays, the future does not look bright and promising, and the time may not be far away when all that we will have to look at when evaluating an ECG will be a few numbers expressing diagnostic probabilities with a few explanatory computer comments.

References

[1]   C. Zywietz and B. Schneider (eds.), Computer application on ECG and VCG analysis. (American Elsevier Publishing Co., Inc., New York, 1973.)

[2]   P. W. Macfarlane and T. D. V. Lawrie, An operational system for routine ECG interpretation on a small digital computer. In: C. Zywietz and B. Schneider (eds.), Computer application on ECG and VCG analysis . (American Elsevier Publishing Co., Inc., New York, 1973), pp. 183-89.

[3]   H. V. Pipberger, Computer analysis of the electrocardiogram. In: R. W. Stacy and B. D. Waxman (eds.), Computers in biomedical research, Vol. I. (Academic Press, New York, 1965), pp. 377-407.

[4]   O. Arvedson, Methods for data acquisition and evaluation of electrocardiograms and vectorcardiograms with the digital computer. Mono-

graph, Department of Clinical Physiology and Computer Center, University of Umea, Sweden, 1968.

[5] K. C. Hu, D. B. Francis, G. T. Gau, and R. E. Smith, Development and performance of Mayo-IBM electrocardiographic computer analysis programs (V 70), Mayo Clin. Proc. 48 (1973) 260–68.

[6] T. A. Pryor, R. Russell, A. Budkin, and W. G. Price, Electrocardiographic interpretation by computer, Comput. Biomed. Res. 2(1969) 537–48.

[7] J. von der Groeben, B. W. Brown, R. S. Crow, J. G. Toole, C. D. Weaver, and R. R. Clappier, The Stanford University computer ECG system. In: C. Zywietz and B. Schneider (eds.), Computer application on ECG and VCG analysis (American Elsevier Publishing Co., Inc., New York, 1973), pp. 171–81.

[8] F. Kornreich and D. Brismee, The missing waveform information in the orthogonal electrocardiogram (Frank leads). II. Diagnosis of left ventricular hypertrophy and myocardial infarction from "total" surface waveform information, Circulation 48 (1973) 996–1004.

[9] F. Kornreich, P. Block, and D. Brismee, The missing waveform information in the orthogonal electrocardiogram (Frank leads). III. Computer diagnosis of angina pectoris from "maximal" QRS surface waveform information at rest, Circulation 49 (1974) 1212–22.

[10] F. Kornreich, P. Block, and D. Brismee, The missing waveform information in the orthogonal electrocardiogram (Frank leads). IV. Computer diagnosis of biventricular hypertrophy from "maximal" surface waveform information, Circulation 49 (1974) 1223–31.

[11] A. S. Berson, Telephone transmission of electrocardiogram. In: C. Zywietz and B. Schneider (eds.), Computer application on ECG and VCG analysis (American Elsevier Publishing Co., Inc., New York, 1973), pp. 83–97.

[12] L. Taback, E. Marden, H. L. Mason, and H. V. Pipberger, Digital recording of electrocardiographic data for analysis by a digital computer, IRE Trans. Med. Electronics 6 (1959) 167–71.

[13] F. W. Stallmann, and H. V. Pipberger, Automatic recognition of electrocardiographic waves by digital computer, Circ. Res. 9 (1961) 1138–43.

[14] H. V. Pipberger, R. A. Dunn, and J. Cornfield, First and second generation computer programs for diagnostic ECG and VCG classification. In: P. Rijlant, I. Ruttkay-Nedecky, and E. Schubert (eds.), Proceedings of the Satellite Symposium of the XXVth International Congress of Physiological Sciences, The Electrical Field of the Heart, and the XIIth International Colloquium Vectorcardiographicum

(Presses Academiques Europeennes, Brussels, 1972).

[15] H. V. Pipberger, D. McCaughan, D. Littmann, H. A. Pipberger, J. Cornfield, R. A. Dunn, C. D. Batchlor, and A. S. Berson, Clinical application of a second generation electrocardiographic computer program, Am. J. Cardiol 35 (1975) 597–608.

[16] E. Simonson, N. Tuna, N. Okamoto, and H. Toshima, Diagnostic accuracy of the vectorcardiogram and electrocardiogram. A cooperative study, Am. J. Cardiol. 17 (1966) 829–78.

[17] J. Cornfield, R. A. Dunn, C. D. Batchlor, and H. V. Pipberger, Multigroup diagnosis of electrocardiogram, Comput. Biomed. Res. 6 (1973) 97–120.

[18] J. Cornfield, Statistical classification methods. In: J. A. Jacquez (ed.), Computer diagnosis and diagnostic methods (Charles C Thomas, Publishers, Springfield, Ill., 1972), pp. 108–30.

[19] L. Crevasse and M. Ariet, A new scalar electrocardiographic computer program. Clinical evaluation, JAMA 226 (1973) 1089–93.

[20] D. W. Romhilt and E. H. Estes, Jr., A point-score system for the ECG diagnosis of left ventricular hypertrophy, Am. Heart J. 75 (1968) 752–58.

[21] C. A. Caceres and H. M. Hochberg, Performance of the computer and physician in the analysis of the electrocardiogram, Am. Heart J. 79 (1970) 439–43.

[22] H. W. Draper, C. J. Peffer, F. W. Stallmann, D. Littmann, and H. V. Pipberger, The corrected orthogonal electrocardiogram and vectorcardiogram in 510 normal men (Frank lead system), Circulation 30 (1964) 853–64.

[23] J. Erikssen and C. Muller, Comparison between scalar and corrected orthogonal electrocardiogram in diagnosis of acute myocardial infarcts, Brit. Heart J. 34 (1972) 81–86.

[24] T. A. Pryor, A. E. Lindsay, and R. W. England, Computer analysis of serial electrocardiograms, Comput. Biomed. Res. 5 (1972) 709–14.

[25] R. A. Dunn, and H. V. Pipberger, Analysis of serial ECG changes in epidemiological studies. Presented at the American Heart Association's Thirteenth Annual Conference on Cardiovascular Disease Epidemiology, New Orleans, La., March 12 and 13, 1973.

[26] P. W. Macfarlane, H. T. Cawood, and T. D. V. Lawrie, A basis for computer interpretation of serial electrocardiograms, Comput. Biomed. Res. 8 (1975) 189–200.

[27] J. L. Willems, P. F. Poblete, and H. V. Pipberger, Day-to-day variation of the normal orthogonal electrocardiogram and vectorcardiogram, Circulation 45 (1972) 1057–64.

[28] P. M. Kini, P. Ginefra, and H. V. Pipberger, Day-to-day variation of the Frank electrocardiogram and vectorcardiogram in heart disease, Am. Heart J. 88 (1974) 698-704.

[29] H. V. Pipberger, R. A. Dunn, and H. A. Pipberger, Automated comparison of serial electrocardiograms. In Proceedings, First International Congress on Electrocardiology, Wiesbaden, Germany, October 14-17, 1974 (in press).

Vectorcardiography 3 I. Hoffman and R.I. Hamby eds.

NEW ECG TECHNIQUES IN THE DIAGNOSIS OF INFARCTION AND HYPERTROPHY

F. Kornreich, J. Holt, Jr., P. Rijlant, A. C. L. Barnard,
J. Tiberghien, J. Kramer, Jr., and J. Snoeck

From the Cardiovascular Research Unit, V.U.B. (Free University Brussels), Belgium, the
Department of Cardiology, V.A. Birmingham, Alabama, U.S.A., the Institute of
Physiology Solvay, U.L.B. (Free University Brusseld), Belgium,
and the University of Antwerp, R.U.C.A., Antwerp, Belgium

As stated by Okada in 1963 [1], recording of potential measurements over the entire body yields the entire information available. Such measurements are the ultimate for empirical diagnosis but the experimental procedures are extremely complex and tedious. The advent of powerful computers, however, has reduced the complexity of this problem and permits handling this bulk of measurements.

But before such an important step is taken, one has to be convinced that the tremendous investment in time, energy and money is really worth while. Since no practitioner would ever agree to place 100 or more electrodes on a patient's torso, the problem has been divided in two closely related aspects: first, to prove that the available lead systems do not account for the total electrical information needed for clinical use, and second to show that "maximal" useful information could be made available for current practice, meaning that no more than $\pm$ 10 electrodes ought to be placed. The first aspect was abundantly proven by Taccardi [2], Horan [3], Spach [4], Holt [5] and many others. The second point was predicted by Geselowitz in 1971 [6] and supported by the experiments of Scher [7], Horan [8] and ourselves [9]. Starting from 126 leads recorded on each patient's torso in a population of 1,200 cases, we reduced this obviously redundant information into 9 ECG waveforms: the main property of these 9 waveforms, recorded in each individual at identical and well-defined anatomical locations is that they were found capable of resynthetizing any ECG waveform on the body surface.

Methods

A. The essence of our method, which actually is in line with generalized cancellation experiments, rests on the empirical evidence obtained by testing each of the 126 surface electrocardiograms for the XYZ (e.g. Frank or McFee leads) content. The results were analyzed by a least-square best fit procedure using a CDC 6500 computer. The poorly fitted curves are considered as additional sources of waveform information (figure 1).

Six such areas were found by superimposing records from more than 1,000 patients. Each area

of poor-fit could be represented by a single waveform accounting for the waveform information of that particular area (figures 2 and 3).

A mixed system consisting of the XYZ leads + 6 additional waveforms was thus created. The XYZ leads could then be replaced by 3 unweighted surface ECGs using the same procedure--testing each of the 126 surface ECGs for the above determined 6 additional leads content. We finally arrived at a 9-lead ECG system, yielding the total available surface electrical waveform information (figure 4). A new independent group of $\pm$ 1,000 patients was then tested with this new lead system; a resynthesis of 97% was achieved, adding support to and confirming the first results. The resynthesis level was not refined further because of the estimated noise ($\pm$ 3 - 4%) (figure 5).

B. The next step was a diagnostic one: a theoretical "complete" lead system does not necessarily yield the best diagnostic results and achieve optimal separation between normals and abnormals. We therefore had to submit our lead system to diagnostic evaluation and compare the results with another widely used lead system. As multivariate statistical procedures were considered optimal for such analysis, we turned to Pipberger's studies on the Frank leads because, to our knowledge, most of the work in that field using these statistical methods has been performed by his group [10, 11, 12, 13]. Our study only deals with the QRS complexes at present. Each time-normalized QRS waveform was divided in 8 equal parts yielding 72 variables for the 9 lead system and 24 variables for the Frank leads. However, an identical number of variables was, of course, retained for both lead systems for comparison of diagnostic performances. In a first step a computer program selected the best discriminators for both lead systems [14]. In a second step a linear discriminant function (DF) was computed using the best (and the same number) of selected variables. This DF permitted the classification of new patients in order to control the quality of the method and the reproductibility of the results [14] using a likelihood ratio test assigning each patient to the category for which his probability was the greatest.

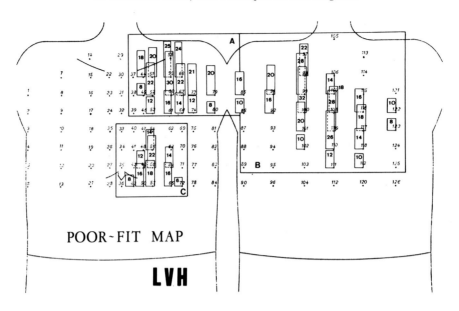

Fig. 1. The figure shows as an example the poorly fitted waveforms with respect to the Frank leads (XYZ) in L.V.H. Out of each area (A, B and C) a representative waveform could be found (usually the poorest one is chosen) as a source of additional information to XYZ. The number in each column or rectangle represents the number of times (in %) a poor fit occurred for the underlying lead in a population of patients with L.V.H.

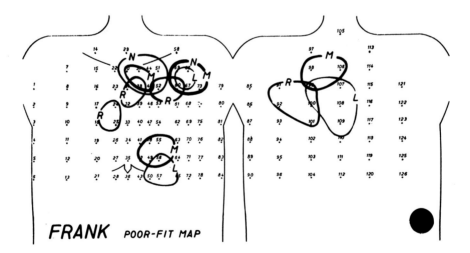

Fig. 2. The areas of poor fit which can be represented by one single waveform are represented for each disease entity considered. N = normals, M = myocardial infarction, L = left ventricular hypertrophy and R = right ventricular hypertrophy. This figure results from the breakdown process of areas as explained in another text [24].

(Reprinted by permission of Circulation, published by the American Heart Association, Inc., 44 East Twenty-third Street, New York 10, N.Y.).

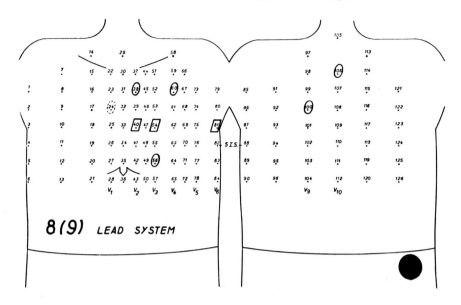

Fig. 3. The solid ovals indicate electrode positions where representative electrocardiograms can be recorded. The dotted oval refers to the RVH group mainly. The solid rectangles represent the leads which can be used together with the previously described ones for achievement of total waveform information, replacing the Frank leads. 5 I.S. = fifth intercostal space; V_1 to V_{10} = standard ECG positions.

(Reprinted by permission of Circulation, published by the American Heart Association, Inc., 44 East Twenty-third Street, New York 10, N.Y.).

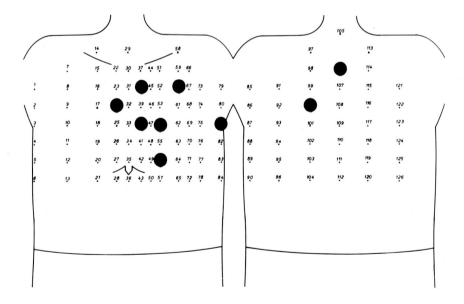

Fig. 4. The electrode sites for the 9-lead system are indicated with large dots.

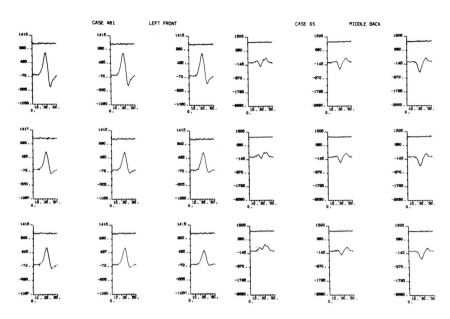

Fig. 5. This figures shows the electrocardiograms recorded on two patients. Samples from the anterior and posterior thoracic surfaces are given. The scale is in microvolts; the abscissa indicates the time (50 = 100 msec.). The lower tracings are the actually recorded waveforms, the upper tracings are the residual time-functions obtained by subtraction of the computed waveforms from the original waveforms. The beginning of the QRS complex is indicated by a small vertical line: at the left of these vertical lines, the terminal part of the PQ (PR) segment is visible, disclosing the noise level. The error or residual curves resulting from the best-fit procedures are clearly within the noise range. (The error curve with an asterisk is a straight line because the corresponding waveform is one of the nine components of the linear combination and consequently perfectly fitted by itself.)

(Reprinted by permission of Circulation, published by the American Heart Association, Inc., 44 East Twenty-third Street, New York 10, N.Y.).

Material

For this particular study on hypertrophy and myocardial infarction 1,196 patients were selected: 295 were normal individuals (N), 292 had proven myocardial infarction (M.I.), 175 had L.V.H., 157 revealed R.V.H., and 114 showed B.V.H.; 163 suffered C.A.D. without evidence of M.I.

The patients were divided into training sets and control sets in order to test the reproducibility of the results (table 1).

Diagnostic Criteria

Normal patients (N). Patients were included if they reported no symptoms and had a normal physical examination and chest X-ray. Moreover, ancillary data and particularly blood pressure, had to be within normal limits. The ages of this group ranged from 20 to 50 years with a mean of 44 years.

Myocardial infarction (M.I.). The criteria for inclusion of individuals in this series were [15]

a. acute cases: typical history of infarction within the past few days and characteristic enzyme changes; all these patients had at least one occluded coronary vessel (occlusion > 70%) as found at autopsy or, by coronary angiography. This group constitutes almost 25% of the 292 patients with M.I.

b. recent or remote cases: typical history of past (more than 6 weeks old) coronary occlusion demonstrated by angiography and/or autopsy. These patients represent about 70% of the total sample.

c. coexisting acute and remote infarctions representing ± 5% of the series of patients with M.I.

Table 1

Material	Training Set	Control Set	Total Number of Patients
N.	195	100	295
M.I.	192	100	292
L.V.H.	95	80	175
R.V.H.	97	60	157
B.V.H.	74	40	114
C.A.D.	83	80	163
	736	460	1,196

Legend
N.   Normal individuals.
M.I.   Myocardial infarction.
L.V.H.   Left ventricular hypertrophy.
R.V.H.   Right ventricular hypertrophy.
B.V.H.   Biventricular hypertrophy.
C.A.D.   Coronary artery disease without
         evidence of M.I.

All the patients also underwent ventriculography. Of the above mentioned cases, 80% demonstrated akinetic and/or dyskinetic areas. The patients with ventricular aneurysm were excluded.

Not enough autopsy material was available to divide the series into subgroups according to the site of the infarction; all the patients with M.I. were therefore pooled in one single group.

Left ventricular hypertrophy (L.V.H.). All patients in this group [16] underwent routine clinical evaluation and cardiac catheterization during which hemodynamic data and biplane angiograms were obtained. Left ventricular volumes were determined using the method of Dodge et al. [17] and left ventricular muscle weight (LVMW) was obtained by the method of Rackley et al. [18]. L.V.H. was defined as LVMW greater than 2 standard deviations above the mean LVMW for adult male subjects, which is 188 gr. $\pm$ 33 gr., as determined by Kennedy et al. [19]; the upper limit is thus 254 grams.
Most of the patients had isolated aortic valve disease (about 80%); the others had congenital heart diseases, cardiomyopathy, hypertension and hypertrophic subaortic stenosis. The right ventricular systolic pressure never exceeded 30 mm Hg.

Right ventricular hypertrophy (R.V.H.).
Patients with a right ventricular systolic pressure (RVSP) exceeding 35 mm Hg [20] were considered as having R.V.H. Frequently this hypertrophy was confirmed by the surgeon's estimate when patients came to surgery. Most of the patients had mitral stenosis

(about 70%); the series was also constituted of patients with cor pulmonale (about 15%), ventricular septal defect with pulmonic stenosis, tetralogy of Fallot, and tricuspid valve disease. None of these patients presented a LVMW above 254 gr.

Biventricular hypertrophy (B.V.H.). The B.V.H. group was classified on the basis of the presence of both a LVMW > 254 gr. and a RVSP > 35 mm Hg. Various heart diseases were encountered but most of them ($\pm$ 90%) were related to multivalvular lesions without evidence of coronary artery disease.

Coronary artery disease without M.I. (C.A.D.). This group first consisted of patients with a typical history of angina pectoris. The group was then limited to only those patients with at least a 70% occlusion in one of the coronary vessels, as determined by angiography, and normal ventricular function by ventriculography. The patients with old, recent or acute myocardial infarction, clinically and biologically assessed, hypertension, valvular disease, congestive heart failure, LVMW > 254 gr. and RVSP > 35 mm Hg. were excluded. Although myocardial infarctions gross enough to produce clinical, biological or electrical evidence are ruled out of this group, the authors are aware that microinfarctions or even larger but "silent" infarctions might have slipped in. However, we believe that this "contamination" is not very important within the scope of this paper as our main goal is to achieve clinical differentiations between C.A.D. with and without gross evidence of M.I. [21].

The E.C.G. was not taken into account in the assessment of normality, nor for the constitution of the other groups except for the QRS duration which was not allowed to exceed 0.12 sec.

Results

The results for both systems are listed in tables 2 and 3, and speak for themselves. The number of variables for each bigroup comparison is kept reasonably low in order not to yield overoptimistic results which could then not be reproduced on new independent samples [22].

The best discriminators can be shown for each bigroup comparison as in figures 6 and 7, as examples for the Frank leads and the 9-lead system respectively. In differentiating N. from M.I. the scores were respectively 76% for the Frank leads and 91% for the 9 leads; a figure of 78% was achieved with the standard 12 lead ECG. The results were also by far superior with the 9 leads when each bigroup classification was considered separately. For the C.A.D. group the specificity was kept at 90%; for all other groups it was constantly kept at 95%.

Table 2

Frank leads	9-lead system	12-lead standard ECG
N-LVH differentiation (sensitivities only) 72%	92%	78%
N-RVH differentiation 60%	80%	73%
N-MI differentiation 76%	91%	78%
N-CAD differentiation 38%	74%	51%
N-BVH differentiation 82%	93%	83%
Mean 66%	86%	73%

The percentages indicate the correctly diagnosed patients.

Table 3

Frank leads	9-lead system	12-lead standard ECG
MI-CAD differentiation 76–83%	82–86%	77–83%
MI-LVH differentiation 88–65%	97–82%	88–73%
MI-RVH differentiation 79–65%	94–90%	90–84%
BVH-LVH differentiation 64–67%	80–78%	75–73%
BVH-RVH differentiation 62–72%	78–85%	77–75%

The percentages indicate the correctly diagnosed patients.

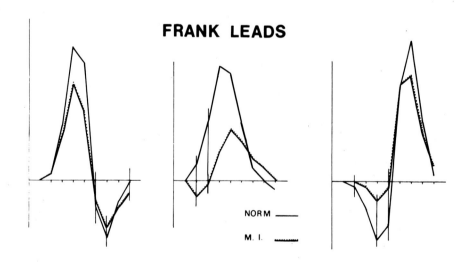

FRANK LEADS

NORM ——
M. I. ········

Fig. 6. The time-normalized Frank XYZ leads represented for the mean normal and M.I. population. The vertical bars indicate the best discriminators between these two groups.

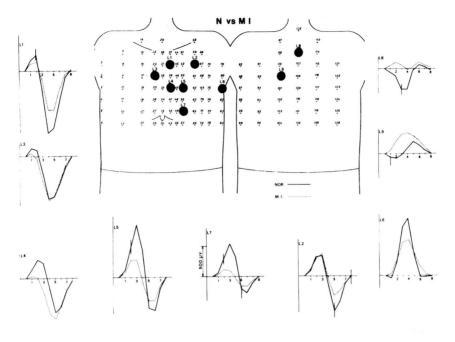

Fig. 7. The time-normalized 9-leads of the newly derived lead system are represented for the averaged normals and individuals with M.I. The best differentiations between these two populations are achieved by linear combination of the discriminators represented on the graph by vertical bars.

Discussion

A new and practical lead system has been devised, providing the total surface electrical waveform information with a limited number (9) well defined electrode positions on the torso of each individual. We now feel that we are entitled to state that this additional information significantly improves upon the results of more classical, routinely used lead systems. Some improvements still being considered are:

1. extending the method to larger samples of well documented patients;
2. using the P and the STT waves;
3. considering more parameters than 8 or 16 instantaneous vectors;
4. taking into account approaches such as those from Pipberger and J. Cornfield using prior possibilities [23].

We finally would like to stress the important fact that computer measurements are not easily performed by the clinician as they mainly involve instants of QRS which are not readily visible or readable by the human eye. Therefore, using similar statistical procedures applied to our lead system, "hand measurements," such as QRS amplitudes and durations will be fed into the computer in order to yield the best, easiest and most practically measurable parameters. This study is about to be finished and will be available soon. The readable measurements refer to QRS amplitudes, durations and ratios. The same will of course be done for the P and STT waves, and for other widely used lead systems.

Our goal in fact is twofold: first, to provide well equipped centers with optimal computer measurements using an optimized lead system, and second, to give the practitioner the tools to perform "ideal" ECG diagnosis by means of practical handmade parameters and a limited number of measurements for correct ECG classification.

Conclusion

A new lead system consisting of 9 ECGs recorded at identical well-defined anatomical positions in each individual has been devised. Its main characteristic is that these 9 leads are capable of resynthesizing in each patient all the thoracic ECG waveforms and, in other words, account in a quantitative sense for the total available electrical waveform information.

The diagnostic performance of this lead system was compared to the more classical and widely used routine systems such as the Frank leads and the 12-lead standard ECG. Multivariate statistical procedures were also involved in this study in seeking optimal discriminators for bigroup comparisons.

The results show an overall increase in the number of correctly classified patients of 21% when compared to the Frank leads and 14% when compared to the 12-lead standard ECG. Only QRS complexes were considered and 8 variables for each QRS waveform were taken into consideration. Some improvement is expected from the addition of STT and P information, but the authors are afraid that although some increase in sensitivity will occur, it might be offset by a decrease in specificity.

The authors believe that the greatest improvements will result from more thoroughly assessed and more sophisticated statistical procedures for class separations. Once these results are achieved and controlled, practical, cheap and reliable tools and parameters will be made available to the clinician for daily utilization. The patient and the physician will both be winners.

References

[1] R. H. Okada, A critical review of vector electrocardiography, IEE Trans. BME 10 (1963) 53.

[2] B. Taccardi, Distribution of heart potentials on the thoracic surface of normal human subjects, Circ. Res. 12 (1963) 341.

[3] L. G. Horan, N. C. Flowers, and D. A. Brody, The limits of information in the VCG: Comparative synthesis of body surface potentials with different lead systems, Am. Heart J. 68 (1964) 362.

[4] J. T. Flaherty, M. S. Spach, J. P. Boineau, R. V. Canent, R. C. Barr, and D. C. Sabiston, Cardiac potentials on body surface of infants with anomalous left coronary artery (Myocardial infarction), Circul. 36 (1967) 345.

[5] J. H. Holt Jr., A. C. L. Barnard, M. S. Lynn, and P. Svendsen, A study of the human heart as a multiple dipole electrical source, I. Normal adult male subjects, Circulation 40 (1969) 687.

[6] D. B. Geselowitz, Some comments on the status of ECG lead systems. In: C. Zywietz and B. Schneider (Eds.), Computer application on ECG and VCG analysis (North-Holland, Amsterdam, 1973), p. 11.

[7] A. M. Scher, A. C. Young, and W. M. Meredith, Factor analysis of the electrocardiogram, Circ. Res. 8 (1960) 519.

[8] L. G. Horan, N. C. Flowers, and D. A. Brody, Principal factor waveforms of the thoracic QRS complex, Circ. Res. 15 (1964) 131.

[9] F. Kornreich, Missing information in different VCG systems. In: S. Rush and E. Lepeschkin (Eds.), Advances in cardiology: Body surface mapping of cardiac fields (S. Karger, Basle, 1974), vol. 10, p. 178.

[10] H. V. Pipberger, Computer analysis of the electrocardiogram. Computers and Biomedical Research (Academic Press, New York, 1965), p. 337.

[11] R. Gamboa, J. D. Klingeman, and H. V. Pipberger, Computer diagnosis of biventricular hypertrophy from the orthogonal electrocardiogram, Circulation 39 (1969) 72.

[12] A. Kerr, Jr., A. Adicoff, J. D. Klingeman, and H. V. Pipberger, Computer analysis of the orthogonal electrocardiogram in pulmonary emphysema, Am. J. Cardiol. 25 (1970) 34.

[13] E. E. Eddleman, Jr., and H. V. Pipberger, Computer analysis of the orthogonal electrocardiogram and vectorcardiogram in 1,002 patients with myocardial infarction, Am. Heart J. 81 (1971) 608.

[14] W. J. Dixon, Biomedical Computer Programs (B.M.D.), University of California Publications in Automatic Computation, No. 2 (University of California Press, Berkeley, 1970).

[15] A. C. L. Barnard, A. J. Merrill, Jr., J. H. Holt, Jr., and J. D. Kramer, Jr., Progress in the evaluation of multiple dipole electrocardiography in a clinical environment (including results in 77 cases of myocardial infarction. In: I. Hoffman (Ed.), Vectorcardiography 2 (North-Holland, Amsterdam, 1971), p. 404.

[16] H. T. Dodge, H. Sandler, D. W. Ballew, and J. D. Lord, Use of biplane angiocardiography for the measurement of left ventricular volume in man, Am. Heart J. 60 (1960) 762.

[17] C. E. Rackley, H. T. Dodge, Y. D. Coble, and R. E. Hay, Method for determining left ventricular mass in man, Circulation 29 (1964) 666.

[18] J. W. Kennedy, W. A. Baxley, M. M. Figley, H. T. Dodge, and J. R. Blackman, Quantitative angiocardiography: Normal left ventricle in man, Circulation 34 (1966) 272.

[19] J. H. Holt, Jr., A. C. L. Barnard, M. S. Lynn, and J. O. Kramer, Jr., A study of the human heart as a multiple dipole electrical source: III. Diagnosis and quantitation of right ventricular hypertrophy, Circulation 40 (1969) 711.

[20] F. Kornreich, P. Block, and D. Brismee, IV. Computer diagnosis of biventricular hypertrophy from "maximal" surface waveform information, Circulation 49 (1974) 1223.

[21] F. Kornreich, P. Block, and D. Brismee, III. Computer diagnosis of angina pectoris from "maximal" QRS surface waveform information at rest, Circulation 49 (1974) 1212.

[22] J. Cornfield, Statistical classification methods. In: J. A. Jacquez (Ed.), Computer Diagnosis and diagnostic methods (Charles C. Thomas, Springfield, Ill., 1972), p. 108.

[23] J. Cornfield, R. A. Dunn, C. D. Batchlor, and H. V. Pipberger, Multigroup diagnosis of electrocardiograms, Comput. Biomed. Res. 6 (1973) 97.

[24] F. Kornreich, The missing waveform information in the orthogonal electrocardiogram (Frank leads). I. Where and how can the missing waveform be retrieved? Circulation 48 (1973) 984.

Vectorcardiography 3 I. Hoffman and R.I. Hamby eds.
© 1976 North-Holland Publishing Company - Amsterdam

ORTHOGONAL ELECTROCARDIOGRAPH CORRELATIVE STUDY OF

100 CHILDREN WITH PURE CARDIAC DEFECTS

Moo Hee Lee, Jerome Liebman, and Wilma Mackay

From the Rainbow Babies and Children's Hospital, Cleveland, Ohio,
and the Departments of Pediatrics and Biometry, Case Western
Reserve University School of Medicine

Our present state of knowledge in electrocardiography indicates tremendous gaps as to what electrocardiographic information is reflected on the surface of the torso [1]. Because of known distortions in standard electrocardiography, "corrected" lead systems were developed, based on the principle that the electrical generator could be considered as a simple dipole. According to these systems, each instant of electrical activity could be described in terms of its X (right-left), Y (superior-inferior) and Z (anterior-posterior) axes, with each axis 90 degrees from the other. In the last few years, excellent work from various groups, utilizing body surface potential mapping, has indicated that the electrical generator does not act as a dipole during much of the activation sequence [2, 3]. In abnormal states, the lack of a simple dipole may be even more important. But, surface mapping as a clinical tool is in its infancy. Correlations with hemodynamics and other pathophysiological states have so far been minimal. Much research needs to be done before its usefulness can be ascertained. It may be, in fact, that surface mapping may always be only a research tool, though we are hopeful that with special recording methods and simple computer techniques, clinical usefulness will be practical. Meanwhile, however, it is incumbent upon us to continue to work with the best methods of practical usefulness today. Therefore, continued studies with the orthogonal electrocardiogram are indicated.

Previous correlative work in our laboratory has clearly demonstrated the superiority of the quantitated Frank lead system [4] orthogonal electrocardiogram over the quantitated non-orthogonal cube system and the quantitated frontal and horizontal plane standard electrocardiogram. This superiority has been demonstrated in many and diverse disease states, including cystic fibrosis [5, 6], sickle cell disease [7] and various congenital cardiac anomalies [8-12]. However, the study of Brody and Arzbaecher [13] provided considerable theoretical evidence that the McFee-Parungao lead system [14] would be more accurate than that of the Frank and many other lead systems. In addition, the study of Gamboa [15] specifically indicated the likelihood of the McFee-Parungao system

being more accurate in children where the hearts are larger in relation to the chest than in adults. Finally, in only the above two "orthogonal" lead systems have significant numbers of quantifications in normal children been obtained [16-25].

Appropriate statistical analyses for electrocardiographic parameters have been developed [26-31], but it is still not known which parameters are most useful in predicting which hemodynamic measurement. Therefore, a study was begun to attempt to determine which of the two most popular orthogonal lead systems can most accurately predict the specific hemodynamics of various congenital cardiac lesions, and to determine which electrocardiographic parameters are most useful in such predictions. This small initial group of patients provides a pilot study.

Methodology

A total of 100 children with "pure" right or left sided cardiac disease were studied. All were patients admitted to the hospital for cardiac catheterization on the basis of their clinical need. In all children, orthogonal electrocardiograms were taken during the day prior to the catheterization. In each case the order of taking the electrocardiograms was that of standard electrocardiography, followed by the Frank system, followed by the McFee-Parungao system. The orthogonal electrocardiograms were recorded on a specially constructed DR-8 Electronics for Medicine machine modified so that the P, QRS and T vectors could be recorded separately. Initial QRS vectors were all well delineated by trace shifting (moving the strip chart recorded during inscription of the loop). In addition, the scalars X, Y and Z could be taken simultaneously with two loops (Horizontal, Frontal and Sagittal). The data were also recorded on a Hewlett-Packard seven-channel tape recorder using half-inch tape.

Two separate programs have been developed. The first is the analysis program and involves measurement of the X, Y and Z parameters at each .001 second. This part is designed to be accomplished either by automatic analysis or by hand, the latter being utilized in this study. The second part of the program is fed by the first part no matter how obtained and involves a computer analysis into multiple measurement groupings as previously described [19].

Supported in part by National Institutes of Health Training Grant #HE 05803 and Research Grant #HE 08286.

Further appropriate statistics then follow as indicated, utilizing the computer. Originally, the computer utilized was the IBM 1620, but the latter has now been replaced by the PDP-11-45. These groupings are:

(1) Total Duration
    (2) Duration Terminal Right
    (3) Duration Terminal Right/Duration Total
    (4) Duration Anterior
    (5) Duration Anterior/Duration Total

Maximal Projections
    (6) X Initial Right (XIR)
    (7) X Left (XL)
    (8) X Terminal Right (XTR)
    (9) Y Initial Superior (YIS)
    (10) Y Inferior (YInf)
    (11) Y Terminal Superior (YTS)
    (12) Z Anterior (ZA)
    (13) Z Posterior (ZP)

Ratios of Maximal Projections
    (14) X Terminal Right/X Left (XTR/XL)
    (15) Y Terminal Superior/Y Inferior (YTS/Y Inf)
    (16) Z Anterior/Z Posterior (ZA/ZP)
    (17) Maximal Spatial Angles and Magnitudes QRS + T
    (18) Angular Deviation of T from QRS

Spatial Magnitudes and Orientations
    (19) Maximal Spatial Magnitude to Right (MSVR)
    (20) Maximal Spatial Magnitude to Left (MSVL)
    (21) Sum of Maximal Spatial Magnitudes to Right (SMSVR)
    (22) Sum of Maximal Spatial Magnitudes to Left (SMSVL)
    (23) Spatial Prevalent Directions α or A and B or β
    (24) Planar vectors and Magnitudes
    (25) Percentile Caps
    (26) Angles and Magnitudes at each .01 Second Vector
    (27) Normalized Angles and Magnitudes into each 1/10 Vector (only portions of the above are to be reported in this report)

Finally, various correlations, simple and multiple, were obtained against multiple hemodynamic measurements:

Hemodynamic Parameters
    (1) Systemic Flow (QS)
    (2) Pulmonary Flow (QP)
    (3) Effective Pulmonary Flow (QEP)
    (4) Pulmonary/Systemic Flow Ratio (P/S)
    (5) L → R Shunt
    (6) R → L Shunt
    (7) % Shunt
    (8) Heart Rate (HR)
    (9) Right Atrial Mean Pressure (RAMP)
    (10) Right Ventricular Pressure (RVP)
    (11) Right Ventricular End-Diastolic Pressure (RVED)

    (12) Pulmonary Artery Pressure (PAP)
    (13) Left Atrial Mean Pressure (LAMP)
    (14) Left Ventricular Pressure (LVP)
    (15) Left Ventricular End-Diastolic Pressure (LVED)
    (16) Arterial Pressure (ARTP)
    (17) Pulmonary Vascular Resistance (PVR)
    (18) Systemic Vascular Resistance (SVR)
    (19) Pulmonic Valve Area
    (20) Right Ventricular Work (RVW)
    (21) Left Ventricular Work (LVW)
    (22) Arterial Pressure/Right Ventricular Pressure Ratio (ATRP/RVP)
    (23) Left Ventricular Work/Right Ventricular Work Ratio (LVW/RVW)
    (24) Systemic Vascular Resistance/Pulmonary Vascular Resistance Ratio (SVR/PVR)

Of the 100 patients there were 27 with congenital valvular pulmonic stenosis (PS), 11 with secundum type atrial septal defect (ASD), 20 with congenital valvular aortic stenosis (AS), 18 with rheumatic mitral valve regurgitation (MR), 7 with coarctation of the aorta (CA), 6 with patent ductus arteriosus (PDA) and 11 with miscellaneous diagnoses but pure lesions. There were 42 patients with "pure" right sided lesions, including 4 from the miscellaneous group. The right volume load group (ASD plus tricuspid regurgitation and total anomalous pulmonary venous return) is 13 patients. The left pressure load group (AS plus CA plus endocardial fibroelastosis) is 30 patients. The left volume load group (MR plus PDA plus aortic regurgitation) totalled 28 patients.

As part of this pilot study the data were statistically examined in multiple ways, only some of which will be reported in the results section.

Results

Not all the data could be put in tables. Tables 1-9 contain some of the most useful for the entire group of 100 patients.

Specific correlations of magnitudes of maximal projections and spatial vectors with simple hemodynamic parameters.

Pulmonic Stenosis (Right ventricular pressure or work vs orthogonal ECG parameters).

Utilizing only simple projections and spatial magnitudes, right ventricular pressure correlated approximately equally in the Frank to Z anterior (ZA) (R = .60) (figure 1), X Terminal R (XTR) (R = .54) (figure 2), and maximal spatial vector to the right (MSVR) (R = .55) (figure 3). There was no significant difference among the three. The sum of maximal

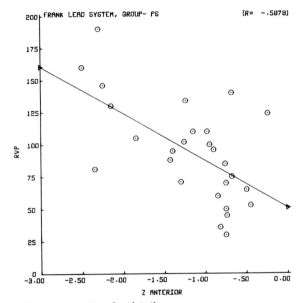

Fig. 1. See text for details.

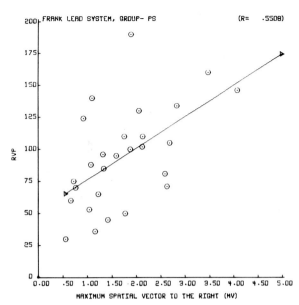

Fig. 3. See text for details.

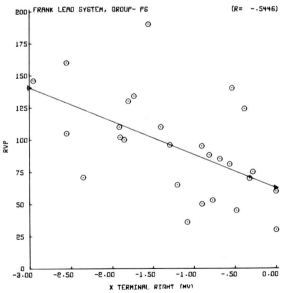

Fig. 2. See text for details.

spatial vectors to the right (SMSVR) had a lower correlation coefficient of .46. For the McFee system, correlation for each of the parameters was lower, at ZA (R = .29) (figure 4), XTR (R = .49) (figure 5), and MSVL (R = .39 (figure 6).

A multiple regression analysis was then performed on the data of 23 patients where all electrocardiographic data were reliably measurable. The data indicated very little improvement.

Frank
ZA (R = .68)	XTR (R = .74)	Mag N.40(R = .74)
p < .005	p < .005	P < .005

McFee
XTR (R = .56)	ZA (R = .67)	Mag N.40(R = .64)
P < .005	P < .01	P < .05

When right ventricular work (RVW) was correlated against vectorcardiographic parameters in pulmonic stenosis there was only a small increase in the correlation coefficient for the Frank system (ZA at R = .68 (figure 7), though XTR (R = .55) and MSVR (R = .56) remained the same.

For the total group of patients with pure right sided lesions, the correlation coefficients for ZA, XTR and MSVR against RVW decreased to .43, .42 and .39 on the Frank system. With McFee, the correlation coefficients were .32, .36 and .33. For this total group, in each system the best correlation was for the SMSVR at .43 for the Frank and .39 for McFee.

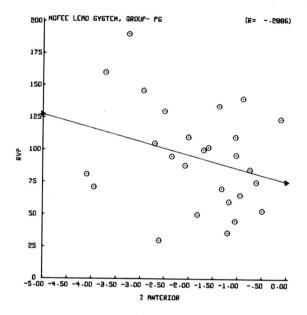

Fig. 4. See text for details.

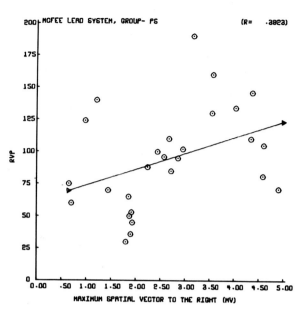

Fig. 6. See text for details.

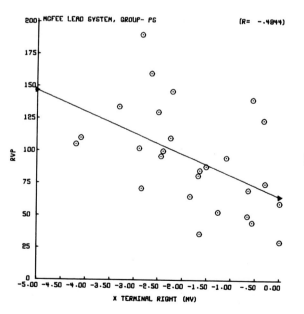

Fig. 5. See text for details.

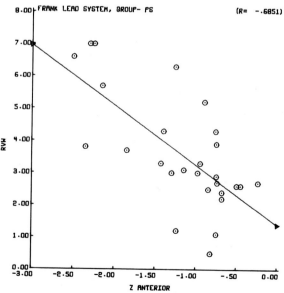

Fig. 7. See text for details.

Aortic Stenosis (Left Ventricular Pressure).

Utilizing only simple projections and spatial magnitudes, left ventricular pressure correlated best with XTR where the coefficient was .68 for the Frank system (figure 8) and .60 for McFee (figure 9). The next best correlation was Z posterior (ZR) at R = .52 for Frank (figure 10) and R = .40 for McFee (figure 11). The MSVL was .48 for Frank (figure 12) and .30 for McFee (figure 13). There was no correlation in either system to X left (XL).

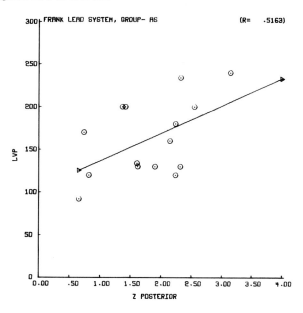

Fig. 10. See text for details.

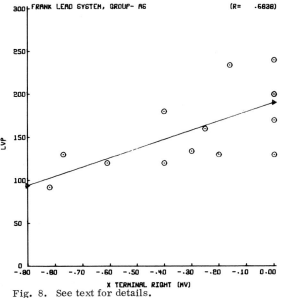

Fig. 8. See text for details.

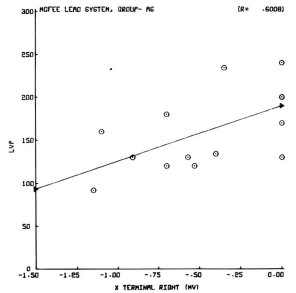

Fig. 9. See text for details.

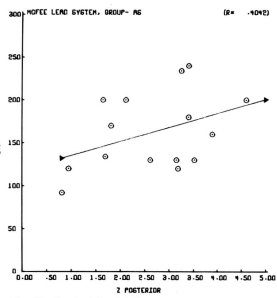

Fig. 11. See text for details.

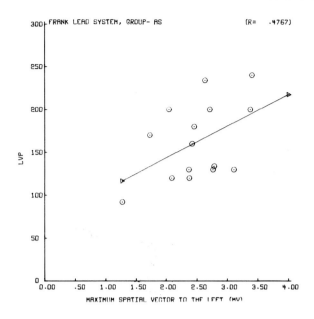

Fig. 12. See text for details.

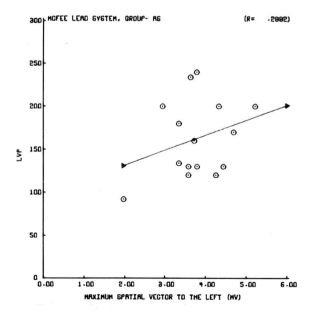

Fig. 13. See text for details.

For the total left pressure load group, the best correlation was also XTR. It was .61 for Frank and .61 for McFee.

A multiple regression analysis was then performed on the data of 15 patients where all possible electrocardiographic data were reliably measurable. The data indicated considerable improvement.

Frank

ZA/ZP (.70)	N.80(.86)	XTR (.92)
$p < .005$	$p < .005$	$p < .005$

McFee

XTR (.60)	N.40(.73)	ZA/ZP (.87)
$p < .025$	$p < .025$	$p < .01$

When the systolic gradient (LVP - systemic arterial pressure) was the hemodynamic variable, the regression was different:

Frank

XTR (.73)	Total duration (.83)	XL (.89)
$p < .005$	$p < .005$	$p < .005$

McFee

XTR (.67)	Total duration (.74)	N.40(.85)
$p < .025$	$p < .005$	$p < .025$

Specific ECG variables in various lesions as compared to the normal.

QRS Durations (table 1)
Both left and right sided lesions caused slightly greater duration of the QRS vector than in the normal, with no difference in the right group versus the left, but with the volume overload group having slightly greater duration. As expected, the right overload patients had a greater duration to the right. Of the left sided group, coarctation of the aorta (CA) had the greatest duration to the right. The durations were essentially the same in both systems attesting to the accuracy of the hand analysis.

Maximal Projections on the X axis (table 2)
Initial X to Right (IXR). The left sided lesions have a greater initial X to the right than normal, while the right sided lesions have a less than normal magnitude. The greatest increase to the right is in the left sided volume overload group. In left pressure overload there is frequently no initial X to the right as is also often the case in the right sided lesions with marked hypertrophy.

X Left (XL). The maximal projection to the left is increased in the left overload group, but not very decreased in the right overload group. In ASD, the X left was normal.

Table 1

QRS Durations (seconds)

	N	Total Duration		Duration Right		Duration Right/ Duration Total	
		Mean	ST.D.	Mean	ST.D.	Mean	ST.D.
Frank Lead System							
Total Normal	341	.097	.030	.027	.016	.28	.13
AS	20	.107	.037	.023	.023	.21	.19
CA	7	.112	.028	.033	.021	.30	.19
MI	18	.118	.035	.021	.023	.17	.17
PDA	6	.072	.038	.020	.025	.19	.20
AS, CA, EFE	30	.107	.034	.026	.022	.24	.19
AI, MI, PDA	28	.111	.039	.021	.021	.17	.16
Total Left	58	.109	.036	.023	.022	.21	.18
PS	27	.107	.035	.049	.025	.45	.19
ASD	11	.118	.033	.056	.020	.47	.09
PS, PPS	28	.107	.034	.049	.025	.45	.19
ASD, TAP	14	.118	.029	.056	.018	.47	.08
Total Right	42	.110	.033	.051	.023	.46	.16
McFee Lead System							
Total Normal	341	.097	.029	.025	.018	.26	.16
AS	20	.109	.037	.024	.022	.21	.19
CA	7	.112	.028	.035	.021	.33	.19
MI	18	.121	.035	.025	.027	.19	.19
PDA	6	.071	.040	.018	.026	.17	.20
AS, CA, EFE	30	.109	.034	.028	.022	.25	.19
AI, MI, PDA	28	.113	.041	.022	.025	.17	.18
Total Left	58	.111	.037	.025	.024	.21	.19
PS	27	.105	.035	.051	.028	.47	.17
ASD	11	.119	.032	.058	.020	.48	.10
PS, PPS	28	.105	.034	.051	.027	.46	.17
ASD, TAP	14	.118	.028	.057	.018	.48	.09
Total Right	42	.109	.033	.053	.024	.47	.14

X Terminal Right (XTR). The magnitude of X terminal right was above normal in the right overload group, particularly for pressure overloads. For the left sided group, the XTR was abnormally to the right in the presence of left sided pressure overload.

Maximal Projections on the Y axis (table 3)
Y initial superior (YIS). There is an increase in Y initial superior in the six patients with PDA in the Frank system and in the left volume overload group in the McFee system. These include mainly the same patients which demonstrated a large magnitude initial X right.
Y Terminal Superior (YTS). There is a moderate increase in YTS in the right sided group, but the largest increase was in mitral regurgitation.

Maximal Projections on the Z axis (table 4)
Z Anterior (ZA). There is an increase in ZA in the right pressure overload group, but not in the right volume overload group. In the left sided group, the large increase in PDA probably reflected associated pulmonary hypertension so that the PDA group was not pure.
Z Posterior (ZP). There was an increase in ZP in the left sided group and a decrease in ZP in the right sided group. The greatest increase in ZP was in the left pressure overload group.

Table 2

Maximal Projections on the X Axis

	N	Frank							McFee						
		Mean Mag.#	ST.D.	P05	P10	P50	P90	P95	Mean Mag.	ST.D.	P05	P10	P50	P90	P95
X Initial Right															
Total Normal	341	.10	.10	0.00	0.00	.08	.23	.30	.17	.16	0.00	0.00	.14	.39	.50
AS	20	.08	.13	0.00	0.00	0.00	.26	.44	.16	.22	0.00	0.00	.08	.55	.74
CA	7	.08	.13	*	*	0.00	*	*	.08	.21	*	*	0.00	*	*
MI	18	.17	.17	*	*	.10	*	*	.28	.36	*	*	.14	*	*
PDA	6	.29	.62	*	*	.04	*	*	.62	1.04	*	*	.10	*	*
AS, CA, EFE	30	.08	.12	0.00	0.00	0.00	.26	.40	.13	.21	0.00	0.00	0.00	.55	.64
AI, MI, PDA	28	.18	.31	0.00	0.00	.10	.38	1.17	.34	.55	0.00	0.00	.14	.87	2.11
Total Left	58	.12	.23	0.00	0.00	.05	.30	.46	.23	.42	0.00	0.00	.10	.61	.83
PS	27	.08	.08	0.00	0.00	.06	.17	.29	.12	.16	0.00	0.00	.05	.38	.53
ASD	11	.05	.04	*	*	.05	*	*	.09	.09	*	*	.08	*	*
PS, PPS	28	.08	.08	0.00	0.00	.06	.16	.28	.11	.16	0.00	0.00	.05	.37	.53
ASD, TAP	14	.04	.04	*	*	.04	*	*	.07	.08	*	*	.03	*	*
Total Right	42	.07	.07	0.00	0.00	.05	.16	.19	.10	.14	0.00	0.00	.05	.31	.48
X Left															
Total Normal	341	1.06	.44	.46	.56	1.04	1.60	1.80	1.60	.57	.80	.93	1.50	2.40	2.60
AS	20	1.41	.66	.34	.81	1.30	2.04	3.39	2.33	.97	.92	1.08	2.22	3.73	4.37
CA	7	1.67	.64	*	*	1.58	*	*	2.23	.90	*	*	2.35	*	*
MI	18	1.25	.64	*	*	1.41	*	*	1.77	.98	*	*	1.85	*	*
PDA	6	1.21	.79	*	*	1.08	*	*	2.24	1.00	*	*	2.00	*	*
AS, CA, EFE	30	1.51	.67	.56	.80	1.46	2.42	3.12	2.37	.93	.82	1.08	2.35	3.69	4.04
AI, MI, PDA	28	1.23	.64	.17	.20	1.23	1.98	2.43	1.97	1.09	.31	.59	1.93	3.37	4.22
Total Left	58	1.37	.66	.20	.70	1.34	2.21	2.51	2.17	1.02	.60	.76	2.20	3.57	4.02
PS	27	.86	.45	.10	.31	.77	1.57	1.69	1.14	.71	.09	.21	1.10	2.24	2.72
ASD	11	1.00	.45	*	*	.86	*	*	1.45	.56	*	*	1.35	*	*
PS, PPS	28	.87	.44	.12	.31	.78	1.56	1.68	1.14	.69	.10	.21	1.14	2.22	2.69
ASD, TAP	14	.92	.44	*	*	.85	*	*	1.33	.56	*	*	1.18	*	*
Total Right	42	.88	.43	.20	.32	.81	1.54	1.73	1.21	.65	.20	.30	1.16	2.24	2.42
X Terminal Right															
Total Normal	341	.23	.19	0.00	0.00	.20	.50	.55	.29	.29	0.00	0.00	.25	.65	.80
AS	20	.27	.34	0.00	0.00	.18	.82	1.13	.41	.44	0.00	0.00	.38	1.15	1.20
CA	7	.48	.40	*	*	.40	*	*	.77	.62	*	*	.75	*	*
MI	18	.09	.15	*	*	.04	*	*	.27	.38	*	*	.03	*	*
PDA	6	.51	.72	*	*	.08	*	*	.73	1.16	*	*	.08	*	*
AS, CA, EFE	30	.38	.40	0.00	0.00	.28	1.12	1.30	.60	.57	0.00	0.00	.52	1.43	1.81
AI, MI, PDA	28	.18	.38	0.00	0.00	.05	.68	1.44	.33	.62	0.00	0.00	0.00	1.22	2.18
Total Left	58	.28	.40	0.00	0.00	.10	.85	1.37	.47	.60	0.00	0.00	.23	1.22	1.80
PS	27	1.21	.82	0.00	.22	1.08	2.55	2.79	1.79	1.19	0.00	.24	1.68	3.47	4.16
ASD	11	.74	.58	*	*	.59	*	*	1.14	.83	*	*	.90	*	*
PS, PPS	28	1.20	.81	0.00	.25	.99	2.55	2.77	1.77	1.17	0.00	.27	1.67	3.39	4.16
ASD, TAP	14	.79	.52	*	*	.79	*	*	1.18	.76	*	*	1.08	*	*
Total Right	42	1.06	.75	.02	.20	.85	2.31	2.55	1.57	1.08	.02	.23	1.46	3.01	3.98

*When less than 20 patients, no percentiles.　　#All magnitudes in millivolts.　　TAP = Total anomalous pulmonary venous return.

Table 3

Maximal Projections on the Y Axis

	N	Frank							McFee						
		Mean Mag.	ST.D.	P05	P10	P50	P90	P95	Mean Mag.	ST.D.	P05	P10	P50	P90	P95
Y Initial Superior															
Total Normal	341	.10	.08	0.00	0.00	.08	.20	.25	.11	.11	0.00	0.00	.10	.25	.32
AS	20	.06	.07	0.00	0.00	.05	.18	.21	.07	.09	0.00	0.00	0.00	.21	.30
CA	7	.09	.10	*	*	.06	*	*	.10	.13	*	*	.05	*	*
MI	18	.10	.12	*	*	.09	*	*	.15	.19	*	*	.05	*	*
PDA	6	.21	.32	*	*	.09	*	*	.24	.33	*	*	.10	*	*
AS, CA, EFE	30	.08	.10	0.00	0.00	.05	.21	.37	.10	.18	0.00	0.00	0.00	.29	.59
AI, MI, PDA	28	.12	.18	0.00	0.00	.08	.28	.69	.16	.22	0.00	0.00	.10	.47	.78
Total Left	58	.10	.15	0.00	0.00	.05	.22	.46	.13	.20	0.00	0.00	.05	.35	.65
PS	27	.13	.15	0.00	0.00	.10	.37	.54	.14	.15	0.00	0.00	.10	.37	.54
ASD	11	.08	.09	*	*	.05	*	*	.11	.14	*	*	.06	*	*
PS, PPS	28	.14	.15	0.00	0.00	.10	.36	.54	.13	.15	0.00	0.00	.10	.36	.53
ASD, TAP	14	.10	.09	*	*	.05	*	*	.14	.14	*	*	.12	*	*
Total Right	42	.12	.13	0.00	0.00	.09	.25	.44	.13	.15	0.00	0.00	.10	.34	.44
Y Inferior															
Total Normal	341	1.15	.40	.58	.65	1.12	1.70	1.88	1.48	.53	.73	.85	1.40	2.19	2.35
AS	20	1.80	.77	.96	.97	1.58	3.10	3.34	2.33	1.01	1.25	1.30	2.01	4.30	4.59
CA	7	1.73	.98	*	*	1.28	*	*	1.85	.78	*	*	1.75	*	*
MI	18	1.05	.63	*	*	.83	*	*	1.44	.79	*	*	1.24	*	*
PDA	6	1.08	.58	*	*	.99	*	*	1.60	.52	*	*	1.61	*	*
AS, CA, EFE	30	1.82	.81	.81	.97	1.58	3.10	3.38	2.25	.97	.96	1.30	2.01	3.55	4.48
AI, MI, PDA	28	1.10	.60	.06	.17	.94	2.04	2.11	1.57	.74	.28	.56	1.48	2.58	2.92
Total Left	58	1.47	.80	.18	.62	1.27	2.60	3.12	1.92	.93	.56	.91	1.71	3.26	3.61
PS	27	1.21	.64	.20	.37	1.20	2.22	2.58	1.64	.89	.37	.49	1.50	2.98	3.74
ASD	11	.79	.35	*	*	.75	*	*	1.18	.49	*	*	1.25	*	*
PS, PPS	28	1.19	.64	.21	.38	1.15	2.20	2.56	1.62	.88	.38	.50	1.48	2.97	3.68
ASD, TAP	14	.78	.35	*	*	.77	*	*	1.15	.47	*	*	1.18	*	*
Total Right	42	1.05	.59	.18	.36	1.02	1.92	2.36	1.46	.79	.47	.51	1.32	2.41	3.04
Y Terminal Superior															
Total Normal	341	.10	.12	0.00	0.00	.07	.26	.32	.17	.19	0.00	0.00	.15	.42	.50
AS	20	.09	.11	0.00	0.00	.03	.29	.35	.17	.21	0.00	0.00	.10	.49	.71
CA	7	.18	.17	*	*	.24	*	*	.23	.19	*	*	.34	*	*
MI	18	.22	.29	*	*	.13	*	*	.34	.50	*	*	.18	*	*
PDA	6	.04	.06	*	*	0.00	*	*	.06	.14	*	*	0.00	*	*
AS, CA, EFE	30	.14	.19	0.00	0.00	.08	.35	.60	.22	.26	0.00	0.00	.15	.50	.89
AI, MI, PDA	28	.15	.25	0.00	0.00	.03	.50	.91	.25	.43	0.00	0.00	.05	.78	1.60
Total Left	58	.14	.22	0.00	0.00	.05	.37	.81	.23	.34	0.00	0.00	.10	.52	1.12
PS	27	.22	.23	0.00	0.00	.18	.62	.70	.26	.31	0.00	0.00	.15	.74	.96
ASD	11	.19	.17	*	*	.18	*	*	.30	.30	*	*	.25	*	*
PS, PPS	28	.21	.23	0.00	0.00	.17	.61	.70	.25	.30	0.00	0.00	.15	.72	.96
ASD, TAP	14	.20	.16	*	*	.19	*	*	.29	.27	*	*	.25	*	*
Total Right	42	.21	.21	0.00	0.00	.18	.56	.67	.27	.29	0.00	0.00	.20	.70	.95

Table 4

Maximal Projections on the Z Axis

		Frank							McFee						
	N	Mean Mag.	ST.D.	P05	P10	P50	P90	P95	Mean Mag.	ST.D.	P05	P10	P50	P90	P95
Z Anterior															
Total Normal	341	.57	.29	.16	.23	.55	.94	1.08	.91	.46	.26	.37	.85	1.50	1.75
AS	20	.53	.35	0.00	.02	.48	1.09	1.29	.98	.65	0.00	.02	.85	2.00	2.10
CA	7	.73	.35	*	*	.76	*	*	1.10	.54	*	*	1.37	*	*
MI	18	.90	.57	*	*	.78	*	*	1.38	.86	*	*	1.23	*	*
PDA	6	1.02	.98	*	*	.84	*	*	2.08	1.47	*	*	2.29	*	*
AS, CA, EFE	30	.63	.40	0.00	.16	.57	1.25	1.39	1.15	.75	0.00	.17	1.21	2.09	2.84
AI, MI, PDA	28	.85	.65	.13	.17	.64	2.16	2.47	1.46	1.01	.14	.40	1.20	3.40	3.62
Total Left	58	.74	.54	.10	.17	.60	1.36	2.15	1.30	.89	.10	.29	1.20	2.73	3.40
PS	27	1.18	.64	.32	.49	.95	2.31	2.44	1.83	1.09	.27	.59	1.60	3.77	4.04
ASD	11	.51	.34	*	*	.42	*	*	.91	.61	*	*	.75	*	*
PS, PPS	28	1.18	.63	.33	.50	.97	2.31	2.48	1.82	1.07	.29	.60	1.65	3.74	4.03
ASD, TAP	14	.63	.44	*	*	.47	*	*	1.09	.78	*	*	.90	*	*
Total Right	42	1.00	.63	.17	.31	.82	2.22	2.34	1.58	1.03	.18	.51	1.26	3.17	3.92
Z Posterior															
Total Normal	341	.97	.40	.32	.48	.94	1.45	1.70	1.42	.62	.44	.64	1.40	2.20	2.55
AS	20	2.07	.86	.66	.75	2.10	3.38	3.83	3.06	1.29	.83	1.02	3.17	4.99	5.29
CA	7	1.38	.84	*	*	1.37	*	*	2.19	1.20	*	*	2.00	*	*
MI	18	1.26	.70	*	*	1.33	*	*	1.77	1.05	*	*	1.72	*	*
PDA	6	1.27	.97	*	*	1.17	*	*	2.07	1.19	*	*	1.73	*	*
AS, CA, EFE	30	1.90	.89	.44	.67	1.96	3.14	3.60	2.89	1.34	.74	1.02	2.91	4.99	5.35
AI, MI, PDA	28	1.30	.72	.11	.42	1.32	2.37	2.82	1.83	1.00	.31	.64	1.69	3.51	3.78
Total Left	58	1.61	.86	.25	.50	1.54	2.96	3.16	2.38	1.29	.64	.81	2.06	4.51	5.02
PS	27	.57	.53	0.00	.01	.40	1.44	1.79	.97	.79	.04	.14	.74	2.29	2.68
ASD	11	.51	.54	*	*	.44	*	*	.81	.87	*	*	.71	*	*
PS, PPS	28	.59	.54	0.00	.01	.47	1.42	1.78	1.02	.83	.05	.15	.78	2.43	2.68
ASD, TAP	14	.46	.49	*	*	.43	*	*	.74	.80	*	*	.66	*	*
Total Right	42	.55	.52	0.00	.00	.43	1.39	1.87	.93	.82	0.00	.11	.73	2.34	2.69

Ratios of Maximal Projections (table 5)

Since the pressure overload group in general demonstrates greater increases in voltages than does the volume overload group, the ratios assume great importance.

XTR/XL. In the right sided group, this is well above normal, though it is not significantly changed from normal in the left group. In coarctation of the aorta, however, XTR/XL is increased above normal.

YTS/Y Inf. The ratio increased markedly in mitral regurgitation and decreased in left pressure loads. It was not changed in the right sided group.

ZA/ZP. For the left sided pressure overload group, the ratio decreased, while in the volume overload, the ratio increased. In the right sided lesions, the ratio increased considerably, but not in ASD.

Maximal Spatial Angles and Magnitudes--QRS and T (table 6)

QRS Orientation. The left sided group is oriented more posteriorly than the right sided group. The left sided pressure overload group is oriented more posteriorly than is the volume overload group. In the right sided group, ASD is not oriented as anteriorly as is the pressure overload group. The spatial magnitudes are greater for pressure overloads than volume overloads.

T Orientation. In left sided pressure overload, the T vector is oriented more anterior than in volume overloads. In the right sided group, the pressure overload causes the T vector to be oriented more anterior than in the volume overload group. The magnitude of the spatial T vector is greater in the pressure overload group than in volume overload.

Angular Deviation of T from QRS (table 7)

A brief explanation is necessary (as previously published). The prevalent direction A is the "average" of the clockwise deviation of T from QRS for the sample. If QRS is 340° and T is 20°, then A is 40°. If T is 340° and QRS is 20°, then A is 320°. The D is a measure of dispersion; the higher the D (maximal 1.0) the less the dispersion of the data. The higher the Ch Square, the better can the D value be trusted.

Clearly, the relation of QRS to T is very different in the right sided from the left sided group. The deviation is greater in the right sided lesions with most of the change from normal being in the QRS.

Maximal Spatial Vector to the Right (MSVR) (table 8)

For right pressure loads, the magnitude of MSVR is greater than for volume loads. It is also oriented more anteriorly. It is of interest that for left sided lesions, MSVR is also increased, especially for left pressure overloads. The MSVR is oriented more posteriorly in left pressure than left volume overloads.

Maximal Spatial Vector to the Left (MSVL) (table 9)

For left pressure loads, the magnitude of MSVL is greater than in left volume overloads. There is no change in MSVL for right sided lesions. However, the orientation is posterior for left sided overloads and anterior for right sided overloads.

Comparison of Change in Specific Projections and Spatial Magnitudes in the Two Lead Systems as Compared to Normal in the Various Groups of Lesions.

For this analysis we were interested in the sensitivity of the system for diagnostic purposes. Thus, if a specific linear parameter increases in magnitude more in the Frank system than in the McFee in response to a disease, then the Frank system is more sensitive diagnostically. There is no attempt here to relate the change in parameter to prediction of hemodynamics. All measurements discussed are mean magnitudes for the group.

Total Right Sided Lesions (42 patients).

The best single measurement for RVH was XTR where in Frank the increase was from .23 to 1.06 and in McFee the increase was .29 to 1.57. The ratio of F/M was 1.06/1.57 = .68 (normal = .79). Thus, the increase in McFee was 442%, while that in Frank was 362%.

An increase in ZA was approximately the same as was the increase in MSVR. For ZA the increase was 75% for Frank and 74% for McFee. For MSVR the increase was 60% for Frank and 100% for McFee. An increase in YTS was 91% for Frank and 59% for McFee.

Pulmonic Stenosis (27 patients).

The best single measurement for RVH was XTR where in Frank the increase was from .23 to 1.21 and in McFee the increase was from .29 to 1.79. The ratio of F/M was 1.21/1.79 = .68 (normal = .79). Thus, the increase in McFee was 517%, while that in Frank was 426%.

An increase in ZA was approximately the same as was the increase in MSVR. For ZA the increase was 104% for Frank and 101% for McFee. For MSVR the increase was 87% for Frank and 110% for McFee.

An increase in YTS was 100% for Frank and 53% for McFee.

Atrial Septal Defect (11 patients).

The best single measurement for RVH was XTR where in Frank the increase was from .23 to .74 and in McFee the increase was from .29 to 1.14. The ratio of F/M was .74/1.14 = .53 (normal = .79). Thus, the increase in McFee was 293% while that in Frank was 221%.

Table 5

Ratios of Maximal Projections

	N	Frank							McFee						
		Mean Mag.	ST.D.	P05	P10	P50	P90	P95	Mean Mag.	ST.D.	P05	P10	P50	P90	P95
X Terminal Right/X Left															
AS	20	.28	.38	0.00	0.00	.13	.93	1.21	.24	.30	0.00	0.00	.20	.81	1.06
CA	7	.42	.53	*	*	.20	*	*	.60	.88	*	*	.25	*	*
MI	18	.07	.10	*	*	.04	*	*	.21	.34	*	*	.01	*	*
PDA	6	.27	.37	*	*	.08	*	*	.31	.49	*	*	.06	*	*
AS, CA, EFE	30	.34	.41	0.00	0.00	.20	.93	1.38	.35	.50	0.00	0.00	.23	.84	1.73
AI, MI, PDA	28	.11	.19	0.00	0.00	.04	.36	.73	.21	.36	0.00	0.00	.13	.92	1.16
Total Left	58	.23	.34	0.00	0.00	.10	.84	.95	.28	.44	0.00	0.00	.13	.86	1.10
PS	27	1.52	1.84	-2.28	0.00	1.57	3.50	5.94	3.50	6.55	0.00	.22	1.57	7.70	25.60
ASD	11	.78	.48	*	*	.63	*	*	.96	.76	*	*	.81	*	*
PS, PPS	28	1.50	1.81	-2.09	0.00	1.51	3.45	5.77	3.40	6.45	0.00	.24	1.51	6.85	24.68
ASD, TAP	14	.99	.66	*	*	.84	*	*	1.07	.71	*	*	.85	*	*
Total Right	42	1.33	1.53	0.00	.16	.99	3.16	3.82	2.62	5.36	.01	.14	1.38	5.28	13.23
Y Terminal Superior/Y Inferior															
AS	20	.06	.08	0.00	0.00	.01	.22	.27	.10	.14	0.00	0.00	.04	.38	.46
CA	7	.17	.21	*	*	.11	*	*	.20	.24	*	*	.12	*	*
MI	18	1.43	4.91	*	*	.08	*	*	.36	.73	*	*	.09	*	*
PDA	6	.03	.07	*	*	0.00	*	*	.06	.14	*	*	0.00	*	*
AS, CA, EFE	30	.11	.19	0.00	0.00	.03	.31	.70	.14	.21	0.00	0.00	.06	.45	.75
AI, MI, PDA	28	.93	3.96	0.00	0.00	.01	1.15	12.45	.25	.60	0.00	0.00	.03	.66	2.19
Total Left	58	.51	2.76	0.00	0.00	.03	.57	1.10	.20	.44	0.00	0.00	.06	.48	.86
PS	27	.37	.79	0.00	0.00	.12	.85	2.97	.27	.42	0.00	0.00	.08	.88	1.51
ASD	11	.25	.25	*	*	.22	*	*	.31	.33	*	*	.23	*	*
PS, PPS	28	.36	.78	0.00	0.00	.11	.78	2.84	.26	.41	0.00	0.00	.07	.80	1.51
ASD, TAP	14	.28	.26	*	*	.23	*	*	.31	.30	*	*	.24	*	*
Total Right	42	.33	.65	0.00	0.00	.13	.70	1.32	.28	.38	0.00	0.00	.12	.73	1.43
Z Anterior/Z Posterior															
AS	20	.31	.23	0.00	.01	.24	.67	.85	.40	.36	0.00	.01	.33	1.07	1.40
CA	7	.84	.94	*	*	.56	*	*	.69	.71	*	*	.47	*	*
MI	18	.82	.41	*	*	.74	*	*	.90	.39	*	*	.86	*	*
PDA	6	1.05	1.01	*	*	.84	*	*	1.03	.80	*	*	.92	*	*
AS, CA, EFE	30	.47	.55	0.00	.07	.36	.85	.08	.52	.51	0.00	.06	.34	1.39	1.92
Total Left	58	.63	.59	.07	.11	.51	1.38	1.83	.69	.53	.05	.16	.54	1.44	1.69
PS	27	6.08	15.72	-12.76	-2.23	1.90	22.83	54.40	2.68	10.50	-23.64	.38	1.81	14.08	23.75
ASD	11	3.16	7.31	*	*	.95	*	*	.51	8.18	*	*	-1.29	*	*
PS, PPS	28	5.89	15.46	-12.73	-.96	1.81	22.75	51.83	2.61	10.31	-21.66	.41	1.69	13.54	23.30
ASD, TAP	14	1.72	8.13	*	*	.86	*	*	2.31	10.73	*	*	1.11	*	*
Total Right	42	4.50	13.51	-12.91	-.58	1.39	19.02	24.78	.97	10.58	-29.09	.12	1.46	9.37	17.57

Table 6

Maximal Spatial Angles and Magnitudes--QRS + T

	N	A	B	D	Chi Sq.	Mean Mag.	ST.D.	P05	P10	P50	P90	P95
Frank Lead System												
QRS												
AS	20	300	130	.91	49.4	2.99	.98	1.29	1.76	2.75	4.76	5.04
CA	7	319	139	.77	12.4	2.65	.95	*	*	2.33	*	*
MI	18	331	120	.76	31.2	1.96	.82	*	*	2.05	*	*
PDA	6	336	135	.62	6.9	2.16	1.17	*	*	2.27	*	*
AS, CA, EFE	30	306	132	.84	63.8	2.96	.95	1.52	1.79	2.68	4.20	4.92
AI, MI, PDA	28	328	124	.75	47.2	2.04	.87	.23	.79	2.02	3.32	3.56
Total Left	58	317	129	.79	107.7	2.51	1.02	.82	1.24	2.44	3.94	4.24
PS	29	139	146	.52	21.8	2.10	.78	.81	1.02	2.11	3.00	3.84
ASD	11	6	134	.76	19.2	1.46	.67	*	*	1.42	*	*
PS, PPS	28	146	148	.51	21.9	2.08	.77	.82	1.03	2.10	2.94	3.81
ASD, TAP	14	18	141	2.65	17.7	1.48	.59	*	*	1.43	*	*
Total Right	42	98	162	.48	28.9	1.88	.77	.74	.96	1.76	2.80	3.39
T Wave												
AS	20	10	115	.65	25.4	.46	.17	.16	.24	.41	.74	.77
CA	7	344	125	.95	18.7	.43	.21	*	*	.36	*	*
MI	18	342	126	.88	41.9	.45	.20	*	*	.46	*	*
PDA	6	315	127	.90	14.4	.30	.16	*	*	.31	*	*
AS, CA, EFE	30	355	120	.69	43.2	.45	.18	.15	.20	.40	.72	.76
AI, MI, PDA	28	339	127	.85	60.9	.39	.19	.05	.14	.39	.60	.79
Total Left	58	347	124	.76	101.4	.42	.19	.14	.17	.40	.68	.74
PS	27	13	130	.77	47.9	.55	.29	.15	.18	.49	1.04	1.23
ASD	10	334	106	.67	13.6	.34	.17	*	*	.36	*	*
PS, PPS	28	14	129	.77	50.0	.55	.28	.15	.18	.49	1.02	1.23
ASD, TAP	13	337	107	.71	19.4	.32	.15	*	*	.35	*	*
Total Right	41	2	123	.71	62.7	.47	.27	.14	.17	.44	.75	1.15
McFee Lead System												
QRS												
AS	20	301	126	.82	40.5	4.34	1.18	2.02	3.00	4.11	5.85	6.91
CA	7	314	128	.68	9.6	3.41	.88	*	*	3.17	*	*
MI	18	326	118	.69	26.0	2.73	1.16	*	*	3.00	*	*
PDA	6	357	137	.45	3.6	3.56	1.23	*	*	3.88	*	*
AS, CA, EFE	30	306	126	.76	52.2	4.22	1.21	2.21	2.73	4.10	5.85	6.76
AI, MI, PDA	28	328	123	.66	36.0	3.04	1.22	.60	1.18	3.30	4.71	5.00
Total Left	58	316	125	.70	85.6	3.65	1.34	1.19	1.96	3.61	5.45	5.89
PS	27	161	137	.51	20.8	3.04	1.27	.84	1.23	2.84	4.94	5.09
ASD	11	6	138	.61	12.2	2.28	.98	*	*	1.88	*	*
PS, PPS	28	167	137	.50	20.9	3.03	1.25	.85	1.26	2.78	4.92	5.09
ASD, TAP	14	21	145	.53	12.0	2.29	.91	*	*	1.89	*	*
Total Right	42	144	159	.42	22.1	2.78	1.19	1.01	1.33	2.63	4.60	5.04
T Wave												
AS	20	9	114	.68	27.5	.69	.25	.16	.38	.69	1.02	1.23
CA	7	343	115	.89	16.6	.67	.17	*	*	.74	*	*
MI	18	352	123	.89	43.0	.60	.24	*	*	.56	*	*
PDA	6	318	138	.67	8.1	.55	.20	*	*	.51	*	*
AS, CA, EFE	29	356	115	.70	42.4	.69	.22	.27	.39	.71	1.02	1.13
AI, MI, PDA	28	351	127	.81	54.5	.58	.25	.12	.25	.56	.96	1.07
Total Left	57	354	121	.75	95.3	.64	.24	.15	.36	.62	.97	1.07
PS	26	23	128	.81	51.8	.69	.33	.19	.23	.68	1.06	1.39
ASD	10	350	116	.84	21.0	.55	.10	*	*	.56	*	*
PS, PPS	27	23	128	.82	54.5	.68	.33	.19	.24	.64	1.05	1.37
ASD, TAP	13	347	116	.84	27.5	.51	.14	*	*	.56	*	*
Total Right	40	10	125	.80	76.3	.63	.29	.20	.28	.59	1.00	1.08

A = α = Horizontal Spatial Angle 0 - 360°
B = β = Superior-Inferior Spatial Angle 0 - 180°
D - Dispersion
Chi Square = ND^2

Table 7

Angular Deviation of T from QRS

Frank Lead System

	N	D	Chi Sq.	A	P05	P10	P50	P90	P95
				Frontal Angular Deviation of T from QRS					
AS	20	.73	21.4	326	180	260	334	3	14
CA	7	.78	8.4	334	*	*	347	*	*
MI	18	.84	25.4	358	*	*	359	*	*
PDA	6	.60	4.3	4	*	*	0	*	*
AS, CA, EFE	30	.71	30.1	332	213	260	338	3	29
AI, MI, PDA	28	.80	35.5	358	246	321	3	27	100
Total Left	58	.73	62.1	345	241	280	351	17	42
PS	27	.39	8.1	284	137	203	282	10	54
ASD	10	.55	6.1	341	*	*	334	*	*
PS, PPS	28	.40	8.9	280	139	208	281	9	51
ASD, TAP	13	.46	5.5	332	*	*	332	*	*
Total Right	41	.38	11.9	298	131	163	294	9	13
				Sagittal Angular Deviation of T from QRS					
AS	20	.45	8.0	41	293	300	31	143	214
CA	7	.75	7.8	6	*	*	1	*	*
MI	18	.69	17.1	19	*	*	24	*	*
PDA	6	.46	2.4	350	*	*	346	*	*
AS, CA, EFE	30	.46	12.4	23	259	298	16	127	168
AI, MI, PDA	28	.62	21.6	18	258	306	24	90	154
Total Left	58	.54	33.3	21	280	302	21	122	147
PS	27	.39	8.1	329	177	220	335	126	141
ASD	10	.49	4.8	304	*	*	298	*	*
PS, PPS	28	.34	6.5	331	180	222	336	130	141
ASD, TAP	13	.51	6.7	314	*	*	299	*	*
Total Right	41	.39	12.4	324	205	223	335	111	139

A decrease in ZP was approximately the same as was the increase in YTS. For ZP the decrease was 43% for Frank and 47% for McFee. YTS the increase was 73% for Frank and 77% for McFee.

The parameters ZA and MSVR were not useful.

Total Left Sided Lesions (58 patients).

The best single measurement for LVH was ZP where in the Frank the increase was from .97 to 1.61 and in the McFee the increase was from 1.42 to 2.38. The ratio of F/M was 1.42/2.38 = .68 (normal = .68). The increase in Frank was 66%, while that in McFee was 68%.

An increase in MSVL was 45% for Frank and 51% for McFee.

An increase in YInf was approximately the same as was an increase in XL. For YInf the increase was 36% for Frank and 33% for McFee. For XL the increase was 29% for Frank and 36% for McFee. An increase in YIR was 20% for Frank and 44% for McFee. An increase in YTS was 27% for Frank and 35% for McFee. Of special interest was an increase of XTR of 23% for Frank and 62% for McFee.

Total Left Pressure Load (AS, CA [coarctation]) and EFE (endocardial fibroelastosis) (30 patients)

The best single measurement was ZP where in the Frank the mean magnitude increase was from .97 to 1.90 while in the McFee the mean increase was from 1.42 to 2.89. The ratio of F/M was 1.90/2.89 = .66 (normal = .68). The increase in Frank was 96% while that in the McFee was 120%.

An increase in MSVL was 69% for Frank and 74% for McFee.

An increase in YInf was 67% for Frank and 52% for McFee. An increase in XL was 42% for Frank and 48% for McFee. Of special interest was an increase in XTR of 65% for Frank and 107% for McFee. Of special interest was a decrease in XIR of 20% for Frank and 19% for McFee.

Table 8

Maximal Spatial Vector to the Right

	N	A	B	D	Chi Sq.	Mean Mag.	ST.D.	P05	P10	P50	P90	P95
Frank Lead System												
Total Normal	341	252	112	.63	406.5	.94	.43	.30	.40	.92	1.51	1.71
AS	15	247	127	.59	15.0	1.70	1.21	*	*	1.35	*	*
CA	7	236	124	.58	7.0	1.44	.97	*	*	1.28	*	*
MI	17	167	67	.16	1.2	.96	.51	*	*	1.05	*	*
PDA	6	157	103	.46	3.8	1.52	1.39	*	*	1.25	*	*
AS, CA, EFE	25	244	124	.62	28.4	1.61	1.06	.35	.40	1.30	3.48	4.18
AI, MI, PDA	27	201	103	.20	3.3	1.06	.78	.09	.17	.87	2.16	3.17
Total Left	52	232	120	.38	22.3	1.32	.96	.16	.34	1.17	2.98	3.46
PS	27	161	124	.67	36.1	1.74	.88	.61	.72	1.60	2.97	3.84
ASD	11	189	115	.79	20.7	1.07	.63	*	*	.85	*	*
PS, PPS	28	164	125	.66	36.4	1.74	.86	.61	.72	1.67	2.91	3.81
ASD, TAP	14	181	119	.71	21.4	1.15	.59	*	*	1.11	*	*
Total Right	42	170	123	.67	56.9	1.54	.83	.54	.65	1.38	2.68	3.38
McFee Lead System												
Total Normal	340	244	103	.45	207.8	1.31	.65	.35	.52	1.25	2.22	2.51
AS	17	232	121	.45	10.4	2.40	1.80	*	*	1.94	*	*
CA	7	247	107	.88	16.3	2.22	.83	*	*	1.91	*	*
MI	16	166	83	.22	2.2	1.69	1.00	*	*	1.77	*	*
PDA	6	168	87	.49	4.2	2.51	1.79	*	*	2.34	*	*
AS, CA, EFE	27	242	114	.61	29.9	2.39	1.49	.53	.57	2.22	4.34	6.01
AI, MI, PDA	26	165	100	.26	5.4	1.84	1.23	.12	.29	1.77	3.97	4.55
Total Left	53	220	113	.37	21.4	2.12	1.38	.29	.52	1.93	3.92	5.05
PS	27	172	120	.62	31.2	2.67	1.24	.68	.93	2.58	4.59	4.78
ASD	11	193	106	.74	17.9	1.64	.82	*	*	1.46	*	*
PS, PPS	28	176	120	.61	31.5	2.67	1.22	.68	.96	2.63	4.59	4.77
ASD, TAP	14	185	112	.65	17.9	1.64	.84	*	*	1.51	*	*
Total Right	42	179	117	.62	48.8	2.36	1.18	.72	.87	2.11	4.36	4.60

Total Left Volume Load (AR, MR and PDA)
(28 patients)

There was no single strong measurement except for an increase in the XTR where in the Frank the increase in mean magnitude was from .10 to .18, while in the McFee the increase was from .16 to .34. The ratio of F/M was .18/.34 = .53 (normal = .63). The increase in Frank was 80% while that in McFee was 112%.

An increase in YTS was 36% for Frank and 47% for McFee. An increase in ZP was 34% for Frank and 29% for McFee. An increase in MSVL was 18% for Frank and 26% for McFee. An increase in XL was 16% for Frank and 23% for McFee.

Aortic Stenosis

The best single measurement for LVH in aortic stenosis was ZP, where in the Frank the increase was from .97 to 2.07 and in McFee the increase was from 1.42 to 3.06. The ratio of F/M was

1.42/3.06 = .68 (normal = .68). Thus, the increase in Frank was 114% while the increase in McFee was 116%.

An increase in MSVL was 70% for Frank and 79% for McFee.

An increase in Y Inf was 65% for Frank and 58% for McFee. An increase in XL was 33% for Frank and 46% for McFee. Of special interest was the XTR which showed a 17% increase in the Frank and a 42% increase in the McFee. Of special interest was the MSVR which showed an 83% increase in both the Frank and McFee.

Mitral Regurgitation

The best single measurement was a surprising finding, the YTS, where in the Frank the increase was from .11 to .22 and in the McFee the increase was from .17 to .34. The ratio of F/M was .22/.34 = .65 (normal = .65). The increases in Frank and McFee were both 100%.

Table 9

Maximal Spatial Vector to the Left

	N	A	B	D	Chi Sq.	Mean Mag.	ST.D.	P05	P10	P50	P90	P95
Frank Lead System												
Total Normal	341	336	136	.88	801.1	1.71	.48	1.00	1.11	1.69	2.31	2.59
AS	20	302	130	.92	50.9	2.89	.99	1.29	1.76	2.68	4.76	5.04
CA	7	329	134	.89	16.5	2.54	1.10	*	*	2.33	*	*
MI	18	331	120	.76	31.2	1.96	.82	*	*	2.05	*	*
PDA	6	321	127	.90	14.6	2.05	1.08	*	*	2.27	*	*
AS, CA, EFE	30	310	132	.88	69.0	2.87	1.00	1.15	1.74	2.60	4.20	4.92
AI, MI, PDA	28	325	123	.81	55.5	2.01	.85	.23	.79	2.02	3.32	3.56
Total Left	58	318	128	.84	122.4	2.46	1.07	.82	1.21	2.38	3.94	4.24
PS	26	52	128	.79	48.7	1.81	.73	.74	.82	1.91	2.74	3.23
ASD	11	6	126	.88	25.4	1.37	.60	*	*	1.35	*	*
PS, PPS	27	51	126	.79	50.3	1.80	.72	.74	.83	1.74	2.72	3.21
ASD, TAP	14	12	129	.83	28.8	1.37	.53	*	*	1.33	*	*
Total Right	41	38	128	.78	73.9	1.65	.69	.73	.80	1.60	2.57	2.86
McFee Lead System												
Total Normal	341	344	132	.87	779.0	2.34	.67	1.37	1.57	2.29	3.15	3.57
AS	20	303	127	.84	42.3	4.19	1.16	2.02	2.99	3.79	5.75	6.90
CA	7	338	124	.80	13.4	3.18	1.30	*	*	3.17	*	*
MI	18	332	122	.82	36.1	2.68	1.18	*	*	3.00	*	*
PDA	6	335	125	.79	11.1	3.32	1.05	*	*	3.60	*	*
AS, CA, EFE	30	314	127	.79	56.3	4.07	1.30	1.44	2.73	3.79	5.75	6.76
AI, MI, PDA	28	330	123	.82	57.0	2.96	1.19	.49	1.16	3.30	4.59	5.00
Total Left	58	322	125	.80	111.7	3.53	1.36	.84	1.85	3.58	5.24	5.81
PS	27	53	127	.72	42.1	2.32	1.27	.42	.70	2.09	4.10	5.09
ASD	11	10	125	.84	23.2	2.11	.94	*	*	1.75	*	*
PS, PPS	28	53	126	.73	44.5	2.32	1.24	.43	.72	2.13	3.98	5.09
ASD, TAP	14	16	127	.80	26.7	2.14	.88	*	*	1.76	*	*
Total Right	42	40	128	.73	66.9	2.26	1.13	.54	.86	1.95	3.85	4.90

An increase in ZP was 30% for Frank and 25% for McFee. An increase in XL was 18% for Frank and 11% for McFee. An increase in MSVL was 15% for Frank and McFee.

Discussion

The data from this pilot study clearly do not answer the question as to which of the two presently most favored orthogonal lead systems is most satisfactory. There are indications from the correlation statistics that the Frank system will be most valuable. On the other hand, in the extensive data presented wherein diagnostic ability and specific electrocardiographic parameters are examined, there may be some indication for superiority of the McFee-Parungao system.

Among the 100 patients studied, there is obviously too much variability of disease to make strong correlations. There are too few patients in each disease group. However, the fact that "pure" lesions could be studied allowed us to test out recently developed statistics and compare a multitude of electrocardiographic parameters with a large number of hemodynamic measurements and calculations.

The largest single group of patients studied was that of pulmonic stenosis, where the simplest hemodynamic measurement to compare was the right ventricular pressure. This correlation data clearly indicated superiority of the Frank system but also showed that simple measurements, possible to make in seconds by eye and hand, were just as useful as the maximal spatial vector to the right. The latter either takes 20 or 30 minutes to measure accurately by hand or needs a computer. The simple measurements were the maximal projections, the magnitude of the terminal X to the right or the Z anterior.

The other group where the methodology was easy to test out was aortic stenosis. Here again the Frank system was superior in the small number of patients to the McFee-Parungao system. And, once again it was indicated that a complex measurement, the maximal spatial vector to the left, was apparently not necessary. A simple maximal projection, the magnitude of Z posterior, was clearly superior, and a surprising measurement, the terminal X to the right, was even better. (The latter measurement presumably indicates posterobasal left ventricular hypertrophy.) For aortic stenosis, a multiple regression appeared to be very useful, bringing out unexpected electrocardiographic variables such as the magnitude of the .40 normalized vector.

The most immediate use of this paper is that by studying the 42 patients with pure right sided lesions and the 58 patients with pure left sided lesions, the "best" parameters for diagnosis could be determined. Furthermore, differences were evident for pressure work and volume work.

For example, for the entire right sided group, the best single measurement for RVH was the magnitude of the terminal X to the right in both lead systems, especially for McFee. However, when pressure load (pulmonic stenosis) was compared with volume load (ASD), there were differences. A useful measurement for pressure load (an increase in Z anterior) was of no use for ASD, though in the latter an increase in Y terminal superior was quite useful. As another example, in the total left sided group, the best single measurement for LVH was an increase in the magnitude of the Z posterior. But, when pressure load was compared to volume loading (mitral regurgitation), it was found that there were differences. For example, the X initial right and the Y terminal superior are both significantly greater in volume loads than pressure loads. In addition, the magnitude of the terminal X to the right was extremely useful for diagnosing left ventricular pressure load hypertrophy. A larger magnitude Y inferior was also useful for pressure loads, but not for volume loads. Obviously, the comparison of pressure and volume loading needs severity matching to make certain that we are not just looking at severe versus milder disease.

Summary

A pilot study comparing multiple hemodynamic measurements with multiple electrocardiographic parameters has been presented. One hundred patients with pure lesions have been studied, 42 with right sided lesions and 58 with left sided lesions. The Frank and McFee-Parungao orthogonal lead systems were utilized.

In the correlation studies involving pure pressure loads, there were indications that the Frank system was superior to the McFee in predicting right or left ventricular pressure.

In studying various parameters for increases or decreases above normal in evaluating their usefulness, there was very little difference between Frank and McFee-Parungao. However, whenever there was any hemodynamic abnormality which caused a large terminal vector to the right (RVH, posterobasal LVH), the McFee appeared to be more useful.

The data are quite preliminary but eventual usefulness appears evident. Therefore, large numbers of patients will be evaluated.

References

[1] J. Liebman and R. Plonsey, Basic principles for understanding electrocardiography, Paediatrician 2 (1973) 251.

[2] R. C. Barr and M. S. Spach, Physiologic correlates and clinical comparisons of Isopotential surface maps with other electrocardiographic methods. In: Schlant and Hurst (eds.), Advances in Cardiology (Grune and Stratton, New York, 1972), pp. 27-36.

[3] Z. G. Horan and N. C. Flowers, Limitation of the dipole concept in electrocardiographic interpretation. In: Schlant and Hurst (eds.), Advances in electrocardiography (Grune and Stratton, New York, 1972), pp. 9-18.

[4] E. Frank, An accurate and clinically practical system for spatial vectorcardiography, Circulation 13 (1956), 737.

[5] J. Liebman, C. F. Doershuk, C. Rapp, and L. Matthews, The vectorcardiogram in cystic fibrosis--diagnostic significance and correlation with pulmonary function tests, Circulation 35 (1967) 552.

[6] J. Liebman, D. A. Krause, C. F. Doershuk, T. D. Downs, and L. W. Matthews, The orthogonal vectorcardiogram in cystic fibrosis--diagnostic significance and correlation with pulmonary function tests. A four-year follow-up, Chest 63 (1973) 218.

[7] M. Ng, J. Liebman, J. Anslovar, and S. Gross, Cardiovascular findings in children with sickle cell anemia, Diseases of the Chest 52 (1967) 788.

[8] R. Agusti, J. Liebman, and T. D. Downs, The orthogonal vectorcardiogram (Frank System) in isolated ventricular septal defect. A correlative

hemodynamic study. Presented by Dr. Agusti at the Inter-American Congress of Cardiology, Lima, Peru, 1968.

[9] J. Liebman, The relation of the standard electrocardiogram to the vectorcardiogram. In: D. E. Cassels and Robert Ziegler (eds.), Electrocardiography in infants and children (Grune and Stratton, New York and London, 1966).

[10] V. V. Sreenivasan and J. Liebman, Posterior mitral regurgitationin girls possibly due to posterior papillary muscle dysfunction, Pediatrics 42 (1968) 476.

[11] J. Liebman, Masked right ventricular hypertrophy in presence of abnormally posterior vector - Unmasked by Frank vectorcardiogram, Proceedings of the American Academy of Pediatrics, Section on Cardiology Meetings, October 1966, Chicago, Illinois.

[12] R. H. Strang, P. G. Hugenholtz, J. Liebman, and A. S. Nadas, The vectorcardiographic reflection of hemodynamic status of pulmonary stenosis with and within intact ventricular septum, Am. J. Cardiol. 12 (1963) 758.

[13] D. A. Brody and R. C. Arzbaecher, A comparison of several corrected vectorcardiographic leads, Circulation 29 (1964) 533.

[14] R. McFee and A. Parungao, An orthogonal lead system for clinical electrocardiography, Am. Heart J. 62 (1961) 93.

[15] R. Gamboa, Applicability of the axial lead system to infants and children, Am. J. Cardiol. 18 (1966) 690.

[16] J. Liebman, T. D. Downs, and A. Priede, The Frank and McFee vectorcardiogram in normal children. A detailed quantitative analysis of 105 children between the ages of two and 19 years. In: I. Hoffman (ed.), Vectorcardiography 2 (North-Holland, Amsterdam, 1971), p. 483.

[17] J. Liebman, H. C. Romberg, T. D. Downs, and R. Agusti, The Frank QRS vectorcardiogram in the premature infant. In: I. Hoffman and Robert Taymor (eds.), Vectorcardiography 1965 (North-Holland, Amsterdam, 1966), p. 256.

[18] P. G. Hugenholtz and J. Liebman, The Orthogonal vectorcardiogram in 100 normal children (Frank system) with some comparative data recorded by the cube system, Circulation 26 (1962) 891.

[19] J. Liebman, M. Lee, P. S. Rao, and W. Mackay, Quantitation of the normal Frank and McFee-Parungao orthogonal electrocardiogram in the adolescent, Circulation 48 (1973) 735.

[20] J. Kan, J. Liebman, and W. Mackay, Quantitation of the normal Frank and McFee-Parungao orthogonal electrocardiogram at ages 2 - 10 years. To be submitted.

[21] R. Gamboa and N. White, The corrected orthogonal electrocardiogram in normal children in the McFee-Parungao lead system, Am. Heart J. 74 (1968) 449.

[22] L. E. Ainger, Digital computer analysis of the vectorcardiogram of the newborn infant, Circulation 36 (1967) 906.

[23] E. P. Namin, R. A. Arcilla, I. A. D'Cruz, and B. Gasul, Evaluation of the Frank vectorcardiogram in normal infants, Am. J. Cardiol. 13 (1964) 757.

[24] E. P. Namin and I. A. D'Cruz, Vectorcardiogram in normal children, Br. Heart J. 26 (1964) 689.

[25] G. H. Khoury and R. S. Fowler, Normal Frank vectorcardiogram in infancy and childhood, Br. Heart J. 29 (1967) 563.

[26] T. Downs, J. Liebman, R. Agusti, and H. C. Romberg, The statistical treatment of angular data in vectorcardiography. In: I. Hoffman and R. C. Taymor (eds.), Vectorcardiography 1965 (North-Holland, Amsterdam, 1966), p. 272.

[27] T. D. Downs and J. Liebman, The analysis of vectorcardiogram angular data. Presented at Fourth Annual Symposium on Biomathematics and Computing, Houston, Texas, March 24, 1966.

[28] T. D. Downs and A. L. Gould, A class of angular distributions related to the normal. Biometrics 24 (1968) 229. Presented at the annual meeting of the American Statistical Association, December, 1967.

[29] J. Liebman and T. D. Downs, Uses and misuses of statistics in analyzing vectorcardiogram directions, Biometrics 23 (1967) 605. Presented at the annual meeting of the American Statistical Association, December 29, 1967.

[30] J. Liebman, T. D. Downs, H. Romberg, and R. Agusti, The statistical treatment of angular data in vectorcardiography. Presented by Dr. Liebman at the American College of Cardiology Fifteenth Annual Scientific Session, 1966.

[31] T. Downs and J. Liebman, Statistical methods for vectorcardiographic directions. IEEE Transactions on Bio-medical Engineering, Vol. BME-16, 87, 1969.

Vectorcardiography 3 I. Hoffman and R.I. Hamby eds.
© 1976 North-Holland Publishing Company - Amsterdam

EVALUATION OF A STATISTICAL DECISION PROGRAM

FOR AUTOMATED ECG PROCESSING

(Pipberger Program)

Harold G. Richman and Christian R. Brohet

From the Department of Internal Medicine and Division of Health Computer
Sciences, University of Minnesota Medical School; and Medical Service,
Cardiovascular Section, Veterans Administration Hospital,
Minneapolis, Minnesota

Introduction

At the present time programs for automated
ECG processing have one of two basic designs. The
first and most familiar is that which involves a deterministic approach and attempts to simulate the interpretative technique ordinarily utilized by the physician. The second is that which utilizes a statistical
decision approach. By selecting best discriminant
measurements and developing a multivariate analysis
this type of program arrives at a probabilistic interpretation.

Generally the evaluation of ECG automated processing programs of the deterministic type have been
accomplished by comparing the computer interpretation with that of the physician. Since these programs
have been developed by use of conventional ECG criteria, it is reasonable that the physician interpretation be regarded as a standard for accuracy and that a
high level of agreement be expected for clinical application of the program. Deterministic programs have
as their purpose a reproduction of the traditional interpretation approach used by the physician and have
been valuable in familiarizing the physician with the
approach to automated ECG processing. However,
these programs, whether they depend on standard 12-
lead or XYZ lead recording, are all vulnerable to the
limited accuracy of the conventional criteria utilized
in analysis and as such have been entitled "First Generation Programs" [1, 2]. In recent years an attempt
to improve the level of accuracy of the ECG has been
approached by use of computer programs involving interpretation by statistical decision. [3-6]. The multivariate probabilistic approach is considered an ad-
vancement in automated ECG processing and as such
has been referred to as a "Second Generation Program"
[1, 2]. This type of program cannot be validated by
the degree of physician agreement in that the logic
utilized to arrive at interpretation is entirely different
than that utilized by conventional criteria. Therefore,
an independent standard should be used to assess the
comparative accuracy of interpretation by traditional
methods. To date the most advanced probabilistic program available for routine use is that developed by
Pipberger and Cornfield at the Research Center for

Cardiovascular Data processing at the Washington,
D.C. VA Hospital. Although determination of the accuracy of this program has been undertaken by the
developers, the results of an overall assessment of
its performance in an independent clinical setting are
not generally available.

Methods

Following successful implementation of the
Pipberger Program on a CDC computer in the Bio-
physical Monitoring Unit at the Minneapolis VA Hospital, an evaluation of ECG processing by this program in a routine clinical setting was undertaken.
This evaluation involved a determination of precision,
agreement, and accuracy all of which were considered important factors in regard to clinical acceptance.

Precision was evaluated by comparison of selected measurement values determined at the Minneapolis VA Hospital to that determined at the Washington, D.C. VA Hospital on the same sample of 200
tracings. Despite considerable differences in A/D
conversion at the two hospitals a quite acceptable level
of differences was observed (table 1). A comparison
can be made with what is considered acceptable for a
deterministic program where considerably less toler-
ance to difference in measurement occurs (table 2).

Table 1

Quantitative Evaluation of the Technical Differences
between WVA and MVA Systems

Measurement Error

Measurement	Mean Difference	Extreme Difference
P (DUR)	0.0035 sec.	0.0130 sec.
QRS (DUR)	0.0021 sec.	0.0420 sec.
P-R INT.	0.0028 sec.	0.0240 sec.
T (AMP) X	0.0417 m V	0.360 m V
(Q/R) Y	0.0341	1.37

Table 2

Required Measurement Precision for Ecan D Program* Compared to the Mean Difference of Measurements between WVA and MVA Systems

Measurement	Precision of Measurement	Mean Difference WVA - MVA
P (DUR)	20 msec.	3.5 msec.
QRS (DUR)	5 msec.	2.1 msec.
T amplitude	50 μV	41.7 μV

*from R. R. Helpi et al., C.M.A. Journal 108 (1973) 1251.

As previously noted, physician agreement cannot be used as a standard for accuracy in evaluating this type of program. However, one cannot avoid the observation that agreement substantially influences physician acceptance. Since the probabilistic program was a particular departure from the conventional approach it was our opinion that an essential aspect of evaluation was an assessment of physician agreement. This was undertaken by a two-step approach. Initially six staff physicians interpreted the standard 12-lead tracing using criteria with which they were most familiar and compared their conclusions to that of the computer printout. At the second step the printout of the same tracing was analyzed by two staff physicians who utilized criteria encompassed by the Minnesota Code [7] for the standard 12-leads and also utilized the XYZ orthogonal lead tracing in arriving at their interpretation.

Initially, considerable difficulty was encountered with the first step analysis since most of the physicians were unfamiliar with XYZ data as well as discriminant function and probability statements (figure 1). The printout was then reprogrammed in a more traditional English language approach for purposes of communication. The posterior probabilities were assigned English language terms based on a categorical division of 30-50% = possible, 50-70% = probable and, greater than 70% = definite as noted in figure 2. If more than one probability value was present, the strength of the shared probabilities was arbitrarily defined as noted on the left side column. Probability values were retained on the printout to familiarize the physician with the values associated with his diagnostic consideration. The original printout was also retained for use by the second step reviewers. The physicians were then requested to grade their own interpretation on the basis of possible, probable or definite before being provided with the modified computer printout (figure 3).

```
                                                                  *** AVA VERSION 3.41  DATE  12/11/74
ID          01025027              DATE        12/10/74
RACE        WHITE                 AGE         50-59
WEIGHT      140                   DIGITALIS   NO

** TIME INTERVAL  (SEC)    AMPLITUDE   (MV)
  P-DURATION      QRS-DURATION    P-R INTERVAL     QT RATIO
    .115             .090           .159             1.3
  Q-DURATION      R-AMPLITUDE     T-AMPLITUDE      POINT-J        Q/R RATIO     R/S RATIO
X   .015            3.15            .77              .01            .04         *******
Y   .022             .61            .36            -0.01            .18         *******
Z   .049             .39          -0.40              .03            .92         *******

HEART RATE   82/MIN          12  QRS
NORMAL SINUS RHYTHM

QRS-T DIAGNOSTIC PROBABILITIES     PRIOR CODE  9.04
        LVH                59.8
        NORMAL             36.9

   LVH    MEAS                    LIMIT     VALUE
        RX+RZ              U      3.10      3.54
        R AMP X            U      1.90      3.15
        R AMP Z            U      1.80       .39
        T AMP X            L       .05       .77

P WAVE PROBABILITIES
        NORMAL             88.0
        RAO                11.5
```

Fig. 1. Standard format of the Pipberger Program printout. Majority of the information is expressed in terms of orthogonal XYZ lead measurements.

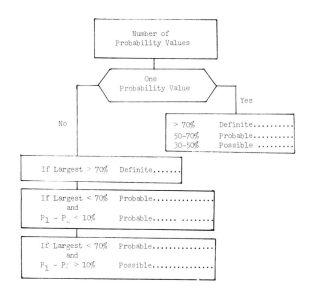

Fig. 2. Algorithm for conversion of probability values to English language statements. Multiple probabilities are required to share the total of 100%. $P_1 - P_2$ represents the percentage difference between the largest probability and any other value.

Subsequently, 1,000 ECGs were reviewed, the tracings being obtained in an unselected manner from an ambulatory in-patient population at the Minneapolis VA Hospital. Both levels of interpretation were then classified as to either complete agreement, minor disagreement or major disagreement. Minor disagreement consisted on one category difference in probability, minor rhythm changes, or minor repolarization changes. Minor disagreements were arbitrarily considered an acceptable diagnosis.

Results

Results of the overall agreement are noted in table 3. Complete agreement at the first step was 57% with 25% minor disagreement and total acceptable diagnoses of 82%. Interestingly, an increase in complete agreement was noted at the second step suggesting that the use of standardized criteria and XYZ data tended to improve the degree of agreement. The comparison with three other ECG analysis programs all of which utilize standard 12-lead information and conventional criteria, is also noted. Complete agreement is less with the probabilistic program at each step most likely due to limitation of the number of traditional diagnostic categories available. No appreciable difference is noted, however, if one allows minor disagreements to be considered as acceptable diagnoses.

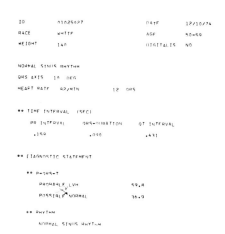

Fig. 3. Modified printout for the Pipberger Program. Measurements and interpretative statements are expressed in a more traditional manner.

Table 3

Physician - Computer Agreement
with Various Programs

	1st Step		2nd Step		
	C	A	C	A	N
PIPBERGER--VA	57%	82%	63%	84%	(1000)
BONNER--IBM	82%	86%	69%	75%	(395)
ECAN E (CEIS)	73%	78%	73%	81%	(346)
TELEMED	76%	79%	71%	77%	(312)

C = Complete agreement
A = Acceptable interpretation
  (complete agreement + minor disagreement)

The comparative interpretation for the primary diagnosis of each ECG is shown by means of a contingency table (table 4). The primary diagnosis for the computer was considered to be that with the greatest probability value when that value was at least 35%. This type of presentation shows the distribution of misclassification but does not presuppose the degree of accuracy of either conventional criteria or of the computer program. On the basis of a single major diagnosis overall agreement was 75%. The categories of "major" and "minor" contained all deterministic interpretations, except for right bundle branch block and left bundle branch block. "Major" consisted of AV conduction disturbances, hemiblocks, frequent premature contractions, arrhythmias and ST-T abnormal-, ities of greater than 1 mm. depression or elevation. "Minor" consisted of occasional premature beats and minimal ST-T changes. The inter-category disagreements in this groups accounted for only 62 tracings (8.8%). Distribution of these misclassifications is shown in table 5. The majority of these misclassifications were failure to recognize marked left axis deviation or significant ST-T abnormalities. Rhythm misclassifications were usually failure to recognize P waves in sinus rhythm with subsequent interpretation as "junctional" or "regular" rhythm.

On the basis of mutual agreement, approximately 40% of the tracings were considered to be normal with most of disagreements in this category being classified as "Major" or "Minor." If one regards the minor disagreements as consistent with acceptable diagnosis, there was agreement of 91% between conventional criteria and computer in regard to normals.

Percentage agreement for major category diagnosis is shown in figure 4. The upper corner represents percentage agreement of computer diagnosis with that of conventional criteria analysis as utilized by the physician. The cross comparison of conven-

tional criteria agreement with the computer diagnosis is noted in the lower corner. There is considerable variation in the degree of agreement for individual categories. However, the greatest disagreement of conventional criteria with the computer program was in the categories of myocardial infarction (MI), left ventricular hypertrophy (LVH), and pulmonary disease (PE). If the deterministic diagnoses were not included and the results analyzed for only the probabilistic categories, the overall agreement was reduced to 57%. This relatively low value seemed to emphasize the need for validation of accuracy by an independent standard.

To evaluate this aspect, 339 of the original 1,000 tracings were selected in which it was felt that clinical diagnosis could be reliably related to pathologic anatomy. The criteria for defining the clinical status is noted in table 6. No attempt was made to analyze the data in terms of localization of infarction. The majority of the patients were categorized as either MI, LVH or no cardiovascular disease.

Overall diagnostic accuracy is noted in figure 5. The overall correct diagnosis for conventional criteria utilized by the physician was 63% while that for the computer interpretation was 72%. Mutual agreement was a poor index of accuracy, being present in only 47%. Analysis by individual diagnostic categories was then assessed for MI, LVH and PE. Figure 6 indicates the results for 66 patients with coronary artery disease diagnosed as having MI. The recognition was significantly greater for probabilistic interpretation than for conventional criteria. Mutual agreement on correct interpretation was present in only 42% which would seem to reflect limited value of this comparison in regard to diagnostic accuracy. The mutual independence of the criteria was evident, however, in that half of those missed by the computer were recognized by conventional criteria. An even greater difference in improved recognition was noted for LVH (figure 7). Here again, half of those missed by the computer were recognized by conventional criteria. For PE (figure 8) correct classification was higher for probabilistic interpretation than for conventional criteria, but in either case it was fairly low. However, the number of patients is much too small adequately to evaluate this category. Of those patients who could not be shown to have any cardiac disease (figure 9), correct classification favored conventional criteria. Twenty-three percent of these tracings were incorrectly classified by the probabilistic program. Of the 33 misclassifications in this group, ten were in the category of posterodiaphragmatic MI, 13 LVH and five PE. This would result in 16% over-diagnosis for each of LVH and MI. This high degree of over-diagnosis suggests either the value for a significant posterior probability is too

Table 4

Comparison of Physician–Computer Program
Diagnostic Classification

CONVENTIONAL CRITERIA

Program	Normal	LVH	RVH	BVH	AMI	LMI	PDMI	PE	LVCD	LVCD & MI	RVCD	RVCD & MI	VH-MI	PE-RVH	Major	Minor	Total
Normal	383	6	2	2	6	1	2	2			1				21	34	460
LVH	15	56		1	3		1						2		10	12	100
RVH	1	1	3				1								3	3	12
BVH	2	1		4									1		2	1	11
AMI	2				35								1		1	1	40
LMI						5											5
PDMI	7			2			81				2	2			4	6	104
PE				1	1			8							6	1	17
LVCD									6								6
LVCD & MI	1	5					1		3	17					1		28
RVCD							1				15	3					19
RVCD & MI											4	5			2		11
VH-MI	3	3	1	2			4						15		7	5	40
PE-RVH	3						1	1						2	5	4	16
Major	3	4													30	5	42
Minor	2	3			1										3	80	89
Total	422	79	6	12	46	6	92	11	9	17	22	10	19	2	95	152	1000

COMPUTER PROGRAM

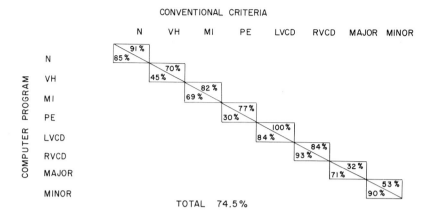

Fig. 4. Cross comparison of computer-physician and physician-computer agreement on the basis of the primary diagnosis. N = normal, VH = right and/or left ventricular hypertrophy, MI = all myocardial infarctions, PE = pulmonary disease, LVCD and RVCD = all left and right ventricular conduction disturbance, major and minor = all other determinant changes (see text).

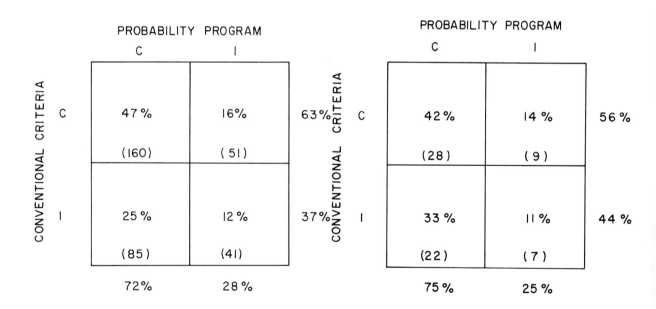

Fig. 5. Overall accuracy as determined by independent clinical data for the primary diagnosis. C = correct, I = incorrect. A definite improvement is noted with the computer program.

Fig. 6. Determination of accuracy for myocardial infarction. The program recognition rate of 75% is markedly increased over that observed for conventional criteria (56%).

Table 5

Distribution of "Major" Category
Misinterpretations (62)

	+	-
ST-T Wave Abnormality	6	21
First Degree AV Block		4
Extreme Axis		
LAD ($\geq$ -30°)		14
RAD ($\geq$ -100°)		1
Rhythm		
Sinus		10
Atrial Fibrillation	2	
PVCs		3
Artificial Pacemaker		1

+ False positive
− False negative

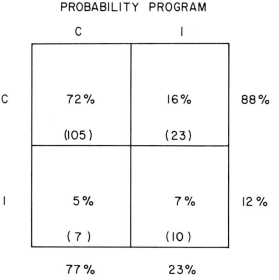

PROBABILITY PROGRAM

	C	I	
C	14 % (3)	14 % (3)	28 %
I	40 % (9)	32 % (7)	72 %
	54 %	46 %	

CONVENTIONAL CRITERIA

Fig. 8. Determination of accuracy for pulmonary disease. Recognition rate, although favoring the computer program, is low by either method. Significance of the results is questionable due to the small number of observations.

PROBABILITY PROGRAM

	C	I	
C	26 % (23)	15 % (13)	41 %
I	43 % (37)	16 % (14)	59 %
	69 %	31 %	

CONVENTIONAL CRITERIA

Fig. 7. Determination of accuracy for left ventricular hypertrophy. The difference in recognition rate favors the computer program to an even greater extent than that observed for myocardial infarction.

PROBABILITY PROGRAM

	C	I	
C	72 % (105)	16 % (23)	88 %
I	5 % (7)	7 % (10)	12 %
	77 %	23 %	

CONVENTIONAL CRITERIA

Fig. 9. Classification of patients with no known cardiovascular disease. Over-diagnosis of ECG abnormality was considerably greater with the computer program than with conventional criteria.

Table 6

Criteria for Clinical Diagnosis
(339 Patients)

LVH (87)
  Hypertension - 2 year history and repeated
    BP $\geq 160/105$

  Valvular Disease
    Aortic stenosis - valve area < 0.8 cm^2
    Mitral insufficiency - 3+ regurgitation
      and/or S3 ↑ LA size

MI (66)
  Clinical history and characteristic enzyme
    abnormality

  Angiographic evidence of poor or non-contractile
    segment

RVH (8)
  PA pressure mean > 40 mm. Hg

PE (22)
  FEV$_1 < 65\%$ p0$_2 < 70$ mm. Hg

LVH + MI (11)

No CV Disease (145)

low or the value of the prior probability too high or
perhaps both. In order to check this, LVH was re-
evaluated by setting the significant posterior probability at 50% instead of 35%. The prior probability
was also lowered from 54% to 42%, a value more representative of our patient population (figure 10). This
result emphasizes the importance of application of
relative probability in evaluating the Pipberger Program.

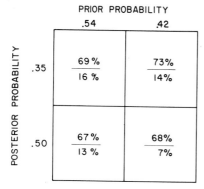

Fig. 10. Effect of adjusting both prior and posterior
probability on recognition rate of left ventricular
hypertrophy. Satisfactory level of specificity was
accomplished without compromise of sensitivity.

Conclusion

A preliminary evaluation of the probabilistic
ECG analysis program developed by Pipberger and
Cornfield has been undertaken in an independent center under conditions of routine in-patient processing.
Our observation to date would indicate that:
  1) A satisfactory level of precision can be obtained.
  2) Despite lack of conventional approach a high
level of physician acceptability can be achieved.
Some problems are related to constraint of the conventional number of diagnostic categories. Greater
educational effort is also required due to lack of
physician familiarity with XYZ criteria and probability terminology.
  3) Comparison with independent clinical data
would indicate considerable potential for improvement
in accuracy in certain diagnostic categories over that
attainable with conventional criteria. In our initial
analysis this seemed to have been accomplished in
part at the expense of increased over-diagnosis.
However, adjustment of probability values resulted
in acceptable specificity without compromise of sensitivity. The ability to adjust for proper conditions
of probability illustrate the flexibility of the probabilistic approach and potentially provides for a diagnostic advantage over the more rigidly structured deterministic approach.

References

[1] H. V. Pipberger, R. A. Dunn, and J. Corn-
     field, First and second generation computer
     programs for diagnostic ECG and VCG classi-
     fication. In: P. Rylandt (ed.), Proceedings of
     the XIIth International Colloquium Vectorcardio-
     graphicum (Presses Academiques Europeenes,
     Brussels, 1972), p. 431.
[2] H. V. Pipberger, Methods of diagnostic ECG
     classification. In: C. Zywietz and B.
     Schneider (eds.), Computer application on ECG
     and VCG analysis (North-Holland, Amsterdam,
     1973), p. 296.
[3] R. A. Dunn, H. V. Pipberger, and J. Corn-
     field, The U.S. Veterans Administration ECG
     analysis system. In: C. Zywietz and B.
     Schneider (eds.), Computer Application on ECG
     and VCG analysis (North-Holland, Amsterdam,
     1973), p. 142.
[4] J. Cornfield, Statistical classification methods.
     In: J. A. Jacques (ed.), Computer diagnosis and
     diagnostic methods (Charles C. Thomas,
     Springfield, Ill., 1972), p. 108.
[5] H. V. Pipberger, J. Cornfield, and R. A.
     Dunn, Diagnosis of the electrocardiogram.
     In: J. A. Jacques (ed.), Computer Diagnosis
     and diagnostic methods (Charles C. Thomas,
     Springfield, Ill., 1972), p. 355.

[6] J. Cornfield, R. A. Dunn, C. D. Batchlor, and
H. V. Pipberger, Multigroup diagnosis of electrocardiograms, Comput. Biomed. Res. 6
(1973) 97.

[7] H. Blackburn, Classification of the electrocardiogram for population studies: Minnesota
code, J. Electrocardiol. 2 (1969) 305-10.

Vectorcardiography 3 I. Hoffman and R.I. Hamby eds.
© 1976 North-Holland Publishing Company - Amsterdam

CHARACTERISTICS OF NORMAL AND ISCHEMIC VCG RESPONSE TO EXERCISE,
QUANTIFIED BY MEANS OF WAVEFORM VECTOR ANALYSIS

G. R. Dagenais, R. B. Villadiego, and P. M. Rautaharju

Institut de Cardiologie de Quebec, Hopital Laval, Quebec
and Biophysics and Bioengineering Research Laboratory,
Faculty of Medicine, Dalhousie University,
Halifax, Nova Scotia, Canada

Several recent studies have shown relatively poor sensitivity and specificity of rest and exercise electrocardiogram (ECG) in the detection of coronary artery disease (CAD). More promising results have been reported from some vectorcardiographic (VCG) studies [1] and investigations with new multiple-lead systems. Kornreich et al. [2] recently reported highly encouraging results from differential diagnosis between normal subjects and patients with ischemic heart disease (IHD), defined as definite CAD and classical angina pectoris. Multivariate analysis of resting QRS complexes of the nine leads of the Kornreich system yielded a sensitivity of 76% at the 70% level of specificity. In the study of Kornreich et al. the results were substantially worse when similar analysis of the Frank leads was performed.

The purpose of this communication is to demonstrate the utility of a novel waveform vector analysis (WVA) method [3, 4] in both classical descriptive VCG analysis and quantitative statistical computer analysis of the Frank lead VCG.

Material and Methods

The group of normal subjects, 375 males aged 50 to 70 years, was described previously [4]. The group of 105 patients with IHD was selected on the basis of clinical examination and findings on coronary arteriography. All patients had a narrowing exceeding 75% in one or more of the coronary arteries. All patients presented a clinical picture of angina pectoris during exercise. There were 101 males and 4 females in this group. The age range was from 27 to 65 years. In all normal subjects and in all but 20 of the patients, a submaximal exercise test was performed on a bicycle ergometer. The initial load was 600 kilogram-force-meters/min for three minutes. Subsequently, the load was increased by 300 kilogram-force-meters/min at two minute intervals until the target heart rate (THR) was reached. Each subject's THR was determined by age, to correspond to 85% of his predicted maximum heart rate (MHR), using the equation: $MHR = 230 - 1.18 \times age$ (yr). When THR was reached, the load was adjusted to maintain THR for the period of recording of the ECG and VCG. In 20 of the patients, the exercise records were made during a treadmill test rather than the standard ergometer exercise. The same THR (85% of MHR) was utilized in both tests.

ECG/VCG Recording and Analysis

The ECG/VCG records were made as seven simultaneous bipolar leads to permit computation of the Frank lead VCG, X, Y, Z components and a set of 12 bipolar leads using a procedure described before [5].

The computer program used to process rest and exercise ECG, and the waveform descriptors used for quantifying P and waveform patterns, have been reported previously [5, 6]. The procedure we use to extract waveform information from scalar components of a vector function produces computational coefficients that are (a) the function's mean value (coefficient C_0); (b) the gradient, or the first order coefficient (C_1); (c) the quadratic coefficient (C_2); and (d) the tertiary coefficient (C_3), using modified Chebyshev polynomials as cardinal functions. (For the modification, even terms are multiplied by $-1/2$ and odd terms by $+1/2$). The coefficient of the linear term, the gradient (C_1), is a measure of the slope of the time-normalized function; that of the quadratic term is an index of convexity, and the tertiary term measures to what extent the function's residual variation (after fitting with the first three terms) is S-shaped, or sigmoid.

When analysis is performed on a vector function of time (e.g., using the three Frank-lead components), these coefficients form components of the four vectors: mean vector ($\tilde{MV}$), gradient vector ($\tilde{GV}$), convex vector ($\tilde{CV}$), and sigmoid vector ($\tilde{SV}$). The magnitude and direction of each vector indicates both the size of the principal waveform features of a vector function of time and in which direction in the orthogonal reference frame the features are most prominent. This VCG information can be used to predict which scalar leads will most prominently display features such as a negative slope or convexity.

The ST-T segment of each lead is defined by identifying time demarcation lines D (estimated end of ventricular excitation) and E (estimated end of ventricular repolarization). ST is considered to extend through the first 7/16, and the T wave through the latter 9/16 of the ST-T segment. Waveform coefficients were determined separately for ST and T of each lead.

Spatial distributions of waveform vectors are described with a reference frame divided into 12 symmetrical regions defined by sides of a rhombododecahedron lattice whose faces are uniformly distributed over 360 degrees in space. These reference regions are identified by a mnemonic code, using positive and negative directions of the Cartesian-coordinate axes; for instance, ILA = inferior, left, anterior, in order of proximity of the reference direction to the X, Y, and Z axes.

Angular mean values, mean angular deviations and the test for significance of differences between mean angles in any two recording states were calculated according to the methods reported by Watson and Williams [7].

For unit vectors distributed on a circle, the mean angle is in the direction of:

$$\left(\sum_{i=i}^{n} \cos\Theta_i, \quad \sum_{i=i}^{n} \right) \sin\Theta_i \quad = \quad \left(\overline{X}, \overline{Y} \right)$$

The magnitude of this resultant vector is given by:

$$R = \sqrt{\overline{X}^2 + \overline{Y}^2}$$

To specify the full hypothesis for the test that a mean angle Θ is equal to a given angle, let the polar vector of the given angle be Θo. Then:

$$\frac{R\,(n-1)\,[1-\cos(\Theta - \Theta o)]}{N - R} \approx F_{2,\,2(n-1)}$$

Letting $r = \dfrac{R}{N}$ this becomes:

$$\frac{r(n-1)\,[1-\cos(\Theta - \Theta o)]}{1 - r} \approx F_{2,\,2(n-1)}$$

For the 'signed' included angle one may set $\Theta o = O$; thus the above test is applicable.

Results

Normal Exercise VCG ST Waveforms. Mean spherical polar coordinates and standard deviations of the first three low order ST waveform vectors are listed in table 1. Figure 1 represents schematically the normal magnitude and spatial relationship of $\widehat{MV}$, $\widetilde{GV}$, $\widehat{CV}$ and $\widetilde{SV}$ in exercise. The elevation angles of these vectors are fairly close to 90°, and thus the horizontal plane display depicts fairly accurately the relationship of these waveform vectors. Figure 1 serves as a good example of the WVA principle. The

average magnitudes of the ST-MV and ST-GV are 0.1 and 0.2 mV. respectively. In the majority of normal subjects, the orientation of these vectors is anterior-left (AL) or inferior-left-anterior (ILA) both in rest and in exercise. Thus, these vectors generate in the majority of normal subjects in AL direction ST segments which are positive and have a positive slope. The ST concave vector ($\widehat{CV}$) points to the right with a magnitude of 0.04 mV generating a convex, 'U-shape' ST with peak to peak convexity of 40 μV in leads oriented to the left. The residual ST waveform variation can be represented with an anteriorly oriented 'S-shaped' sigmoid vector ($\widetilde{SV}$). The average magnitude of SV is only 0.02 mV. It is evident that although these higher order vectors are important for exact representation of minor morphological details of ST waveforms, their actual information content may be quite insignificant in comparison with the prominent role of ST-$\widetilde{MV}$ and ST-$\widetilde{GV}$.

Normal and Abnormal Response to Exercise. Tables 1 and 2 reveal some interesting differences between VCG response to exercise in normals and the IHD group. There was a highly significant decrease in the magnitude of the ST mean vector in normals and an opposite change, a highly significant increase in the IHD group. In fact, ST-$\widehat{MV}$ magnitude decreased as a response to exercise in 75% of the normals, and increased in 80% of the IHD patients.

The clockwise rotation (to the right) of ST-$\widehat{MV}$ was quite substantial in both groups, and considerably more pronounced in IHD patients. It is noted (table 1) that the mean azimuth of ST-MV at rest of the IHD group (-82°) is equal to the mean azimuth of the exercise $\widehat{MV}$ in the normal group. This indicates that the orientation of the ST vectors of the IHD group tends to be abnormal at rest, and undergoes a further substantial abnormal clockwise rotation in exercise. This rotation to the right and posterior, is accompanied by an upward shift.

The contrasting orientation differences in rest and exercise VCG of these two groups are summarized in table 2. The fairly narrow spatial orientation distribution of $\widehat{MV}$ and $\widetilde{GV}$ in normals in rest and exercise contrasts a wider spatial dispersion in the IHD group. The orientation of ST-$\widehat{MV}$ in the IHD group is outside the four normal reference regions (AL, AR, SA, ILA) in 63%. However, the $\widehat{MV}$ orientation is abnormal in the resting VCG in 50% of the patients. In close to one-third of the IHD group, the rest as well as the exercise ST-$\widehat{GV}$ lie outside AL and ILA, the normal orientation reference regions for this vector.

Table 1. Mean Values (standard deviations in brackets) of azimuth (H) and elevation (V) angles, (degrees) and magnitudes (MAG, microvolts) of ST waveform vectors of rest and exercise VCG of 135 normal male subjects and 105 patients with ischemic heart disease (IHD). Azimuth angle is positive posterior and negative anterior. An increase in azimuth implies a shift counterclockwise. Elevation is determined with respect to the positive direction of the Y lead; 0 degrees = straight down, 90 degrees = horizontal, and 180 degrees = straight up. An increase in elevation indicates a shift upwards. Methods of computation of angular statistics is described in the methods section. MV = mean vector, GV = gradient vector, CV = concave vector.

		ST – MV			ST – GV			ST – CV		
		H	V	MAG	H	V	MAG	H	V	MAG
Normals (N=135)	Rest (R)	−55(18)	69(12)	137(52)	−47(17)	68(11)	192(67)	−171(39)	116(26)	40(19)
	Exercise (E)	−80(35)	86(27)	104(54)	−34(18)	60(13)	211(77)	170(39)	116(23)	44(22)
	E−R	−24(31)#	17(26)#	−33(53)#	13(13)#	−7(10)#	18(61)#	−14(44)	0(30)	3(23)*
IHD (N=105)	Rest	−82(53)	71(31)	72(33)	−63(37)	73(27)	97(41)	−132(57)	123(32)	31(17)
	Exercise	−158(53)	107(32)	133(74)	−57(40)	65(26)	137(66)	−147(75)	104(37)	35(20)
	E−R	−76(60)#	36(37)	61(73)#	6(31)	−7(19)	39(56)#	−15(64)	−18(38)#	4(22)

= p<0.001,   * = p<0.01.

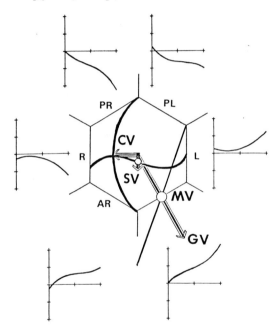

Fig. 1. Normal exercise VCG ST waveform vectors and resulting ST waveform patterns in horizontal plane reference frame. The average magnitudes of the ST-Mean Vector (MV) and Gradient Vector (GV) are 0.1 and 0.2 mV, respectively, and they are both oriented towards anterior-left (AL). These vectors generate in AL direction ST segments with a mean amplitude of 0.1 mV and a positive gradient of 0.2 mV from the beginning to the end of the ST segment. The ST-Concave Vector (CV) points right (R) with a magnitude of 0.04 mV, generating a convex 'U-shape' ST in leads oriented to left (L).

The waveform vector orientation changes as a mechanism in the generation of so-called ischemic ST patterns in the left chest leads is illustrated in figure 2. This scheme reveals that orientation changes alone, without ST vector magnitude changes, can produce characteristic ischemic ST patterns in the left chest leads. The degree of ischemic depression depends primarily on the magnitude of ST-$\widetilde{MV}$ and ST-$\widetilde{GV}$.

Maximum QRS and T Vectors in Rest and Exercise. Table 3 indicates a notable lack of significant changes in maximum QRS and T spatial vectors in the IHD group. The sole exception is a 15° increase in the spatial angle between QRS and T which is significant at p = 0.01 level. Although not statistically significant, the increase of T magnitude in IHD group is of interest in view of the fact that the maximum T magnitude in the normal group decreased from its mean value of 507 µV at rest to 348 µV during exercise (p<0.001).

Discriminant Analysis of ST and T Waveforms. A comprehensive multivariate analysis was performed to identify waveform features which produce the best diagnostic discrimination between the normal and IHD groups. The performance of various waveform combinations in diagnostic discrimination was judged on the basis of sensitivity at a 90% level of specificity. Two waveform vectors at a time (i.e., six X, Y, Z coefficients of two waveform vectors) were permitted in the discriminant function analysis program.

Table 2. Contrasting directional distributions and magnitude changes of ST mean vector (ST-MV) and gradient vector (ST-GV) in rest and exercise VCG of 375 normal men and 105 patients with ischemic heart disease (IHD). The 12 spatial orientation reference regions are described in figure 3. AL = anterior-left, ILA = inferior-left-anterior, AR = anterior-right, SA = superior-anterior.

	Waveform Vector		Directional Distribution	Vector Magnitude Change
Normals	ST-MV	Rest	95% within AL, ILA	MV Magnitude decrease
		Exercise	91% within AL, AR, SA, ILA	in exercise in 75%
	ST-GV	Rest	94% within AL, ILA	
		Exercise	89% within ILA, AL	
IHD Group	ST-MV	Rest	50% outside AL, ILA	MV Magnitude increase
		Exercise	63% outside AL, AR, SA, ILA	in exercise in 80%
	ST-GV	Rest	30% outside AL, ILA	
		Exercise	31% outside ILA, AL	

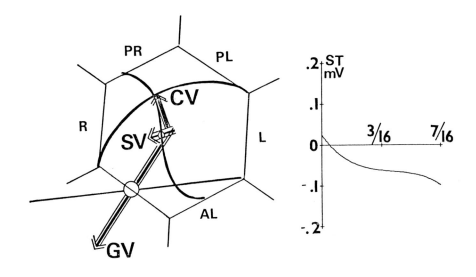

Fig. 2. Waveform vector orientation changes as a mechanism in generation of ischemic ST patterns. A 60° clockwise rotation of ST waveform vectors in relation to their normal orientation (figure 1) as a response to exercise produces an ischemic ST segment in the ECG with lead vectors oriented to the left (L).

Table 3. QRS and T maximum spatial magnitudes (microvolts), azimuth and elevation angles (defined in table 1) and the spatial angle between maximum QRS and T vectors in rest and exercise VCG of 105 patients with ischemic heart disease.

	Rest (R)		Exercise (E)		E-R	
	M	SD	M	SD	M	SD
QRS Spatial Mag.	1218	339	1239	348	20	184
T Spatial Mag.	282	116	309	174	27	180
QRS Max Azimuth	21	36	23	39	2	29
QRS Max Elevation	64	21	65	23	1	16
T Max Azimuth	-54	50	-63	58	-9	52
T Max Elevation	62	33	73	37	11	33
QRS/T Spatial Angle	71	42	94	48	15*	44

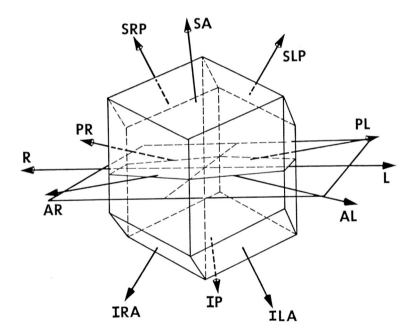

Fig. 3. Spatial reference regions for categorizing directions of waveform vectors. The 12 reference vectors shown are normals of the sides of a rhombodecahedron lattice. The direction code indicates, in order of prominence, the Cartesian directions left (L), right (R), posterior (P), superior (S), and inferior (I). (Reproduced from Circulation 48 (1973) 543, by permission of the publisher and the American Heart Association.)

The best separation from the exercise VCG was obtained using ST-$\widetilde{\text{MV}}$ and ST-$\widetilde{\text{GV}}$, which yielded 87% sensitivity. When the same analysis procedure was performed with the resting VCG, 97 of the 105 IHD patients (92%) were discriminated from the normal group, with 10% false positives (i.e., 90% specificity). The best discriminators from the resting VCG were T-$\widetilde{\text{CV}}$ and ST-$\widetilde{\text{MV}}$. Finally, when discriminant analysis was done on changes in waveform features induced by exercise, a sensitivity of 88% (92 of 105 HD patients) using ST-$\widetilde{\text{MV}}$ and T-$\widetilde{\text{MV}}$ as discriminators.

Discussion

There are relatively few quantitative reports on exercise VCG analysis in the vast literature on exercise testing. In many instances, good results from diagnostic analysis of the exercise VCG are highly misleading because patients with classical ischemic ECG response were selected for the VCG analysis test group [1]. The meaning of highly significant differences reported from such VCG analyses can be questioned. Some novel approaches to quantitative exercise VCG analysis hold promise, however, such as the studies of Ascoop [8] and Blomqvist [9].

Results from WVA indicate that the orientation and magnitudes of the waveform vectors at rest deviate from normal in a substantial fraction of the IHD group. Thus, it can be questioned whether any useful conclusions can be drawn from the analysis of the exercise records if the resting VCG ST and T already deviate from normal. This fact was verified through discriminant function analysis of the resting VCG ST and T waveform vectors: combined use of T-$\widetilde{\text{CV}}$ and ST-$\widetilde{\text{MV}}$ permitted discrimination of 92% (97 out of 105) of IHD patients from the normal group with 90% specificity. It is thus not surprising that exercise VCG analysis performance was so good. The real issue then is whether the VCG changes induced by exercise are adequate diagnostic discriminators. In this respect the analysis of changes from rest to exercise yielded as good results as analysis of the exercise VCG alone. This is perhaps the most significant result of this study. It is emphasized that not too much attention should be paid to the actual values of sensitivity achieved (88%); this is clearly an optimistic estimate of the performance of the program, and considerably worse performance can be expected when these criteria are used on other test groups.

No attempt was made here to stratify the IHD group on the basis of the severity of CHD etc. The group is fairly small, and is used here mainly to demonstrate the WVA principle in clinical VCG investigation. It should also be noted that the group of 375 normals used in this study was drawn from a large rural working total population sample of men, and thus they

may substantially differ from groups sometimes called "hospital normals," including groups of patients with negative coronary arteriography.

WVA principle is one of several possible approaches to quantify VCG analysis [10]. It is by no means limited to ST-T analysis as in the present study; it is equally applicable to P and QRS analysis and can be used for analysis of any set of ECG leads, not necessarily orthogonal.

Comprehensive analysis was performed, although not reported here, on atrial waveform vectors in our IHD group. It suffices to mention here that although substantial changes are induced by exercise in atrial waveform patterns in IHD, we have thus far been unable to find any systematic differences in the exercise P waves of normal subjects and IHD patients.

Summary and Conclusions

Waveform vector analysis (WVA) was performed of the rest and submaximal exercise VCG of 375 normal elderly men and of 105 patients with ischemic heart disease (IHD) manifested as angina pectoris during exercise and over 75% angiographic narrowing of at least one of the coronary arteries.

The characteristic VCG response to exercise in this group of elderly normal subjects was a 24° clockwise shift of the ST mean vector and a ST mean vector magnitude decrease in 75% of the subjects. As a contrast, the ST mean vector magnitude increased in 80% of the patients in IHD group with a much more pronounced clockwise shift, averaging 76°.

In the normal and in the IHD group, the clockwise rotation of the ST mean vector was associated with an increased elevation (shift up) by an average of 17° and 36°, respectively.

The orientation of the ST mean vector was abnormal in the exercise VCG in 63% of the IHD patients. However, in one-half of the IHD group, the ST mean vector orientation was already abnormal in the resting VCG. The ST gradient vector orientation was abnormal in close to one-third of the IHD group in rest as well as exercise.

Discriminant analysis of major WVA parameters revealed that the deviations from normal VCG repolarization patterns were present in 92% of IHD patients of this study. Consequently, exercise VCG analysis alone reveals little useful diagnostic information. However, it was found that efficient WVA of changes induced by exercise offer at least potentially an adequate diagnostic discrimination in spite of the high prevalence of minor repolarization abnormalities in patient groups derived from coronary arteriography population samples.

It is concluded that WVA suitably quantifies VCG waveform features for computer analysis. A careful stratification of test populations regarding rest VCG repolarization patterns appears necessary in testing the diagnostic value of the exercise VCG.

Acknowledgments

The authors wish to acknowledge the contributions of Mr. James Warren, B.Sc., and Mr. James Middleton, B.Sc., and Mrs. Marlene Corye, B.Sc., to statistical analysis of the data, design and implementation of ECG analysis programs for this study.

References

[1] G. E. Dower, R. A. Bruce, J. Pool, M. L. Simoons, M. W. Niederberger, and L. J. Meilink, Ischemic polarcardiographic changes induced by exercise. A new criterion, Circulation 48 (1973) 725.

[2] F. Kornreich, P. Block, and D. Brismee, The missing waveform information in the orthogonal electrocardiogram (Frank Leads). III Computer Diagnosis of Angina Pectoris from "Maximal" QRS Surface Waveform Information at Rest, Circulation 49 (1974) 1212.

[3] P. M. Rautaharju, J. Warren, and H. Wolf, Waveform vector analysis of orthogonal electrocardiograms: quantification and data reduction, J. Electrocardiol. 6 (1973) 102.

[4] P. M. Rautaharju, S. Punsar, H. Blackburn, J. Warren, and A. Menotti, Waveform patterns in Frank-Lead rest and exercise electrocardiograms of healthy elderly men, Circulation 48 (1973) 541.

[5] P. M. Rautaharju, J. Warren, and H. Wolf, Computer analysis of orthogonal and multiple scalar lead exercise electrocardiograms. In: C. Zywietz and B. Schneider (eds.), Computer application on ECG and VCG analysis. Proc. 2nd IFIP TC-4 Working Conference, Hannover, Germany 1971 (North-Holland, Amsterdam, 1973), p. 517.

[6] H. D. Wolf, P. J. MacInnis, S. Stock, R. K. Helppi, and P. M. Rautaharju, The Dalhousie program: A comprehensive analysis program for rest and exercise electrocardiograms. In: C. Zywietz and B. Schneider (eds.), Computer application on ECG and VCG analysis. Proc. 2nd IFIP TC-4 Working Conference, Hannover, Germany 1971 (North-Holland, Amsterdam, 1973), p. 231.

[7] G. S. Watson and E. J. Williams, On the construction of significance test on the circle and the sphere, Biometrika 43 (1956) 344.

[8] C. A. Ascoop, ST forces during exercise (Grafisch Bedrijf Schotanus & Jens Utrecht BV - Utrecht, 1974).

[9] G. Blomqvist, The Frank lead exercise electrocardiogram. A quantitative study based on averaging technic and digital computer analysis (Tryckeri Balder AB, Stockholm, 1965).

[10] P. M. Rautaharju, H. W. Blackburn, H. K. Wolf, and M. Horacek, Computers in clinical electrocardiology. Is vectorcardiography becoming obsolete? Adv. in Cardiol. 16 (1975) 1.

AUTHOR INDEX

SUBJECT INDEX